Artificial Intelligence in Dentistry

Kaan Orhan • Rohan Jagtap
Editors

Artificial Intelligence in Dentistry

Springer

Editors
Kaan Orhan
Faculty of Dentistry
Ankara University
Ankara, Türkiye

Rohan Jagtap
School of Dentistry
University of Mississippi Medical Center
Jackson, MS, USA

ISBN 978-3-031-43826-4 ISBN 978-3-031-43827-1 (eBook)
https://doi.org/10.1007/978-3-031-43827-1

This Springer imprint is published by the registered company Springer Nature Switzerland AG
The registered company address is: Gewerbestrasse 11, 6330 Cham, Switzerland

Paper in this product is recyclable.

Contents

1 **Introduction to Artificial Intelligence** 1
Kaan Orhan and Rohan Jagtap

2 **Understanding of AI in Dental Field with Technical Aspects** 9
Nurullah Akkaya, Gürkan Ünsal, and Kaan Orhan

3 **Artificial Intelligence from Medicine to Dentistry** 33
Kaan Orhan and Hakan Amasya

4 **Applications of Artificial Intelligence in Dentistry** 43
Prashant P. Jaju, Ibrahim Sevki Bayrakdar, Sushma Jaju, Vidhi Shah, Kaan Orhan, and Rohan Jagtap

5 **Applications of AI in Endodontics and Restorative Dentistry** 69
Kaan Orhan, Umut Aksoy, and Seçil Aksoy

6 **Artificial Neural Networks for the Design Optimization of Implants** 83
Jason A. Griggs

7 **Outlook for AI in Oral Surgery and Periodontics** 97
Sevda Kurt-Bayrakdar, Kaan Orhan, and Rohan Jagtap

8 **AI in Orthodontics** 131
Kaan Orhan and Hakan Amasya

9 **AI on Oral Mucosal Lesion Detection** 143
Gaye Keser, Filiz Namdar Pekiner, and Kaan Orhan

10 **Impact of AI in Obstructive Sleep Apnea** 177
Kaan Orhan and Seçil Aksoy

11 **Artificial Intelligence in Temporomandibular Joint Disorders** 187
Rohan Jagtap, Ibrahim Sevki Bayrakdar, and Kaan Orhan

12 **Artificial Intelligence for 3D Printing and Bioprinting** 203
Isil Yazgan, Utku Serhat Derici, Burak Barıs Altunay, Osama Ali Hindy, and Pinar Yilgor Huri

13 Artificial Intelligence in Dental Education 223
Ibrahim Sevki Bayrakdar, Kaan Orhan, and Rohan Jagtap

14 Advantages, Disadvantages, and Limitations of AI in Dental Health 235
Rohan Jagtap, Sevda Kurt Bayrakdar, and Kaan Orhan

15 Applications of Machine Learning and Artificial Intelligence in the COVID-19 Pandemic 247
Ingrid Różyło-Kalinowska and Kaan Orhan

16 Medico-Legal Problems of Artificial Intelligence 259
Kaan Orhan, Melis Mısırlı Gülbeş, Aniket Jadhav, and Rohan Jagtap

17 Deep Learning in Image Processing: Part 1—Types of Neural Networks, Image Segmentation 283
Ruben Pauwels and Alexandros Iosifidis

18 Deep Learning in Image Processing: Part 2—Image Enhancement, Reconstruction and Registration 317
Ruben Pauwels and Alexandros Iosifidis

19 Future Perspectives of Artificial Intelligence in Dentistry 353
Gürkan Ünsal and Kaan Orhan

Introduction to Artificial Intelligence

1

Kaan Orhan and Rohan Jagtap

What Is AI?

Artificial intelligence (AI) is a rapidly growing field of computer science that aims to create intelligent machines capable of performing tasks that typically require human intelligence. These tasks can include recognizing speech, making decisions, solving problems, playing games, and even translating languages. AI systems are designed to mimic human cognition and behavior, making them powerful tools for automating complex and repetitive tasks.

There are two main categories of AI: narrow or weak AI, and general or strong AI. Narrow AI is designed to perform a single task, such as playing chess or recognizing speech, and has been widely adopted in various industries, including finance, healthcare, and retail. On the other hand, general AI has the potential to perform any intellectual task that a human can, but it is still in its early stages of development.

AI technologies are driven by algorithms, which consist of sets of instructions that guide a computer's actions. Some of the most widely used algorithms in AI include decision trees, neural networks, and deep learning algorithms. Decision trees are employed for decision-making, neural networks for pattern recognition, and deep learning algorithms for tasks like image and speech recognition.

K. Orhan (✉)
Faculty of Dentistry, Department of Dentomaxillofacial Radiology, Ankara University, Ankara, Turkey

R. Jagtap
Division of Oral and Maxillofacial Radiology, University of Mississippi Medical Center, Jackson, MS, USA

Department of Care Planning and Restorative Sciences, University of Mississippi Medical Center, Jackson, MS, USA

Department of Radiology, School of Medicine, University of Mississippi Medical Center, Jackson, MS, USA

K. Orhan, R. Jagtap (eds.), *Artificial Intelligence in Dentistry*,
https://doi.org/10.1007/978-3-031-43827-1_1

Machine learning, a subset of AI, enables computers to learn from data and improve their performance over time. This is achieved by utilizing algorithms to analyze vast datasets, identify patterns, and make predictions or decisions without explicit programming. Deep learning, another subset of machine learning, leverages deep neural networks to process and analyze large datasets, enabling computers to recognize intricate patterns and perform complex tasks.

Natural language processing (NLP) is another critical area of AI that centers around teaching computers to understand and process human language. This encompasses tasks like speech recognition, sentiment analysis, and language translation and is widely applied in virtual assistants and customer service chatbots.

Similarly, computer vision is another important field of AI that concentrates on instructing computers to recognize and comprehend images and videos. This technology finds applications in object recognition, image classification, and even autonomous vehicles.

Robotics is another significant area of AI that involves designing and constructing robots capable of performing tasks that typically require human intelligence. These robots can be programmed to carry out activities in industries such as manufacturing and logistics, automating repetitive tasks, and enhancing overall efficiency.

AI has the potential to revolutionize the way we live and work, and it is already making a profound impact across numerous industries. However, like any technology, AI raises ethical and societal concerns, including job displacement, privacy issues, and bias in decision-making. It is essential for researchers, policymakers, and the general public to carefully consider these issues and cultivate responsible AI practices as the field continues to advance and mature.

How Does AI Work?

The term artificial intelligence (AI) describes the creation of computer systems capable of performing activities that typically require human intellect, such as speech recognition, visual perception, decision-making, and language translation. AI programs can learn from data, discern patterns, and arrive at conclusions or predictions. AI comes in various forms, including:

Machine learning, a branch of artificial intelligence, focuses on teaching algorithms to make predictions or judgments using data. Depending on the type of problem they are designed to address, machine learning algorithms can be supervised, unsupervised, or semi-supervised.

Artificial neural networks, also known as "artificial neural networks," are utilized in deep learning and are designed to mimic the structure and operations of the human brain. Deep learning algorithms, powered by these networks, have been successfully applied to tasks such as image recognition.

Natural language processing (NLP) is another branch of AI that aims to provide computers with the ability to understand and analyze human language. NLP algorithms can handle various tasks, including machine translation, sentiment analysis, and text categorization.

Robotics is an area of artificial intelligence that concentrates on developing robots capable of performing activities that would typically require human intellect. To create robots that can interact with the real environment, robotics combines AI with other technologies such as computer vision and mechanical engineering.

Computer vision is another branch of artificial intelligence that seeks to enable machines to comprehend and analyze visual data from the outside world, including images and videos. Computer vision algorithms can be employed for various tasks such as object detection, scene comprehension, and image recognition.

Examples of predictive modeling for disease spread and resource allocation include the use of machine learning algorithms to create models that predict the spread of the virus. These models enable healthcare systems to allocate resources more effectively and prepare for potential outbreaks. For instance, predictive models have been developed to estimate the number of hospital beds and intensive care units needed for treatment.

Additionally, machine learning and artificial intelligence have been valuable in rapidly and accurately tracking cases of the virus. These technologies assist in identifying hotspots and potential outbreaks. For example, machine learning algorithms analyze data from various sources, such as news reports, social media, and official health reports, to identify potential outbreaks and monitor the virus's spread.

Machine learning algorithms have been utilized to analyze radiographical scans and other imaging data quickly and accurately.

Drug discovery and repurposing using AI-assisted techniques: Machine learning and artificial intelligence have been employed to identify potential drugs and repurpose existing drugs for treatment. For example, algorithms have been developed to analyze vast datasets of chemical compounds to identify those with potential antiviral properties and predict which existing drugs may be effective against the virus.

Providing chatbot and virtual assistants for answering common questions about the virus and offering guidance on self-care: Machine learning and natural language processing have been leveraged to develop chatbots and virtual assistants capable of answering common questions about the virus and providing self-care guidance. For instance, chatbots have been created to furnish information on symptoms, transmission, and treatments.

What Are the Different Approaches of AI?

There are several approaches to AI, mainly listed below:

Supervised learning: A supervised learning algorithm is one that has been provided with the correct answers, and it uses this knowledge to learn how to solve its problem.

Unsupervised learning: An unsupervised learning algorithm learns without being given any information about the data or its features. For example, if you want to recognize images of cats in photos, an unsupervised machine-learning algorithm could use similarities between images as the basis for recognizing patterns that might contain cats, without being told whether or not there are any actual cats within each photo being classified.

Reinforcement learning: This form of machine intelligence combines both supervised and unsupervised techniques simultaneously, allowing it to improve its performance through trial-and-error experimentation with new behaviors learned from experience over time, if necessary. In other words, instead of having preprogrammed rules guiding its actions (like those used by traditional computer programs), reinforcement learning allows for flexibility based on feedback from past experiences. This means there won't always be clear answers when attempting something new because sometimes things will work out better than expected based on trial and error rather than predetermined rulesets.

Why Is AI Important to Dental Professions?

AI has the potential to significantly advance dentistry and improve patient treatment. In the dental field, artificial intelligence is applied in the following ways:

Precise diagnoses and treatment recommendations: AI systems can be trained using vast amounts of dental data, including radiographs and patient histories, to produce accurate diagnoses and treatment recommendations. This assists dental practitioners in making informed judgments and offering their patients better treatment options.

Predictive modeling for dental issues: AI systems can forecast the likelihood of dental problems, such as tooth decay or gum disease, and suggest preventive treatments using predictive modeling. This empowers dental practitioners to take preventive actions, enhancing patient outcomes and reducing the need for invasive procedures.

Digital dental impressions: AI algorithms can process dental digital photos to create precise digital imprints, which can be used for treatment planning, orthodontics, and dental restorations. Compared to traditional impressions, digital impressions are faster and more accurate, enhancing patient comfort and reducing the number of required consultations.

Dental image analysis: AI algorithms can analyze radiographs and other dental images to detect issues and provide accurate diagnoses. Dental experts can achieve more precise diagnoses and deliver better treatment to their patients as a result.

Predictive maintenance: AI algorithms can be utilized to predict potential equipment failures in dental tools, enabling dental professionals to take preventive measures and avoid equipment downtime. This ensures that patients receive the best care possible without disruptions.

Why Is AI Important to Medical Professions?

Medical professionals value AI because of its potential to greatly enhance healthcare in various ways, including the following:

Diagnosing and treatment: AI algorithms can analyze diverse patient data, including medical records, images, and test results, to aid medical personnel in diagnosing illnesses more reliably and quickly.

Predictive analytics: By analyzing data from various sources, such as wearables and electronic health records, AI can assist medical personnel in identifying patterns and predicting health outcomes. This can lead to cost savings in healthcare while improving patient outcomes.

Personalized medicine: AI algorithms can create personalized treatment plans for patients by considering their unique characteristics, such as genetics and lifestyle.

Clinical decision support: AI algorithms can provide real-time guidance to medical experts during diagnosis and treatment, helping them make optimal decisions.

Drug research and discovery: AI systems can evaluate vast amounts of data and efficiently identify potential new medications, accelerating the drug discovery process.

Clinical trials: By examining data from earlier studies and patient records, AI algorithms may assist medical practitioners in designing and carrying out clinical trials that are more successful and efficient. AI has the potential to revolutionize healthcare by enhancing the precision, effectiveness, and timeliness of diagnoses and treatments, as well as by offering patients individualized care. Medical practitioners can improve patient outcomes and develop medicine by harnessing the potential of AI.

Image analysis: AI algorithms are capable of analyzing medical images such as X-rays, MRIs, and CT scans to find patterns and anomalies that could indicate the presence of a disease. This can aid doctors in making more accurate diagnoses, particularly when manually interpreting images is challenging.

Predictive modeling using AI algorithms trained on a vast amount of patient data can forecast a patient's likelihood of developing a certain ailment, such as cancer or heart disease. This ability allows medical practitioners to adopt preventative actions and make early diagnoses, potentially leading to better patient outcomes.

Diagnoses made in real time: AI algorithms can assist doctors in diagnosing and treating patients in real time. For instance, AI systems can assess patient data and offer healthcare providers instant suggestions for the best course of action based on the most recent evidence-based research.

Treatment planning: By taking into consideration a patient's unique traits, such as genetics and lifestyle, AI algorithms may be utilized to create individualized treatment plans. This can aid healthcare practitioners in choosing the optimal course of action for each patient, improving results, and lowering the chance of adverse consequences.

Clinical decision support: AI algorithms can provide real-time guidance to medical professionals during diagnosis and treatment, helping to ensure that they make the best decisions for their patients. For example, AI algorithms can analyze patient data and provide medical professionals with recommendations for the best course of action based on the latest evidence-based research.

Predictive modeling: AI algorithms can be trained on large amounts of patient data, such as electronic health records, to predict the likelihood of a patient developing a certain condition, such as heart disease or cancer. This can help medical professionals take preventive measures and make earlier diagnoses, leading to better patient outcomes.

AI algorithms can be used to predict when medical equipment is likely to fail, enabling medical professionals to take preventive measures to avoid equipment downtime and ensure that patients receive the best possible care.

Moreover, AI algorithms can analyze large amounts of data from various sources, such as electronic health records, wearables, and social media, to predict population health trends and identify populations at risk of certain conditions. This can help medical professionals implement preventive measures to improve population health.

Additionally, AI algorithms can provide real-time guidance to medical professionals during diagnosis and treatment by analyzing patient data and predicting the best course of action based on the latest evidence-based research. Predictive analytics has the potential to significantly improve healthcare by allowing medical professionals to make predictions about future health outcomes and take preventive measures to enhance patient outcomes. By leveraging the power of AI, medical professionals can advance the field of medicine and provide better care for patients.

Conclusions

In general, AI systems work by processing large amounts of data, identifying patterns and relationships within the data, and using this information to make predictions or decisions. AI systems can improve over time as they are exposed to more data and experience, allowing them to make better predictions and decisions. AI has the potential to significantly improve the field of dentistry by enabling dental professionals to make more accurate diagnoses, provide better care for their patients, and improve overall efficiency. By leveraging the power of AI, dental professionals can advance the field of dentistry and provide better care for their patients.

Bibliography

Agrawal P, Nikhade P. Artificial intelligence in dentistry: past, present, and future. Cureus. 2022;14(7):e27405. https://doi.org/10.7759/cureus.27405.

Fatima A, Shafi I, Afzal H, Diez IT, Lourdes DRM, Brenosa J, Espinosa JCM, Ashraf I. Advancements in dentistry with artificial intelligence: current clinical applications and future perspectives. Healthcare (Basel). 2022;10(11):2188. https://doi.org/10.3390/healthcare10112188.

Hsu LP, Huang YK, Chang YC. The implementation of artificial intelligence in dentistry could enhance environmental sustainability. J Dent Sci. 2022;17(2):1081–2. https://doi.org/10.1016/j.jds.2022.02.002.

Nie Y, Wei J, Sun J. Machine learning models for predicting the number of confirmed COVID-19 cases in different regions. Chaos, Solitons Fractals. 2021;140:110610.

Orhan K, Bayrakdar IS, Celik O, Ayan B, Polat E. Can the blockchain-enabled interplanetary file system (block-IPFS) be a solution for securely transferring imaging data for artificial intelligence research in oral and maxillofacial radiology? Imaging Sci Dent. 2021;51(3):337. https://doi.org/10.5624/isd.20210144.

Orhan K, Bilgir E, Bayrakdar IS, Ezhov M, Gusarev M, Shumilov E. Evaluation of artificial intelligence for detecting impacted third molars on cone-beam computed tomography scans. J Stomatol Oral Maxillofac Surg. 2021;122(4):333–7. https://doi.org/10.1016/j.jormas.2020.12.006.

Orhan K, Shamshiev M, Ezhov M, Plaksin A, Kurbanova A, Unsal G, Gusarev M, Golitsyna M, Aksoy S, Misirli M, Rasmussen F, Shumilov E, Sanders A. AI-based automatic segmentation of craniomaxillofacial anatomy from CBCT scans for automatic detection of pharyngeal airway evaluations in OSA patients. Sci Rep. 2022;12(1):11863. https://doi.org/10.1038/s41598-022-159201.

Russell SJ, Norvig P. Artificial intelligence: a modern approach. Englewood Cliffs, N.J.: Prentice Hall; 1995.

Thurzo A, Urbanova W, Novak B, Czako L, Siebert T, Stano P, Marekova S, Fountoulaki G, Kosnacova H, Varga I. Where is the artificial intelligence applied in dentistry? Systematic review and literature analysis. Healthcare (Basel). 2022;10(7):1269. https://doi.org/10.3390/healthcare10071269.

Understanding of AI in Dental Field with Technical Aspects

2

Nurullah Akkaya, Gürkan Ünsal, and Kaan Orhan

Introduction

For diagnostic radiologists, deciphering and interpreting medical images is a critical cognitive task. It has historically been difficult to automate these tasks effectively, despite numerous advances in the field of computer vision, which entails teaching computer programs to interpret and comprehend the visual world.

A branch of AI known as DL has recently made substantial advancements in challenging tasks such as image classification, object identification, speech recognition, language translation, and natural language processing. This breakthrough is particularly important as DL with convolutional neural networks (CNNs) has entirely transformed pattern recognition.

The extraordinary achievement of DL using CNNs in nonmedical fields has created considerable excitement and research interest in changing the computerized processing of medical images. This development has also highlighted how urgent it is for radiology specialists to become familiar with this quickly developing technology. AI researchers have hypothesized that DL algorithms may soon exceed radiologists in some radiological reports. Recent advances in DL algorithms have been made in the field of diagnostic imaging, including the detection of breast cancer on mammograms, the segmentation of liver metastases using CT, the segmentation of

N. Akkaya
Faculty of Engineering, Department of Computer Engineering, Near East University, Nicosia, Cyprus
e-mail: nurullah@nakkaya.com

G. Ünsal (✉)
Faculty of Dentistry, Department of Dentomaxillofacial Radiology, Near East University, Nicosia, Cyprus

K. Orhan
Faculty of Dentistry, Department of Dentomaxillofacial Radiology, Ankara University, Ankara, Turkey

K. Orhan, R. Jagtap (eds.), *Artificial Intelligence in Dentistry*,
https://doi.org/10.1007/978-3-031-43827-1_2

brain tumors using MRI, and the classification of interstitial lung disease using a high-resolution chest CT.

By defining important AI terms and outlining the background that led to the development of DL systems, this chapter reviews the potential of DL. CNN architecture and the basic structure of neural networks (NNs) will be outlined and various emerging clinical applications will be explored. A summary of the technical and data requirements for DL will be provided and the field's current limitations and potential future perspectives will be discussed.

Artificial Intelligence

The goal of AI is to create computer systems that can carry out activities that traditionally require human intelligence. This is a comprehensive phrase that covers a wide variety of approaches and subfields. ML, which includes learning algorithms to recognize patterns and make predictions based on data, is one of the most well-known subdisciplines of AI. As a result, tremendous progress has been made in fields including autonomous cars, computer vision, and natural language processing. Robotics is a crucial topic that deals with building intelligent devices that can communicate with the real world. Manufacturing, healthcare, and space exploration are just a few industries where robotics is used. Expert systems, which are computer programs created to overcome complicated issues in specialized disciplines, and evolutionary computation, which simulates natural selection to address optimization issues, are other subfields of AI. Overall, as scientists continue to create new approaches and technology to create intelligent systems, the area of AI is continually growing and evolving (Fig. 2.1).

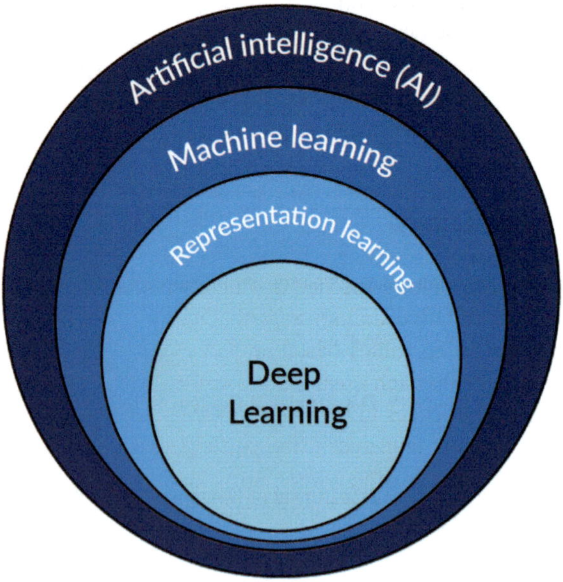

Fig. 2.1 The link between AI, ML, representation learning, and DL is shown by a Venn diagram

Machine Learning

ML is a branch of AI that includes teaching algorithms to carry out tasks by inferring patterns from data rather than having them programmed directly. In traditional ML statistical techniques are used to categorize or separate the data based on features, where human specialists discover and encode features that are singular in the data (Fig. 2.2). For instance, a specialist in image processing could develop an algorithm to deconstruct incoming images into its fundamental elements, such as edges, gradients, and textures, in order to analyze them. To categorize or interpret an image, one can statistically examine the presence of certain features in the image.

Complex computer vision tasks often lack a clear definition of optimal image features for ML algorithms, even for experts in the field. For instance, teaching a computer to recognize an anatomic landmark based solely on pixel brightness (Fig. 2.3) might not be immediately obvious. Consequently, it may be preferable for computer systems to learn and optimize feature combinations themselves, in addition to learning the mappings of features to desired outputs.

One type of ML that doesn't involve feature engineering is representation learning. Instead, the algorithm decides which attributes are most important for categorizing the input data on its own. A representation learning-based system has the ability to produce better classification outcomes than one that depends on manually engineered features when there are enough training examples available. The challenge is allowing an ML system to learn complex structures directly from raw data.

In this chapter, we will focus on DL, a kind of representation learning that involves the algorithm learning a series of features that capture a hierarchy of structures within the data. The representations become progressively more complex by being built up from simpler representations. These DL systems take an end-to-end approach, where they learn basic features such as signal intensity, edges, and textures as building blocks for more intricate features like shapes, lesions, or organs. This enables DL systems to exploit the compositional nature of images.

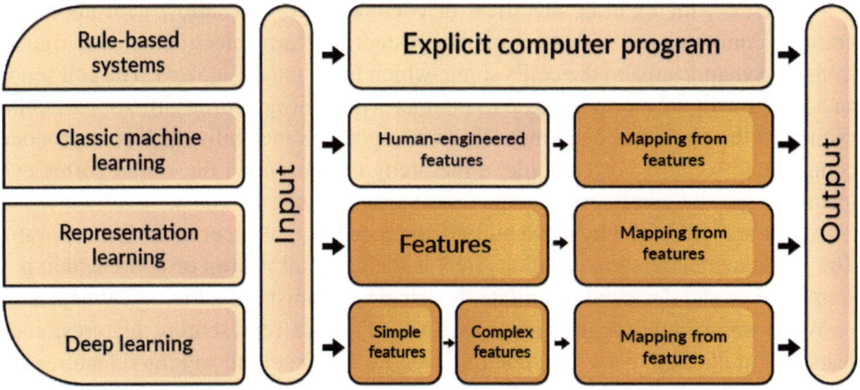

Fig. 2.2 Evolution of various AI systems. From classical rule-based systems to DL

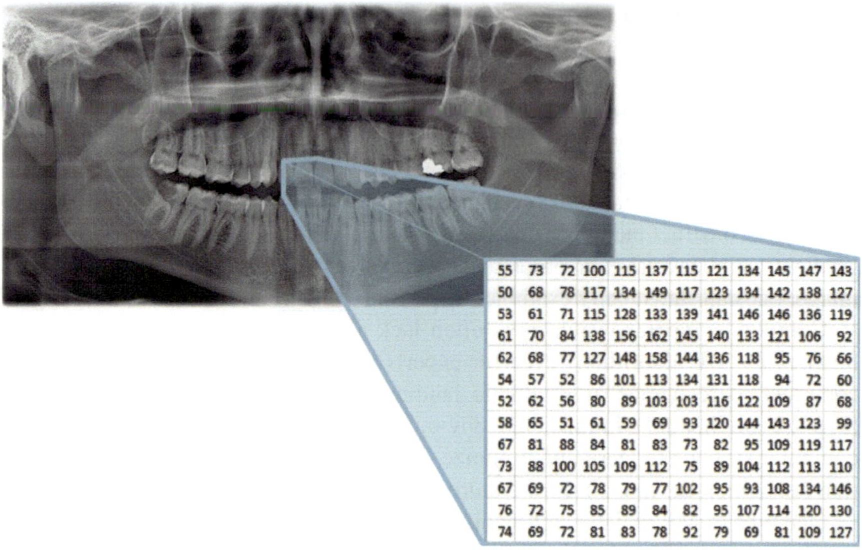

Fig. 2.3 Comparison between how a human interprets the image versus how a machine sees the image

Artificial Neural Networks

Many of the earliest known learning algorithms were developed as computer models of biological learning; that is, they were intended to mimic how learning could or might not occur in the brain.

NNs, which are also referred to as ANNs or neural nets, are a subfield of ML and play a central role in DL algorithms. These networks derive their name and structure from the human brain, emulating how biological neurons communicate with each other.

Synapses, which can be electrical or chemical, are what allow neurons in the brain to communicate with one another. Dendrites carry electrochemical signals from the synaptic area to the cell's soma, which is its body (Fig. 2.4). The cell sends an activation signal along its axon to interact with nearby neurons after a particular excitation threshold has been met. This idea underlies the ability of NNs to encode complicated signals. For example, a hierarchy of neurons in the visual cortex can identify edges by combining signals from various visual receptors.

ANNs are influenced by these biological processes that occur in the human brain. The fundamental component of an ANN is the artificial neuron or node, which is a simplified model designed to imitate the basic mechanism of a biological neuron.

When an artificial neuron receives a set of values representing features, each feature is multiplied by a corresponding weight. The resulting weighted features are then added together and passed through a nonlinear activation function. This process enables an artificial neuron to make decisions by evaluating a set of evidence.

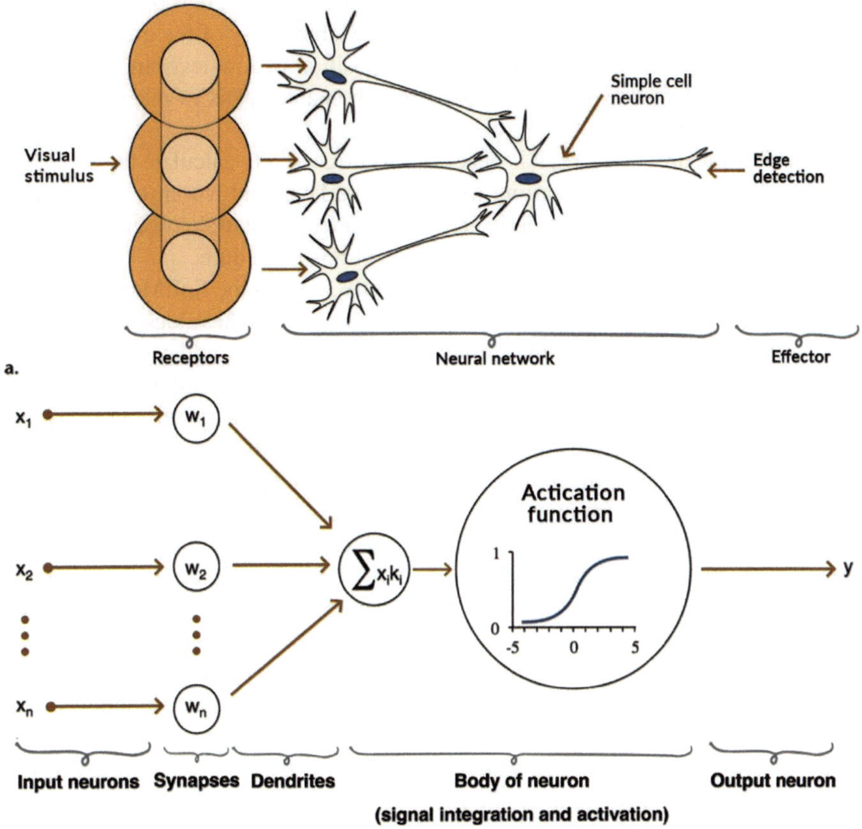

Fig. 2.4 Comparison between biological and artificial neurons

The design of a neural network can be quite complicated, as opposed to the simplicity of a single artificial neuron. Multilayer perceptrons, for example, are composed of hundreds of neurons and can express nonlinear functions. These multilayer perceptrons are built by stacking layers created by numerous neurons connected in series, with the input of one layer feeding into the output of the next.

Deep Learning

The multilayer architecture of a perceptron with more than one hidden layer is regarded as "deep" in DL. The output layer of the network generates goal values, such as a target value for classification, whereas the input layer corresponds to the input data, which can be individual pixel intensities, like the first layer. The intermediate layers, frequently referred to as hidden layers, calculate intermediate representations of the input characteristics that are beneficial to the inference procedure instead than producing visible outputs immediately.

A neural network may successfully simulate increasing degrees of abstraction in the data by stacking numerous layers to generate a hierarchy of features that represents a progressively more sophisticated composition of low-level input information. Deep architectures' compositional strength enables NNs to make judgments based on intangible ideas.

By using a neural network, it is necessary to successively calculate the activation of each node of each layer, starting from the input layer and working your way up to the output layer, in order to derive a prediction from a sample observation, such as an image. Forward propagation is the name of this procedure.

The activation of the output layer is frequently sent via the SoftMax function, a normalized "squashing" function that converts a vector of real values to a probability distribution, while performing classification tasks. The output layer's raw activation signals are converted into target class probabilities via the SoftMax algorithm.

The weights and biases of each node, which together make up millions of parameters in current architectures, must be changed in order to train a neural network. Gradient descent is an optimization procedure that is used to find a set of parameters that perform well on a training dataset. The process begins with a random initial configuration. Predictions are created for a specific data sample during forward propagation, and the network's performance is assessed using a loss function that gauges forecast inaccuracy. The network's parameters are then individually small-adjusted via back-propagation in the direction that minimizes loss.

A random portion of the training data is chosen at each cycle to alter the parameters according to memory constraints and the benefits of specific techniques. This strategy is a common optimization method known as stochastic gradient descent. The variables will move toward values that maximize the model's accuracy as it is trained repeatedly on each sample in the training dataset.

Deep Convolutional Neural Networks

Since local properties and regularities frequently predominate in natural pictures, deep NNs are able to build features as a result. This makes it possible to build complex pieces from tiny local characteristics. This characteristic enables CNNs to process bigger and more complex inputs than multilayer perceptrons. Nevertheless, since they must store redundant representations for all conceivable feature combinations, multilayer perceptrons typically perform badly on pictures where the object of interest fluctuates in shape, location, or orientation.

However, a CNN deals with those variances by performing a convolution operation and running each kernel across the whole image. This is appropriate for natural pictures because it enables each feature detector to find local features in its immediate input. Deep CNNs take advantage of this compositional structure of real pictures to continue to perform well even when objects in the images shift or change shape. Using a simplified model architecture that contains convolutions, activation functions, pooling, and SoftMax function, they are able to complete challenging tasks like image classification.

Convolutions

This particular network utilizes convolution operations which involve applying a filter or kernel linearly to local areas of points in an input. Such as in PACS workstations, typical image filters, such as those for image smoothing and sharpening, operate through such operations. These filters generally represent features and are defined by a grid of small weights, typically 3 × 3 × 3. If the input comprises of n channels (e.g., different color channels), then the filter size would be $n \times 3 \times 3 \times 3$.

The weights of the filters are distributed throughout all image positions to enable accurate modeling of features that could exist anywhere in an image. By using this method, the model is more effective, and less parameters are needed to model picture features. For each layer, typically several convolutional filters are learned, producing a variety of feature maps. The locations where various characteristics of the input image or the previous hidden layer have been recognized are highlighted on these maps.

Activation Function

The activation function is a crucial element in deep NNs. It is a nonlinear function that is applied to the outputs of linear operations like convolutions. By stacking these functions, the input can be transformed into a representation that is linearly separable by a linear classifier. The activation function is inspired by biological neurons and typically acts as a selection function in a neural network layer. It enables some features to be propagated to the output.

Previously, activation functions such as sigmoidal or hyperbolic tangent were popular as they were believed to be biologically plausible. However, today, most CNNs employ the rectified linear unit (ReLU) activation function in their hidden layers. This function is linear for positive inputs, transmitting them as is, while blocking negative inputs. This activation function has been proven to be effective in various computer vision applications.

Downsampling

CNNs employ downsampling (or pooling) operation as an additional component. This operation groups activations of feature maps into a lower-resolution feature map. Downsampling enhances the effective scope, also known as the receptive field, of subsequent filters. Furthermore, in conjunction with convolutions, this operation minimizes the model's sensitivity to small shifts of objects. This is because deeper layers depend increasingly on spatially low resolution yet contextually rich information.

In addition to its effectiveness in increasing the receptive field, downsampling also reduces the memory footprint of the model. For example, every time a 2 × 2 pooling operator is used, the size of each feature map will decrease by 4.

Max pooling is a commonly used form of downsampling. It works by transmitting the maximum activation within a region transforming it into a lower-resolution feature map. By repeating this process successively, we obtain maps that have increasingly lower resolution yet represent richer information on the region of interest.

Convolutional Neural Networks (CNN)

Early back-propagation CNNs were created for the purpose of reading handwritten digits. The Neocognitron, an early network architecture that could recognize visual patterns by layering simple and complex cells, served as an inspiration for the initially developed CNNs. The study of Hubel and Wiesel, which won them the 1981 Nobel Prize in Physiology or Medicine, on the two distinct cell types found in the primary visual cortex served as the foundation for the creation of the Neocognitron.

CNNs may combine characteristics to acquire progressively more spatial information. Only local characteristics collected by convolutional kernels are significant at the input layer, whereas weak interactions exist between distant pixels. Each layer of representation in the network maintains this pattern. The kernels analyze features over bigger and larger spatial scales as we go further into the network, which leads to downsampling and pooling layers that produce a coarser definition of the feature's geographical location. The downsampling and pooling layers diminish spatial resolution while the convolutional layers and activation functions alter the feature maps. A standard network that has been trained for classification often transforms the coarse feature representation close to the output into a vector form through fully connected layers, where each neuron is linked to every neuron in the layer before it. Layers that are fully linked allow for inference about the entire image's content. In classification tasks, the output nodes of a model can be thought of as a vector of log probabilities for each target class. The output of a neural network may be normalized using a SoftMax function at the final layer to parameterize a categorical distribution for class probabilities (Fig. 2.5).

With their sophistication and capacity for learning characteristics, NNs are sometimes referred to as opaque "black boxes." Yet, there are several techniques that may be used to enhance comprehension of the thought process that goes into a

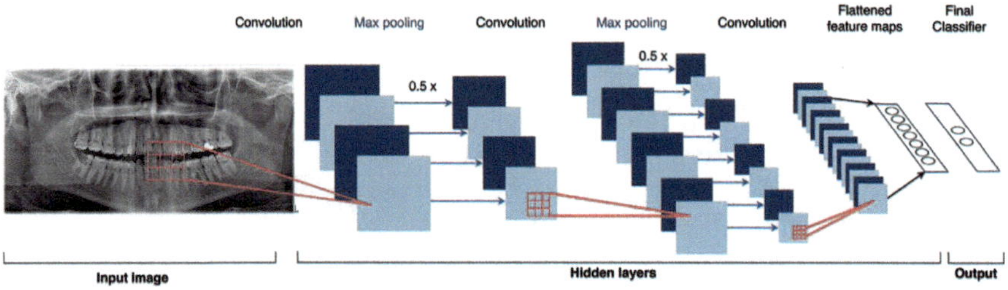

Fig. 2.5 How building blocks outlined in this chapter is organized into deep neural architectures

trained CNN. Examining the related receptive field in the image that resulted in the maximum activation for a particular feature map is one such technique that can provide light on the function that the map serves. One might observe, for instance, that low-level feature maps are activated when their receptive field overlaps with different kinds of edges and corners, whereas mid-level feature maps are activated on organ parts, and high-level feature maps contain information about whole organs and large structures.

An alternative method for gaining insight into a CNN is to examine the pre-SoftMax layer, which precedes the final classification layer. This layer represents the image as an N-dimensional feature vector, which can be difficult to visualize directly. To overcome this challenge, dimensionality-reduction techniques, such as t-stochastic neighbor embedding (t-SNE), can be applied to project the N-dimensional vectors onto a 2D space that is easier to visualize. t-SNE is a common technique that tends to preserve the Euclidean distances, meaning that close vectors in the high-dimensional space are projected to be close to each other in the 2D projection.

Recurrent Neural Networks

Recurrent neural networks (RNNs) are a type of ANN that has the ability to process sequential data by utilizing feedback loops. This allows RNNs to take into account past information when making predictions or classifications, making them particularly useful in tasks such as natural language processing, speech recognition, and time series analysis. In the field of dentistry, RNNs have been applied to tasks such as dental diagnosis, treatment planning, and prediction of treatment outcomes. For example, RNNs have been used to analyze dental images and predict the risk of caries or periodontitis as well as to identify features of tooth morphology for orthodontic treatment planning. Additionally, RNNs have been employed to analyze electronic dental records and predict the success of dental implants or the outcome of orthognathic surgery. The ability of RNNs to handle sequential data and incorporate past information makes them a valuable tool in the field of dentistry for improving diagnosis, treatment planning, and patient outcomes.

Generative Adversarial Networks (GANs)

A type of DL technique known as GANs creates new data that closely resembles a given dataset using two NNs: a discriminator and a generator. When the discriminator network determines whether the samples are genuine, the generator network creates fabricated samples. In a two-player minimax game, these two networks are trained concurrently to maximize their individual goals. GANs have demonstrated promise in a number of dental applications. For instance, they can create fake images of dental components like teeth and gums to train and evaluate dental imaging algorithms. GANs can also be used to generate patient-specific dental models for use in treatment planning, such as in the design of dental implants or orthodontic appliances. Additionally, GANs have been used to generate realistic simulations of dental procedures, which can be used to train dental students or assist in virtual dental surgeries. Overall, the use of GANs in dentistry has the potential to enhance the accuracy and efficiency of dental procedures and training, ultimately improving patient outcomes. However, further research is needed to fully explore the potential of GANs in this field and to address any ethical considerations related to the generation of synthetic patient data.

Training the Model

Data

Data is necessary to create an ML model. Unsupervised learning and supervised learning are two categories of ML methodologies that differ in the kind of data utilized for training. Each instance in the dataset is given a matching output label in supervised learning. For instance, a particular tumor picture can be tagged with the appropriate tumor kind, such as "oncocytoma," in an ML system made to categorize kidney malignancies.

Unsupervised learning doesn't employ annotated data in the dataset, in contrast to supervised learning. Conversely, the algorithm looks for commonalities or patterns among the data points before clustering them. While the generated structure could help with some problems, such tumor segmentation or classification, it is still difficult to implement totally unsupervised learning in real-world applications. Semi-supervised learning, which trains the model using both labeled and unlabeled data, is a more practical method that often employs more unlabeled data than labeled data.

The complexity and nature of the job at hand define the ideal amount of a dataset for training DL models, which might vary. Larger datasets tend to improve the performance of DL models, allowing them to learn more intricate features and correlations. To get high-quality labeled data, though, may be a difficult and expensive operation. Two specialists may need to labor full time for a month to annotate 1000 medical photos for a 20-min image segmentation assignment, for instance. Notwithstanding these difficulties, having a bigger dataset frequently has advantages over disadvantages, particularly when it comes to doing well on challenging tasks.

Data augmentation is a technique which can be used to increase the size of a dataset by applying random transformations to the data while maintaining the validity of the label assignments. This approach is useful when a limited amount of good-quality data is available. Examples of transformations that can be used on images include rotation, flipping, zooming, translation, skewing, and elastic deformation. By generating image variants using data augmentation, the size of the training dataset can be increased, which improves the performance of DL models.

Three subsets of the available data are frequently used in ML: training, validation, and test sets. By continuously analyzing the training images and modifying the weights of the network connections depending on the errors, the training set is used to optimize the parameters of the neural network. For doing model selection and keeping track of the model's performance throughout training, the validation set is used. It is also the best proxy for estimating how well the model will perform on the test set. Finally, the test set is used only at the end of the study to report the final model performance after all parameters have been fixed. It is important to note that using a separate test set ensures an unbiased evaluation of the model's performance on unseen data.

Learning

Hyperparameters, or parameters that are defined by the user rather than learned by the model, are crucial for building efficient neural network architectures. The network architecture, the number of filters used in each layer, and the optimization parameters are a few examples of hyperparameters. In order to find the optimum performing architecture, many configurations are tried and trained before being used to pick the hyperparameters. While time-consuming, this procedure is essential to ensuring the model performs at its best.

After obtaining an appropriate dataset and neural network architecture, the next step is to learn the model parameters. However, it is important to avoid overfitting, which occurs when the model learns unique statistical variations in the training set rather than generalizable patterns for the given task. Overfitting can be detected by analyzing the accuracy of the model on both the training and validation sets. If the model scores high accuracy on the training set but scores poorly on the validation set, it is said to have overfit the training data.

The risk of overfitting the training and validation sets, which would result in the model performing well on these sets but scores poorly on the test set, exists if we thoroughly test the model on the validation data. A model that has too many parameters overfits itself by memorizing the training data while failing to adapt to new data. We can think about reducing the model's capacity or flexibility, like by decreasing the amount of parameters, or adding additional data by using more rigorous data augmentation, to solve overfitting.

Technical Requirements

Hardware

Modern DL models frequently require a substantial amount of computing to train from beginning to conclusion. Deep CNNs have proven successful in part due to the introduction of inexpensive parallel computing capability in the form of graphical processing units (GPUs). Although GPUs were primarily intended for gaming, they have proven to be efficient for parallel processing of operations on matrices and are frequently seen as essential for quickly training huge, complicated DL models. In comparison to traditional central processing units, GPUs may dramatically speed up performance, enabling the training of complicated models containing billions of trainable parameters to be finished in a matter of days compared to several months or weeks it would take for CPU-based training.

Software

Convolutional networks and other multilayer NNs may now be constructed and trained using a variety of software frameworks. Popular frameworks like Theano, Torch, and TensorFlow provide developers with effective low-level functions that can define neural network designs with just a few lines of code. As contrast to becoming mired down in low-level minutiae, this enables developers to concentrate on higher-level architectural challenges. Moreover, these libraries give researchers quick access to processing tools like GPUs. Also, a majority of these software tools are open-source and free, making it possible for anybody to see and edit their codebases. The academic and industry research groups are working together on ML issues at an accelerating rate because to the open nature of these technologies, exchanging code, models, data, and papers without restriction.

Benefits of Artificial Intelligence

As it has the potential to revolutionize several industries, including dentistry, AI has drawn a lot of interest. AI is capable of carrying out jobs that were previously handled by humans, but more accurately, quickly, and effectively. We will examine some of the possible advantages of AI for dentists in this setting, such as its capacity to automate workflows, lessen human error, and enhance decision-making. These advantages could enhance patient results and general dentistry practice effectiveness. Some of these advantages include but not limited to the following:

- **Automation**: AI has the capacity to function freely from a human team, automate workflows. This can lower labor expenses, boost productivity, and enhance accuracy while doing routine activities. Aspects of dental treatment that may be automated include appointment scheduling, reminding patients of their visits, and processing insurance claims. Digital imaging and 3D printing technology may be utilized to design and create dental restorations such as crowns or implants.
- **Reduce human error**: AI may improve decision-making, increase safety, and improve outcomes by removing manual errors from data processing, analytics, industrial assembly, and other processes. Algorithms that consistently adhere to pre-programmed procedures can aid in lowering the possibility of human error. By giving dentists real-time feedback while doing operations, AI can assist lower human error. For instance, AI can examine photos taken during dental operations and notify clinicians of any potential problems or places that need further attention.

- **Eliminate repetitive tasks**: AI may be used to automate monotonous operations, freeing up human resources to concentrate on issues with a bigger impact. Productivity, job happiness, and general workplace effectiveness may all benefit from this. Data input, appointment scheduling, and patient reminders are all repetitive processes that AI may automate in dental clinics.
- **Fast and accurate**: AI is capable of processing more data more quickly than a person, seeing links and patterns in data that a human could overlook. This can help improve decision-making and enable organizations to respond more quickly to changes in their environment. AI can process large amounts of patient data quickly and accurately, allowing dentists to make informed decisions about patient care. For example, AI can analyze patient data to identify risk factors for oral diseases and develop personalized treatment plans.
- **Infinite availability**: AI is not limited by the hours of the day, the requirement for breaks, or other human limitations. AI and ML can be "always on" and working on their assigned duties when operating in the cloud. By virtual consultations and remote monitoring, AI can give patients access to dental treatment around the clock. Patients who reside in rural places or have trouble getting to the dentist's office may find this to be extremely helpful.
- **Accelerated research and development**: Research and development breakthroughs can happen more quickly if huge amounts of data can be promptly analyzed. AI has been used, for example, to measure the human genome or to anticipate potential new medicinal treatments. To find trends and patterns relevant to oral health, AI can be used to examine big datasets. For instance, AI can examine patient records to find oral disease risk factors or genetic data to find possible targets for novel dental treatments.
- **Personalization**: AI can be used to personalize experiences, from recommending products or services based on customer data to tailoring educational content based on an individual's learning style. AI can be used to personalize treatment plans based on individual patient needs and preferences. For example, AI can analyze patient data to determine the most effective treatment options for a particular patient based on factors such as age, medical history, lifestyle, and genetic makeup.
- **Cost savings**: Savings: By automating repetitive processes, removing the need for human data input, and boosting efficiency, AI can help lower the cost of dental treatment. For instance, by evaluating consumption trends and placing orders for supplies automatically as needed, AI may assist dentists in streamlining their supply chain.
- **Improved decision-making**: By analyzing large amounts of data and identifying patterns and trends, AI can help organizations make better decisions, reduce risk, and optimize performance. AI can be used to support decision-making in various industries by providing data-driven insights and recommendations. For example, in finance, AI can be used to analyze market data and provide investment recommendations to financial advisors.
- **Increased efficiency**: AI may assist businesses in streamlining operations and reducing inefficiencies, which leads to cost savings, increased productivity, and higher client happiness. By automating repetitive procedures and offering

real-time data insights, AI can increase productivity in dentistry clinics. For instance, AI may use data on patient flow to assess appointment scheduling, resulting in shorter wait times and more patient satisfaction.

- **Enhanced safety**: AI can be used to monitor and respond to potential safety risks, such as detecting and alerting to hazards in the workplace or predicting and preventing equipment failures. AI can be used to enhance safety in various industries, such as manufacturing and transportation, by identifying potential safety hazards, and providing real-time alerts to workers. For example, AI can be used to analyze sensor data from machinery in a factory to identify potential safety risks and alert workers to take action.
- **Improved customer service**: AI can help improve customer service by automating responses to simple inquiries, providing personalized recommendations, and identifying and resolving customer issues in real time. AI can be used to improve customer service by providing personalized recommendations, answering customer questions, and resolving customer issues quickly and efficiently. For example, AI-powered chatbots and voice assistants can help dental practices communicate with patients and provide support 24/7. These tools can help patients schedule appointments, ask questions about procedures, and receive reminders about their treatment plans.
- **Sustainability**: AI can be used to optimize resource usage, reduce waste, and promote sustainability, such as by optimizing energy usage in buildings or predicting crop yields in agriculture.
- **Predictive maintenance**: AI can be used to predict when equipment or machinery is likely to fail, allowing for preventative maintenance and reducing downtime and maintenance costs. AI can be used to provide predictive analytics to dentists, helping them to identify patients at high risk for oral diseases and develop preventative treatment plans. For example, AI can analyze patient data to identify risk factors for oral diseases such as periodontal disease and develop personalized treatment plans to prevent the onset of the disease.
- **Fraud detection:** By examining data trends and spotting probable anomalies or suspicious activity, AI can be used to both detect and prevent fraud. AI can be used to identify and stop dental insurance claim fraud. AI, for instance, can examine claims data to spot patterns of fraud or abuse, assisting insurance companies in identifying and preventing false claims.
- **Improved medical diagnosis and treatment**: AI can assist healthcare professionals in making more accurate diagnoses and treatment plans by analyzing medical images, patient data, and other relevant information. AI can analyze dental X-rays or scans to help dentists accurately diagnose and develop treatment plans for oral diseases or conditions. For example, AI can analyze images to detect cavities or bone loss that may not be visible to the naked eye.
- **Language translation**: AI may be used to translate text or speech from one language to another automatically, facilitating cross-cultural interaction and collaboration. AI can assist dentists in communicating with clients that are linguistically diverse. For instance, AI-powered language translation

technologies may assist dentists in communicating with clients who speak a different language and making sure they comprehend the steps and instructions.

- **Improved supply chain management**: AI can be used to optimize supply chain management by analyzing data on inventory levels, transportation routes, and demand patterns, resulting in cost savings and improved efficiency. AI can help dental practices optimize their supply chain by analyzing inventory levels, ordering patterns, and demanding patterns to ensure that necessary supplies are always available.
- **Improved education and learning**: AI may be used to customize educational content and give students real-time feedback and support, which can help to enhance learning results. Dental students can benefit from personalized learning experiences that employ AI to adapt the learning materials and feedback to their particular requirements and learning preferences.
- **Improved cybersecurity**: AI can be used to detect and respond to potential cybersecurity threats, such as identifying and blocking malicious activity or analyzing data for potential vulnerabilities. AI can be used to protect patient data and prevent cyberattacks on dental practices. For example, AI-powered cybersecurity tools can monitor network traffic and detect and respond to potential threats in real-time.

AI Methods in Dental Field

The clinical use of DL has demonstrated outstanding performance, especially for jobs using real imagery like pictures. This has prompted the medical image processing community to quickly adopt it. The latest uses of DL for classification, semantic segmentation, object identification, clustering, prediction modeling, and anomaly detection tasks will be the main emphasis of this section.

Classification

Predicting the class or category of an input is the goal of the supervised ML process known as classification. In radiology, classification tasks may entail predicting lesion type or condition given a patient image. This method can be used to determine the kind of cancer or to determine the existence of a disease, among many other issues. Convolutional neural networks (CNNs), in particular, are frequently utilized in DL to handle classification problems in radiology. After forward propagation of the input images, the softmax layer generates a vector of class probabilities, where the predicted class is represented by the greatest value. DL methods are more data-hungry than conventional computer vision and ML techniques. The lack of labeled medical imaging datasets, however, is a serious problem for the community. Millions of nature photographs can be tagged via crowdsourcing, but precisely categorizing medical images is difficult and costly. A balanced and representative

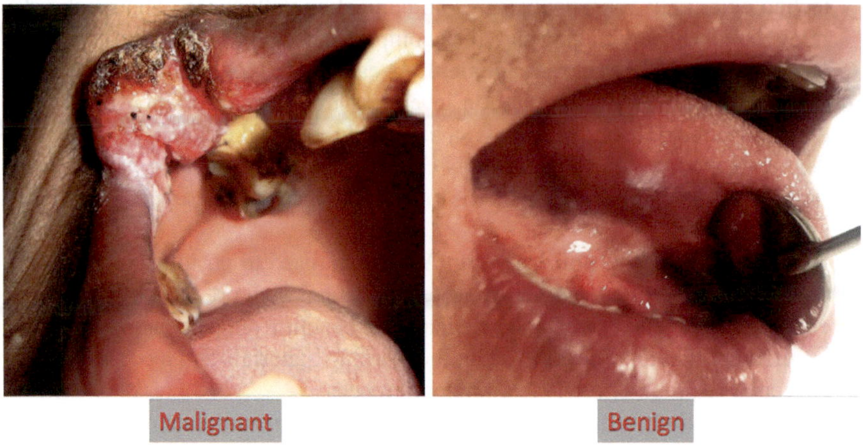

Fig. 2.6 Classification of two oral lesions. Squamous cell carcinoma (left) is classified as malignant, and frictional keratosis of the tongue (right) is classified as benign by the algorithm

training dataset might be difficult to put together given the large range of pathologic states seen in clinical practice.

Transfer learning is a popular method for dealing with the shortage of labeled pictures. This method entails pre-training a CNN on a job for which there is ample data before fine-tuning the network's final layers to match a relatively small and specialized dataset. Numerous authors have obtained a high performance by reusing pre-trained generic architectures since algorithms pre-trained on the well-known ImageNet challenge dataset are freely accessible. Accuracy, which is the proportion of properly predicted samples over all predictions, is often used to evaluate these models' performance. In image classification contests, top-five accuracy is a frequent criterion used for problems with several target classes. This measure evaluates whether the right label falls among the five classes with the greatest expected probability. By providing anticipated and true labels, a confusion matrix is a common method used to visualize the model performance.

For instance, ML algorithms can be taught to categorize dental radiographs as healthy or affected to help with early identification and treatment or to diagnose oral lesions as either benign or malignant based on criteria such as size, shape, and texture (Fig. 2.6).

Semantic Segmentation

Semantic segmentation is a subfield of computer vision that involves dividing an image into different regions or segments and assigning each segment a semantic label. The goal of semantic segmentation is to extract a rich and meaningful understanding of the visual content of an image. It is an important problem in many fields, including autonomous driving, medical imaging, and robotics. In recent years, semantic segmentation has also become increasingly important in dentistry, where it is used to analyze and diagnose various oral diseases. One of the key challenges in semantic segmentation is the accurate delineation of object boundaries. This requires not only identifying the object in question but also being able to separate it from its surrounding background. To achieve this, researchers have developed various DL models based on CNNs, which have proven highly effective for semantic segmentation tasks.

As the majority of pixels do not correspond to the target class, segmentation quality cannot be determined by pixel-wise classification accuracy. Metrics such as intersection over union (IoU) or Dice score are frequently used these metrics measure the overlap between ground truth and segmentation mask. Their values range from 0 for no overlap to 1 complete overlap.

One popular approach to semantic segmentation is the fully convolutional network (FCN) architecture. FCN is a CNN that replaces the fully connected layers of a traditional CNN with convolutional layers, enabling it to produce a dense pixel-wise output. FCN is trained end to end on large datasets of annotated images, enabling it to learn the complex relationships between image features and their corresponding semantic labels. Another popular approach to semantic segmentation is the U-Net architecture, which was developed specifically for biomedical image segmentation. The U-Net architecture consists of an encoder network that downsamples the input image and a decoder network that upsamples the feature maps to produce a pixel-wise segmentation map. The U-Net architecture has been shown to be highly effective for segmenting a wide range of biomedical images, including dental radiographs and 3D dental scans.

In dentistry, semantic segmentation is used for a variety of applications, including the diagnosis and treatment planning of dental diseases. For example, in the case of periodontitis, a common oral disease that affects the supporting tissues of the teeth, semantic segmentation can be used to segment the periodontal ligament, alveolar bone, and gingival tissues. This segmentation can then be used to measure the thickness of the periodontal ligament, which is a key indicator of the severity of the disease. Semantic segmentation can also be used in the diagnosis of dental caries, a common dental disease caused by bacterial infection. By segmenting the teeth and the carious lesions, dentists can accurately assess the extent of the caries and plan the appropriate treatment. Additionally, semantic segmentation can be used to segment dental implants and surrounding tissues, enabling the assessment of the implant stability and the diagnosis of implant-related complications. In Figs. 2.7 and 2.8, automatic segmentation of crown/bridge restorations and automatic segmentation of lichen planus are seen, respectively.

Object Detection

Object detection is the process of finding possible lesions or abnormalities in images, e.g., lung nodules. This is frequently accomplished by projecting these lesions' locations as bounding boxes. Sampling potential patches near areas of

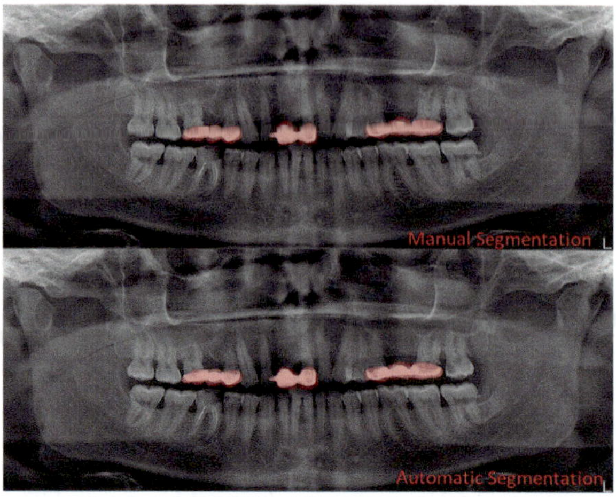

Fig. 2.7 Automatic segmentation of the crown/bridge restorations on an OPG. Manual segmentations of the clinicians (above) and automatic segmentation of the algorithm (below) have a high spatial overlap that shows that algorithm is successful in that task

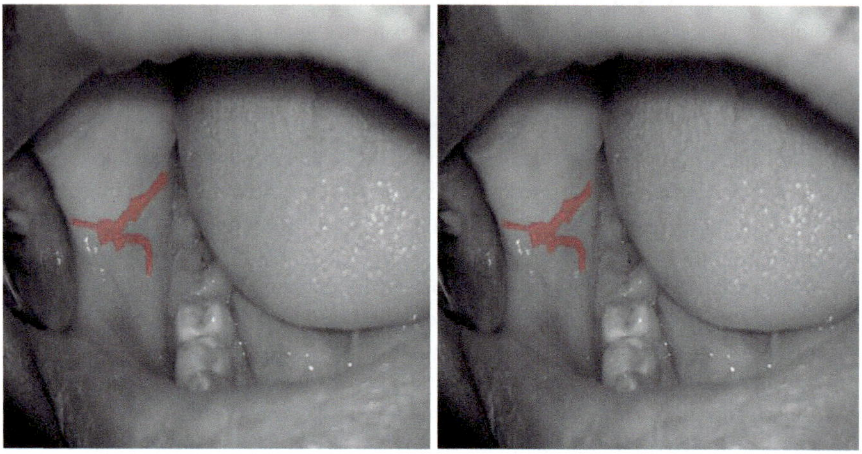

Fig. 2.8 Automatic segmentation of the reticular lichen planus lesion on an intraoral photograph. Manual segmentations of the clinicians (left) and automatic segmentation of the algorithm (right) have a high spatial overlap that shows that algorithm is successful in that task

interest and categorizing them as positive or negative samples is one method for finding lesions. Another strategy is to execute segmentation directly, with detection implicit in the linked sections that arise. A third strategy involves directly deriving the bounding box coordinates surrounding the target items from the input image. In medical imaging, the first method is often applied.

The fact that the target class often has fewer instances than the background class, which might have more examples and be more variable, is a frequent problem when training a network for detection or segmentation. In order to overcome this, patches from the target and background classes are sampled in an equal amount to create a

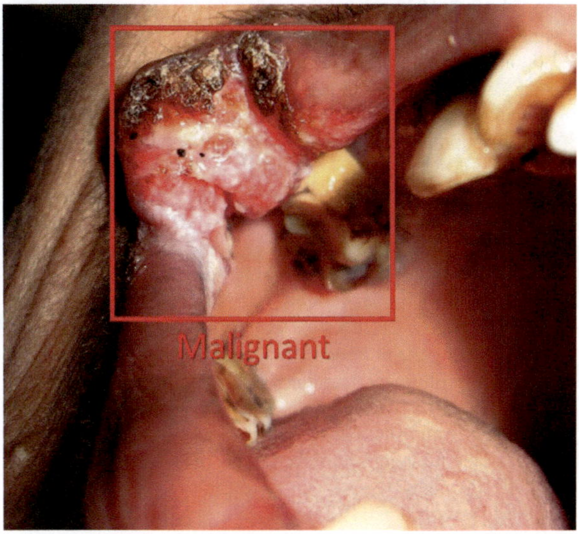

Fig. 2.9 Squamous cell carcinoma (malignant lesion) of the oral commissure is automatically detected by the algorithm in a red square box

surrogate dataset. This lessens the normally existing class imbalance in detection tasks.

As most of the images often comprises normal tissue (true negative), relying on accuracy as the primary performance metric is not very instructive for detection tasks and may obscure missed lesions (false negative). Instead, other assessment criteria such as sensitivity, precision, and F1 score are frequently provided, which do not take real negatives into consideration.

Using object detection, it is possible to detect oral lesions, including oral cancers. Dental practitioners can use this technology to enhance patient outcomes by utilizing earlier diagnosis and treatment by teaching ML models to distinguish the distinct visual features of these lesions (Fig. 2.9).

Clustering

An ML technique called clustering involves assembling related data points into clusters based on their characteristics. Clustering can be used in dentistry for a variety of tasks, including locating patient groups who share similar oral health issues, classifying teeth according to their properties, and grouping radiographic pictures according to their attributes. The selection of appropriate features or attributes that can capture the similarities or contrasts between data points is part of the clustering training pipeline in dentistry. Clustering methods can be used to organize the data points into clusters after the features have been retrieved. K-means clustering, hierarchical clustering, and DBSCAN are examples of clustering techniques frequently used in dentistry.

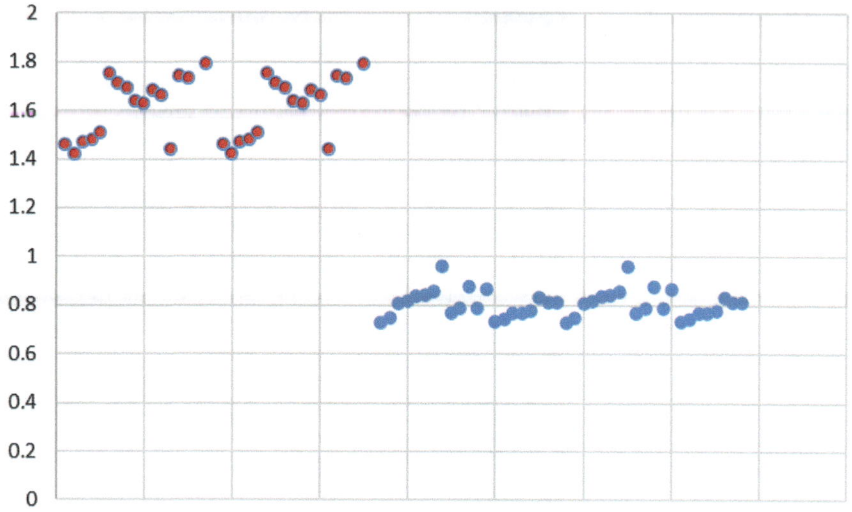

Fig. 2.10 Comparison of mean apparent diffusion coefficient (ADC) values for benign (red dots) and malignant lesions (blue dots), showing a clear separation between the two groups based on AI-powered clustering algorithm

Dental clustering methods are evaluated using criteria such the Davies-Bouldin index, Dunn index, and silhouette score. Based on the similarity and dissimilarity of the clusters, these metrics rate the quality of the clusters. Patient stratification for individualized treatment plans, tooth grouping for orthodontic treatment planning, and radiographic image clustering for diagnostic and treatment planning are all examples of clustering's dental applications (Fig. 2.10). Using clustering in dentistry research can help discover groupings of patients or teeth based on their features, which could help create novel technologies and treatment plans.

Prediction Modeling

A subset of ML known as predictive modeling makes predictions about the future based on historical data. In order to forecast new, unforeseen data, a model based on known inputs and outputs must be constructed. Predictive modeling can be used in dentistry to examine huge databases of patient records, including clinical and imaging data, to spot trends and forecast the course of a disease or the success of a therapy. There are various steps in the training pipeline for predictive modeling. To guarantee that the data is correct, comprehensive, and in a format that the model can use, it must first be gathered and preprocessed. Next, features are selected based on their relevance to the prediction task, and the model is trained using various algorithms, such as linear regression, decision trees, or NNs. The trained model is then evaluated using a test dataset to measure its accuracy and generalizability. Finally, the model can be deployed for use on new data.

The performance of a predictive model can be evaluated using various metrics, including accuracy, precision, recall, F1 score, and area under the curve (AUC). These metrics help to measure the model's ability to correctly predict outcomes and to balance false positives and false negatives. In dentistry, these metrics can be used to evaluate the performance of models for predicting disease progression, treatment outcomes, or the likelihood of developing certain conditions. Predicting the results of orthodontic or prosthodontic procedures is just one use of predictive modeling in dentistry. Moreover, imaging data may be analyzed to identify potential problems of certain treatments or to forecast the chance of acquiring caries. Predictive modeling may also be used to examine huge datasets of medical records in order to spot patterns and trends that can help guide clinical decision-making and enhance patient outcomes.

Anomaly Detection

Anomaly detection, commonly referred to as the outlier detection, is a method for locating data patterns that deviate from predicted behavior. It is especially helpful in finding uncommon or rare situations that might be a sign of abnormal or flawed circumstances. Building a model that can distinguish between normal and abnormal data points is the aim of anomaly detection. The process of training a model for anomaly detection entails locating and gathering pertinent data, choosing pertinent features, and training the model with a suitable algorithm. Unsupervised learning techniques like clustering or density estimation are frequently used to find patterns in the data.

Evaluation metrics for anomaly detection depend on the specific application and the nature of the data. Common metrics include precision, recall, and F1-score. Precision measures the proportion of detected anomalies that are truly anomalous, while recall measures the proportion of true anomalies that are detected. F1-score is a weighted average of precision and recall. Anomaly detection has a wide range of applications in dentistry, including identifying rare or unusual cases of disease or abnormal conditions in radiographic images, detecting outliers in patient data, and identifying patterns of drug interactions or adverse events that may be indicative of an underlying problem. Anomaly detection can also be used to identify fraudulent or malicious behavior, such as unauthorized access to patient records or other security breaches.

Bibliography

Alotaibi G, Awawdeh M, Farook FF, Aljohani M, Aldhafiri RM, Aldhoayan M. Artificial intelligence (AI) diagnostic tools: utilizing a convolutional neural network (CNN) to assess periodontal bone level radiographically-a retrospective study. BMC Oral Health. 2022;22(1):399. https://doi.org/10.1186/s12903-022-02436-3.

Amasya H, Cesur E, Yildirim D, Orhan K. Validation of cervical vertebral maturation stages: artificial intelligence vs human observer visual analysis. Am J Orthod Dentofac Orthop. 2020;158(6):e173–9. https://doi.org/10.1016/j.ajodo.2020.08.014.

Baur C, Wiestler B, Muehlau M, Zimmer C, Navab N, Albarqouni S. Modeling healthy anatomy with artificial intelligence for unsupervised anomaly detection in brain MRI. Radiol Artif Intell. 2021;3(3):e190169. https://doi.org/10.1148/ryai.2021190169.

Birkenbihl C, Ahmad A, Massat NJ, Raschka T, Avbersek A, Downey P, Armstrong M, Frohlich H. Artificial intelligence-based clustering and characterization of Parkinson's disease trajectories. Sci Rep. 2023;13(1):2897. https://doi.org/10.1038/s41598-023-30038-8.

Buyuk C, Akkaya N, Arsan B, Unsal G, Aksoy S, Orhan K. A fused deep learning architecture for the detection of the relationship between the mandibular third molar and the mandibular canal. Diagnostics (Basel). 2022;12(8) https://doi.org/10.3390/diagnostics12082018.

Buyuk C, Arican Alpay B, Er F. Detection of the separated root canal instrument on panoramic radiograph: a comparison of LSTM and CNN deep learning methods. Dentomaxillofac Radiol. 2023;52(3):20220209. https://doi.org/10.1259/dmfr.20220209.

Ezhov M, Gusarev M, Golitsyna M, Yates JM, Kushnerev E, Tamimi D, Aksoy S, Shumilov E, Sanders A, Orhan K. Clinically applicable artificial intelligence system for dental diagnosis with CBCT. Sci Rep. 2021;11(1):15006. https://doi.org/10.1038/s41598-021-94093-9.

Galante N, Cotroneo R, Furci D, Lodetti G, Casali MB. Applications of artificial intelligence in forensic sciences: current potential benefits, limitations and perspectives. Int J Legal Med. 2023;137(2):445–58. https://doi.org/10.1007/s00414-022-02928-5.

Gomes RFT, Schmith J, Figueiredo RM, Freitas SA, Machado GN, Romanini J, Carrard VC. Use of artificial intelligence in the classification of elementary oral lesions from clinical images. Int J Environ Res Public Health. 2023;20(5):3894. https://doi.org/10.3390/ijerph20053894.

Hung KF, Yeung AWK, Bornstein MM, Schwendicke F. Personalized dental medicine, artificial intelligence, and their relevance for dentomaxillofacial imaging. Dentomaxillofac Radiol. 2023;52(1):20220335. https://doi.org/10.1259/dmfr.20220335.

Keser G, Bayrakdar IS, Pekiner FN, Celik O, Orhan K. A deep learning approach for masseter muscle segmentation on ultrasonography. J Ultrason. 2022;22(91):e204–8. https://doi.org/10.15557/jou.2022.0034.

Keser G, Bayrakdar IS, Pekiner FN, Celik O, Orhan K. A deep learning algorithm for classification of oral lichen planus lesions from photographic images: A retrospective study. J Stomatol Oral Maxillofac Surg. 2023;124(1):101264. https://doi.org/10.1016/j.jormas.2022.08.007.

Kim KS, Kim BK, Chung MJ, Cho HB, Cho BH, Jung YG. Detection of maxillary sinus fungal ball via 3-D CNN-based artificial intelligence: fully automated system and clinical validation. PLoS One. 2022;17(2):e0263125. https://doi.org/10.1371/journal.pone.0263125.

Li X, Liu X, Deng X, Fan Y. Interplay between artificial intelligence and biomechanics modeling in the cardiovascular disease prediction. Biomedicine. 2022;10(9):2157. https://doi.org/10.3390/biomedicines10092157.

Mori Y, East JE, Hassan C, Halvorsen N, Berzin TM, Byrne M, von Renteln D, Hewett DG, Repici A, Ramchandani M, Al Khatry M, Kudo SE, Wang P, Yu H, Saito Y, Misawa M, Parasa S, Matsubayashi CO, Ogata H, et al. Benefits and challenges in implementation of artificial intelligence in colonoscopy: world endoscopy organization position statement. Dig Endosc. 2023;35:422. https://doi.org/10.1111/den.14531.

Mutasa S, Sun S, Ha R. Understanding artificial intelligence based radiology studies: CNN architecture. Clin Imaging. 2021;80:72–6. https://doi.org/10.1016/j.clinimag.2021.06.033.

Orhan K, Bayrakdar IS, Ezhov M, Kravtsov A, Ozyurek T. Evaluation of artificial intelligence for detecting periapical pathosis on cone-beam computed tomography scans. Int Endod J. 2020;53(5):680–9. https://doi.org/10.1111/iej.13265.

Salastekar NV, Maxfield C, Hanna TN, Krupinski EA, Heitkamp D, Grimm LJ. Artificial intelligence/machine learning education in radiology: multi-institutional survey of radiology residents in the United States. Acad Radiol. 2023;30:1481. https://doi.org/10.1016/j.acra.2023.01.005.

Saravi B, Hassel F, Ulkumen S, Zink A, Shavlokhova V, Couillard-Despres S, Boeker M, Obid P, Lang GM. Artificial intelligence-driven prediction modeling and decision making in spine surgery using hybrid machine learning models. J Pers Med. 2022;12(4):509. https://doi.org/10.3390/jpm12040509.

Schwendicke F, Chaurasia A, Wiegand T, Uribe SE, Fontana M, Akota I, Tryfonos O, Krois J, IADR e-oral health network and the ITU/WHO focus group AI for health. Artificial intelligence for oral and dental healthcare: Core education curriculum. J Dent. 2023;128:104363. https://doi.org/10.1016/j.jdent.2022.104363.

Shahnavazi M, Mohamadrahimi H. The application of artificial neural networks in the detection of mandibular fractures using panoramic radiography. Dent Res J (Isfahan). 2023;20:27. https://doi.org/10.4103/1735-3327.369629.

Xu IRL, Van Booven DJ, Goberdhan S, Breto A, Porto J, Alhusseini M, Algohary A, Stoyanova R, Punnen S, Mahne A, Arora H. Generative adversarial networks can create high quality artificial prostate cancer magnetic resonance images. J Pers Med. 2023;13(3):547. https://doi.org/10.3390/jpm13030547.

Artificial Intelligence from Medicine to Dentistry

3

Kaan Orhan and Hakan Amasya

Introduction

In 2020, global spending on healthcare reached to a high of US$ 9 trillion, or 10.8% of global gross domestic product (GDP), according to the Global Health Expenditure Report 2022 released by the World Health Organization (WHO) (Organization WH 2022). According to RBC Capital Market, approximately 30% of the data volume produced today is health data, and this ratio is expected to reach 36% by 2025 (Wiederrecht et al. n.d.).

Healthcare providers around the globe often have one common challenge: increasing patient benefits at an affordable cost. With the digital transformation in healthcare, the amount of data produced per patient is increasing day by day. Analyzing large medical data with the machine learning (ML) tools can contribute to increase the patient experience and service quality while reducing the costs (Gopal et al. 2019).

Gopal et al. reported four maturity stages of digitalization in a healthcare provider setting, as paper-based (patient data is recorded on papers), digitized (paper-based recordings are digitized), intelligent (fully implemented), and value-based healthcare (payment based on patient health outcome). The higher the stage of digital transformation, the greater the integration potential and effectiveness of ML tools (Gopal et al. 2019).

The beginning of artificial intelligence (AI) technologies with its modern definition begins in the early 1950s. This section of the book contains information about some of the milestones in the development of AI and their uses in medicine and

K. Orhan
Faculty of Dentistry, Department of Dentomaxillofacial Radiology, Ankara University, Ankara, Turkey

H. Amasya (✉)
Faculty of Dentistry, Department of Dentomaxillofacial Radiology, Istanbul University-Cerrahpaşa, Istanbul, Turkey

K. Orhan, R. Jagtap (eds.), *Artificial Intelligence in Dentistry*,
https://doi.org/10.1007/978-3-031-43827-1_3

dentistry. Although there is no definite information about the start and end dates of the projects realized in some periods, it would be appropriate to consider it as an example reflecting the technology of the relevant period, reminding that there may be slight deviations in the given years.

AI in the 1950s

In 1943, Warren S. McCulloch and Walter Pitts suggested that neural events and the relations among them can be processed by means of propositional logic, because of the "all-or-none" characteristics of nervous activity. The researchers developed a logical calculus model to imitate the working mechanism of the neurons (McCulloch and Pitts 1943). The proposed concept can be considered as a pioneering element of the modern architecture of artificial neural network (ANN) or deep learning (DL) models.

British mathematician and computer scientist Alan Turing considered the question "Can machines think?" and introduced "The Imitation Game" in 1950 (Fig. 3.1). The Turing test evaluates a machine's ability to imitate human and involves three components, a human interrogator, a machine, and a human. The interrogator is in an isolated environment and can only communicate the others by sending or receiving texts. A machine competes with a human to convince an interrogator that it is human. In this sense, if the interrogator decides who is machine and who is human mistakenly, the machine can be considered to surpass the human intelligence. Machines not only imitate the highly intelligent functions of humans to pass the test but also mimics the human behavioral patterns such as delaying the responses or making intended mistakes. Hence, the claim of "machines cannot make mistakes" is questioned. Turing test is often considered as the beginning of AI; however, the exact term "artificial intelligence" is not defined yet (Turing 1950).

American computer scientist John McCarthy used the term "artificial intelligence" during the Dartmouth Summer Research Project in 1956. In this project, features of human learning and intelligence were studied to be described precisely, so that the answers for how a machine can simulate the human intelligence were

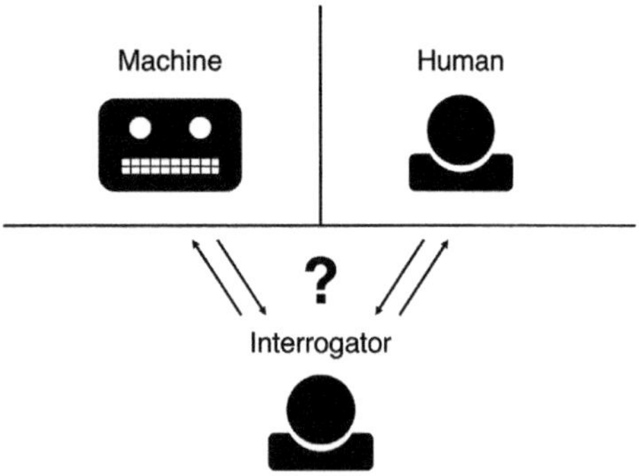

Fig. 3.1 "The Imitation Game," a.k.a. Turing test. The interrogator decides who is human or computer based on text conversation. If the machine can convince the interrogator to be the human, one can speak of an intelligent machine

searched. AI problems are discussed on topics such as automated computers or how to make machines use language, and this project is often attributed as the beginning of AI as a research discipline. The choice of the terms "artificial" and "intelligence" to describe such technologies is still controversial. It is interesting to speculate on the possible effects on the field if another label such as "computer intelligence" was adopted at that time (McCarthy et al. 2006; Moor 2006).

In 1958, Canadian-born psychologist and computer scientist Franck Rosenblatt from Cornell Aeronautical Laboratory developed the theory of "perceptron" by questioning how information is perceived, stored, remembered, or influenced behavior in the biological systems (Fig. 3.2). The proposed hypothetical nervous system was demonstrated by photo-perception analogy, and predicting learning curves from neurological variables became possible (Rosenblatt 1958). The concept of perceptron and further improvements are contributed to the development of the ANNs and other machine learning (ML) techniques.

In 1959, Robert S. Ledley and Lee B. Lusted released an article in Nature and analyzed the steps of reasoning in medical diagnosis with the disciplines of symbolic logic, probability, and value theory. In their article, the symbolic logic was described as each "feature" of patient, such as a sign of "swelling" or a disease of "osteoporosis" is represented by symbols such as x, y, … The symbols of X + Y represent that the patient has feature x and/or y, while the symbols of X → Y represent that if the patient has feature x, then the feature y is present. Symbolic logic provides a fundamental framework for logical reasoning. Probabilistic concepts emphasize that the statement of "there is a chance" instead of "it must" in the sentence of "if the patient has feature x, then 'it must/there is a change' that the patient has feature y" may be used in assessing the likelihood of different diagnoses or patient outcomes. "Value theory" contributes to optimizing the treatment options by analyzing parameters such as therapeutic, moral, ethical, social, and economic status of the patient. Medical professionals may enhance their diagnostic reasoning and decision-making abilities employing such techniques (Ledley and Lusted 1959).

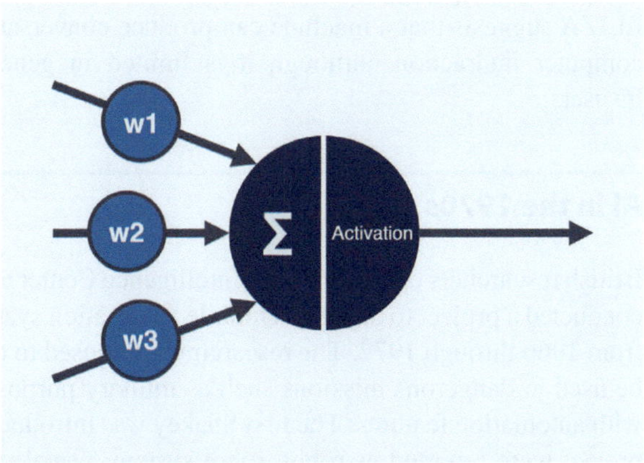

Fig. 3.2 A simple model for the perceptron concept defined by Franck Rosenblatt, similar to human neural elements

AI in the 1960s

In 1962, Frank Rosenblatt described the design of a multilayer perceptron, with three layers: an input layer, a hidden layer with randomized weights that do not learn, and an output layer with learning connections (Rosenblatt 1962). The proposed system was not a "deep learning" model; however, it was defined as "extreme machine learning" in the future.

Unimate was invented by George Devol as the first industrial robotic arm in 1962 and marketed by Joseph Engelberger. The first product was installed at an assembly line at General Motors plant in Terstedt, New Jersey, and performed automated die casting (Moran 2007). Just as the other humanoid robots described previously, like the "mechanical knight" of the Leonardo da Vinci in 1495, the Unimate was a forerunner and a source of inspiration for today's more advanced machines like da Vinci's robotic arm (Bogue 2020).

In 1965, Edward Feigenbaum and his team began the DENDRAL project in the Stanford University to develop an automated system to identify the unknown organic molecules, by analyzing their mass spectra of amino acids and knowledge of chemistry (Lederberg 1966). The project was conducted as two main programs, Heuristic DENDRAL and Meta-DENDRAL. The Heuristic DENDRAL use algorithms and rules in the system to analyze the mass spectrometry data and determine the structure of organic molecules. Meta-DENDRAL was published in 1978, with the aim of improving the system by knowledge directly from electronic libraries of mass spectral data (Feigenbaum and Buchanan 1993; Buchanan and Feigenbaum 1978; Buchanan et al. 1969).

Joseph Weizenbaum from Massachusetts Institute of Technology (MIT) developed an early example of a natural language conversation program, named ELIZA, to mimic human conversation in 1966. Input texts are analyzed on the basis of decomposition rules and the keywords to generate a response by reassembly rules using the pattern matching technique. The limitations for this early chatbot example were reported as the definition of keywords, the discovery of minimal context, the choice of appropriate transformation technique, the generation of keyword-independent responses, and the capacity to edit ELIZA "texts" (Weizenbaum 1966). ELIZA suggests that a machine can produce conversations in the sense of human-computer interaction, although it is limited in generating unique responses to its user.

AI in the 1970s

British researchers of the Artificial Intelligence Center at Stanford Research Institute conducted a project to develop a mobile automation system with the name "Shakey," from 1966 through 1972. The research was focused to develop a mobile machine to be used in dangerous missions such as military purposes or planetary exploration, with automation features. The first Shakey was introduced in 1969. Keywords of the project were reported as robot, robot system, visual processing, problem-solving, question answering, theorem proving, models of the world, planning, scene analysis, and mobile automation. The three primary required abilities for the system were reported as problem-solving, modelling, and perception. The first version of the Shakey was completed in 1969. The main parts of the device were an all radio-controlled SDS-940 time-shared computer system, TV, camera, and other sensors. The basic workflow of the device was to process the sensory data, store the perceived environment, and plan the sequence of motor actions accordingly. Pushing an object was a typical task for Shakey (Nilsson 1969; Nilsson 1984). In 1971, the development of an improved version of the Shakey was completed. In this version, the SDS-940 was replaced with a Digital Equipment Corporation PDP-10/PDP-15 facility, and seven tactile sensors, called "cat-whiskers," are used to perceive if the Shakey bumps into something, with other improvements. The Shakey is one of the pioneering research projects containing visual, tactile, and acoustic sensors, signal processing and pattern-recognition equipment, and computer programming for automated robotics (Nilsson 1984).

WABOT-1 (WAseda roBOT) was a pioneering humanoid robot developed in Japan at Waseda University between 1970 and 1973. The system features bipedal walking for mobility, stereovision, speech recognition, artificial ears and mouth, distance, and tactile sensors. An improved version of the first humanoid, WABOT-2 was produced in 1984, with the ability of playing musical instrument (Bogue 2020).

SUMEX-AIM (Stanford University Medical Experimental Computer for Artificial Intelligence in Medicine) was established in 1974. The project was based on a nationally shared computing resource for developing AI applications in biomedical science, using nationwide networks like ARPANET or TYMNET. In 1980, 16 research and three pilot projects were active on SUMEX-AIM, such as DENDRAL, INTERNIST, MYCIN, CASNET, EXPERT, MOLGEN, PUFF, and more (Freiherr 1980).

In 1970s, INTERNIST was developed by Jack D. Myers and Harry E. Pople as a consultative diagnostic program in internal medicine. About 3,000 different manifestations of the diseases were assigned to 400 disease entities with an "importance" from 1 to 5, and the system suggested the "evoking strength" and "frequency" of a disease, with a value from 1 to 5. The physicians were able to enter the manifestations of a clinical problem as present or absent, and the system confirm or deny the diseases and provide expert diagnostic consultative aid (Myers and Pople 1977).

MYCIN was a rule-based expert system for selecting the proper antimicrobial therapy for patients with bacterial infections. The system was running on a DEC PDP-10 computer and programmed with INTERLISP, a dialect of the LISP language. The MYCIN system consisted of consultation, explanation, and knowledge-acquisition subprograms and developed with some 350 rules, each intended to be a single, modular chunk of medical knowledge (Van Melle 1978). The consultation system used the knowledge database, the consultation system produced a therapeutic suggestion based on the patient data and knowledge base, and the explanation system was a question-answerer and explained the reasoning behind the suggestions, and the knowledge-acquisition system enabled experts to update MYCIN's static knowledge base without requiring the knowledge of computer programming

(Shortliffe 1977). The system was also used for educational purposes (Van Melle 1978).

Causal-associational network (CASNET) was an expert system for consulting the diagnosis, prognosis, and therapy of glaucoma. The system was developed using time-shared PDP-10 computers at Rutgers University and SUMEX-AIM project of Stanford University. In the development, experts from Mt. Sinai School of Medicine, Johns Hopkins University, Washington University, the University of Illinois at Chicago, and the University of Miami accessed to the SUMEX-AIM through a nationwide computer communication system. The decision-making strategy of the system was based on three main components: observations, states, and classification. Observations of patients are associated with the pathophysiological states and patterns of states in the network indicated an appropriate disease classification (Weiss et al. 1977). The major new features of CASNET system were reported as making generalizations from the disease qualitative model, reasoning the follow-up management, suggesting alternative expert opinions on subjects under debate and its testing and updating by glaucoma researchers using computed-based network (Weiss et al. 1978).

Expert systems developed at that time were generally limited to a specific field. Some systems, such as CASNET or MYCIN, have been further updated into a more generalizable model. EXPERT was developed as a general system for developing and testing such expert systems, independent of the specific application. The consultation system was an improved version of the CASNET/Glaucoma model and was used to develop new models in endocrinology (thyroid diseases), rheumatology, and ophthalmology, employing CASNET-like rules. The main motivation for the development of EXPERT was reported as expanding access to consultation of specialists, which was in shortage at that time (Weiss 1979).

Stephen G. Pauker et al. developed a computer program in MIT to study the clinical cognition of the patients with edema, named Present Illness Program (PIP) around 1975. The cognitive insights of the clinician's decisions were used to develop a computer program, and then the program was tested with a series of prototypical cases to be refined by analyzing the discrepancies between the results of the program and the clinicians. The authors stated that their study was possible by the advancements in the field of AI and computer science, such as "goal-directed" programming, pattern-matching and a large associative memory. The system was described as a program which uses knowledge of diseases and pathophysiology, along with the "common sense," to reach its goals (Pauker et al. 1976).

In 1976, Tomas Lozano-Perez at MIT published a paper describing the development of a simple LISP program for medical diagnosis, named PSUDOC. The required features of a good baseline program were listed as simplicity, flexibility, and effectiveness, while the three primary strategies to reach these goals were reported as Bayesian decision analysis, feature intersection, and tree traversal strategies. Bayesian decision analysis was defined to be working well on well-constrained problems, but more general problems violate the rules, and the explanation of the results is lacking. Feature intersection was described as finding the matches in the set of diseases with the present symptoms; however, the method reported to be not favorable for medical diagnosis because of the complexity. Tree traversal strategies were suggested as the simplest of the three and described as a tree whose internal nodes are test/questions and linked until a leaf (diagnosis) is reached, similar to the decision tree algorithms (Lozano-Perez 1976).

The Association for the Advancement of Artificial Intelligence was established as a nonprofit scientific society with the name, American Association for Artificial Intelligence, in 1979 (About the Association for the Advancement of Artificial Intelligence (AAAI) Member Organization n.d.).

AI in the 1980s

EMYCIN was described as "MYCIN without infectious disease diagnosis" by Edward A. Feigenbaum in the 1980s. The idea was to remove the knowledge base of MYCIN and configure new rules for another task. EMYCIN was not an expert system for an end user, but a software tool for developing expert systems (Feigenbaum 1981). For example, PUFF was developed using the EMYCIN tool, to analyze the laboratory measurements of pulmonary function to evaluate the pulmonary disease of the patient. Just as the MYCIN or EMYCIN, PUFF was written in INTERLISP language and runs on a DEC KI-10 at the SUMEX-AIM facility. The authors developed a second version of PUFF to run on a PDP-11 at the Pacific Medical Center, using BASIC language. The expert system analyzed about 50 quantitative parameters and generated an automatic report for three types of pulmonary disease, following the knowledge-based rules (Feigenbaum 1981; Aikins et al. 1983).

In 1986, Fikret Ulug developed the EMYCIN-Prolog expert system shell. In their study, the interference engine of MYCIN was translated into PROLOG language, and built-in pattern matching and backtracking ability were reported to be two important features of the system. The idea was to produce a tool for developing expert systems, and two different concepts are studied. One system (CAR) was developed for diagnosing engine problems in a car, while the other (FINANCE analysis system) was giving financial advices. The authors reported that it was possible to build an expert system with the developed shell quickly (Ulug 1986).

In 1986, David E. Rumelhart et al. defined a new learning procedure with the name back-propagation, for networks of neurone-like units. The procedure was defined as minimizing the variance in the desired and the actual output, by adjusting the weights of the hidden units. Hidden units are in the layers independent of the input and the output and play an important role in the learning process (Rumelhart et al. 1986). The origins of this technique go back to the 1960s, and the concept has been partially described in different ways by a few researchers such as Franck Rosenblatt, Paul Werbos, or Seppo Linnainmaa (Werbos 1990; Linnainmaa 1970).

In 1987, DXplain was developed as a computer-based diagnostic decision-support system for physicians with no computer expertise. The developed system was distributed through AMA/NET, a nationwide computer network, and the physicians interacted with the system by answering the questions regarding the patient data and the medical terms. The system reported the results separately as common and rare diseases. The authors suggested six important criteria for a decision-support system such as ease of use without computer knowledge, based on comprehensive medical information, provide correct and accurate results, justify the results, easy access from different locations such as home and hospital, and evolve and improve with the user interactions (Barnett et al. 1987).

Introduction of the Deep Learning Models

In 1998, Yann Lecun et al. developed the LeNet-5, the convolutional neural network (CNN) architecture, a multilayer neural network trained with the back-propagation algorithm using gradient-based learning technique. The system was developed for classifying the patterns in handwritten characters and suggested to provide adequate record accuracy on business and personal checks (LeCun et al. 1998). LeNet-5 achieved a high accuracy in recognizing handwritten digits and played a pivotal role in the development of deep learning for image classification tasks.

In 2009, the ImageNet was introduced as a large-scale dataset designed for training and evaluating computer vision models. It consists of millions of labeled images, with a wide range of object classes, including animals, objects, vehicles, and more. The dataset was created with the goal of promoting the experiments of training the deep neural networks with supervised learning, to lead significant improvements in object recognition and image classification (Deng et al. 2009).

In 2012, a CNN model was developed by Alex Krizhevsky, Ilya Sutskever, and Geoffrey Hinton named AlexNet. The system consisted of eight layers, including five convolutional layers and three fully connected layers, and introduced innovative features such as ReLU activation functions, overlapping pooling, local response normalization, and dropout regularization (Krizhevsky et al. 2017). AlexNet won the ImageNet LSVRC-2012 competition.

In 2015, Olaf Ronneberger, Philipp Fischer, and Thomas Brox presented the U-Net, a convolutional neural network architecture designed for biomedical image segmentation tasks. The U-shaped structure of the algorithm consists of an encoder path and a decoder path and enables efficient feature extraction and accurate localization. Numerous medical imaging applications, including tumor segmentation, cell identification, and organ segmentation, make extensive use of U-Net.

AlphaGo, developed by DeepMind, made history in 2016 by defeating the world champion Go player, Lee Sedol, in a five-game match. This victory marked a significant milestone in the field of artificial intelligence and demonstrated the power of deep learning and reinforcement learning techniques. AlphaGo's success showcased its ability to analyze complex board positions and make strategic moves that surpassed human expertise (Wang et al. 2016). This is not the first time a machine has surpassed a human, but it is one of the pioneering events that has made a worldwide impact.

AI's Past and Future

In this section, information about the origin and development of AI systems in the modern sense and their pioneering use in the medical field have been compiled. Especially with DL and advanced automation features, AI or ML has reached an incredible place from its original point of view. However, we would like to emphasize that at the beginning of such systems, the goal was to transfer the human mind and decision-making process to a machine. While trying to define the human intelligence and decision-making process mathematically, data about biological processes were obtained; on the other hand, the concept of transferring the obtained data to a machine led to the development of robotic systems. Today, although DL models are providing marvelous results with their outstanding achievements, their inadequacies in matters such as the explainability of the results contradict the principles of the period when the systems in question emerged.

References

About the Association for the Advancement of Artificial Intelligence (AAAI) Member Organization. https://aaai.org/about-aaai/.

Aikins JS, Kunz JC, Shortliffe EH, Fallat RJ. PUFF: an expert system for interpretation of pulmonary function data. Comput Biomed Res. 1983;16(3):199–208.

Barnett GO, Cimino JJ, Hupp JA, Hoffer EP. DXplain: an evolving diagnostic decision-support system. JAMA. 1987;258(1):67–74.

Bogue R. Humanoid robots from the past to the present. Ind Robot Int J Robot Res Appl. 2020;47(4):465–72.

Buchanan BG, Feigenbaum EA. DENDRAL and meta-DENDRAL: their applications dimension. Artif Intell. 1978;11(1–2):5–24.

Buchanan B, Sutherland G, Feigenbaum EA. Heuristic DENDRAL: A program for generating explanatory hypotheses. Org Chem. 1969;30

Deng J, Dong W, Socher R, Li L-J, Li K, Fei-Fei L. Imagenet: A large-scale hierarchical image database. 2009 IEEE conference on computer vision and pattern recognition, IEEE; 2009.

Feigenbaum EA. Expert systems in the 1980s. State of the art report on machine intelligence Maidenhead: Pergamon-Infotech. 1981.

Feigenbaum EA, Buchanan BG. Dendral and meta-Dendral. Artif Intell. 1993;59:233–40.

Freiherr G. The seeds of artificial intelligence: SUMEX-AIM: US Department of Health, Education, and Welfare, Public Health Service…; 1980.

Gopal G, Suter-Crazzolara C, Toldo L, Eberhardt W. Digital transformation in healthcare–architectures of present and future information technologies. Clin Chem Lab Med (CCLM). 2019;57(3):328–35.

Krizhevsky A, Sutskever I, Hinton GE. Imagenet classification with deep convolutional neural networks. Commun ACM. 2017;60(6):84–90.

LeCun Y, Bottou L, Bengio Y, Haffner P. Gradient-based learning applied to document recognition. Proc IEEE. 1998;86(11):2278–324.

Lederberg J. Systematics of organic molecules, graph topology and Hamilton circuits. A general outline of the Dendral system Interim report; 1966.

Ledley RS, Lusted LB. Reasoning foundations of medical diagnosis: symbolic logic, probability, and value theory aid our understanding of how physicians reason. Science. 1959;130(3366):9–21.

Linnainmaa S. The representation of the cumulative rounding error of an algorithm as a Taylor expansion of the local rounding errors: Master's thesis (in Finnish), Univ. Helsinki; 1970.

Lozano-Perez T. PSUDOC-A simple diagnostic program. 1976.

McCarthy J, Minsky ML, Rochester N, Shannon CE. A proposal for the Dartmouth summer research project on artificial intelligence, august 31, 1955. AI Mag. 2006;27(4):12.

McCulloch WS, Pitts W. A logical calculus of the ideas immanent in nervous activity. Bull Math Biophys. 1943;5:115–33.

Moor J. The Dartmouth College artificial intelligence conference: the next fifty years. AI Mag. 2006;27(4):87.

Moran ME. Evolution of robotic arms. J Robot Surg. 2007;1(2):103–11.

Myers J, Pople HE, editors. INTERNIST: A consultative diagnostic program in internal medicine. Proceedings of the Annual Symposium on Computer Application in Medical Care. American Medical Informatics Association; 1977.

Nilsson NJ. A mobile automaton: an application of artificial intelligence techniques. Sri International Menlo Park Ca Artificial Intelligence Center; 1969.

Nilsson NJ, editor Shakey the Robot; 1984.

Organization WH. Global spending on health: rising to the pandemic's challenges. Geneva: World Health Organization; 2022.

Pauker SG, Gorry GA, Kassirer JP, Schwartz WB. Towards the simulation of clinical cognition: taking a present illness by computer. Am J Med. 1976;60(7):981–96.

Rosenblatt F. The perceptron: a probabilistic model for information storage and organization in the brain. Psychol Rev. 1958;65(6):386.

Rosenblatt F. Principles of neurodynamics, vol. 10. New York: Spartan; 1962. p. 318–62.

Rumelhart DE, Hinton GE, Williams RJ. Learning representations by back-propagating errors. Nature. 1986;323(6088):533–6.

Shortliffe EH, editor Mycin: A knowledge-based computer program applied to infectious diseases. Proceedings of the Annual Symposium on Computer Application in Medical Care. American Medical Informatics Association; 1977.

Turing AM. I.—Computing machinery and intelligence. Mind. 1950;LIX(236):433–60.

Ulug F. Emycin-Prolog expert system shell. Monterey, CA: Naval Postgraduate School; 1986.

Van Melle W. MYCIN: a knowledge-based consultation program for infectious disease diagnosis. Int J Man Mach Stud. 1978;10(3):313–22.

Wang F-Y, Zhang JJ, Zheng X, Wang X, Yuan Y, Dai X, et al. Where does AlphaGo go: from church-turing thesis to AlphaGo thesis and beyond. IEEE/CAA J Automat Sin. 2016;3(2):113–20.

Weiss S. The EXPERT and CASNET consultation systems. 情報処理学会研究報告医療情報処理 (MED). 1979;1979(15 (1979-MED-001)):1–5.

Weiss SM, Kulikowski CA, Safir A, editors. A Model-Based Consultation System for the Long-Term Management of Glaucoma. IJCAI; 1977.

Weiss S, Kulikowski CA, Safir A. Glaucoma consultation by computer. Comput Biol Med. 1978;8(1):25–40.

Weizenbaum J. ELIZA—a computer program for the study of natural language communication between man and machine. Commun ACM. 1966;9(1):36–45.

Werbos PJ. Backpropagation through time: what it does and how to do it. Proc IEEE. 1990;78(10):1550–60.

Wiederrecht G, Darwish S, Callaway A. The healthcare data explosion. https://www.rbccm.com/en/gib/healthcare/episode/the_healthcare_data_explosion.

Applications of Artificial Intelligence in Dentistry

4

Prashant P. Jaju, Ibrahim Sevki Bayrakdar, Sushma Jaju, Vidhi Shah, Kaan Orhan, and Rohan Jagtap

P. P. Jaju (✉)
Department of Oral Medicine and Radiology, Rishiraj College of Dental Sciences and Research Centre, Bhopal, India

I. S. Bayrakdar
Division of Oral and Maxillofacial Radiology, Department of Care Planning and Restorative Sciences, School of Dentistry, University of Mississippi Medical Center, Jackson, MS, USA

Department of Oral and Maxillofacial Radiology, School of Dentistry, Center of Research and Application for Computer-Aided Diagnosis and Treatment in Health, Eskisehir Osmangazi University, ESOGÜ Meşelik Yerleşkesi, Eskisehir, Turkey

S. Jaju
Department of Conservative Dentistry and Endodontics, Rishiraj College of Dental Sciences And Research Centre, Bhopal, India

V. Shah
Velmeni Inc., Sunnyvale, USA

K. Orhan
Faculty of Dentistry, Department of Dentomaxillofacial Radiology, Ankara University, Ankara, Turkey

R. Jagtap
Division of Oral and Maxillofacial Radiology, Department of Care Planning and Restorative Sciences, School of Dentistry, University of Mississippi Medical Center, Jackson, MS, USA

Department of Radiology, School of Medicine, University of Mississippi Medical Center, Jackson, MS, USA

K. Orhan, R. Jagtap (eds.), *Artificial Intelligence in Dentistry*,
https://doi.org/10.1007/978-3-031-43827-1_4

Introduction

Dave Waters said, "Predicting the future is not magic, its artificial intelligence."

What is 'artificial intelligence'? The field of computer science known as artificial intelligence (AI) is focused on creating intelligent machines that can think and behave like humans. Examples of AI applications include speech recognition, problem-solving, learning, and planning. Artificial intelligence (AI) is demonstrated by machines, as opposed to the natural intelligence displayed by humans. At its core, AI comprises computer-trained algorithms that aim to mimic human intelligence (HI). HI refers to the biologically formed congenital intelligence capability of humans, which includes various skills such as perception, learning, problem-solving, decision-making, language comprehension, and social interaction. Human intelligence can be improved through experience and learning over the lifespan. Artificial intelligence (AI) is the field of computer science that focuses on producing machines capable of performing tasks that typically require human intelligence. AI can be trained by analyzing enormous amounts of data, which results in better and more accurate outcomes for medical diagnosis and treatment. Machine learning (ML) is a subset of AI that involves the development of algorithms capable of learning and improving from experience without explicit programming. ML algorithms are designed to identify patterns and relationships in large datasets, making them useful in various applications such as image recognition, natural language processing, and predictive analytics. Deep learning (DL) is a type of ML that utilizes artificial neural networks (ANN), inspired by the structure and function of the human brain. DL algorithms are designed to learn and improve from experience by analyzing massive amounts of data, enabling them to perform complex tasks (Shan et al. 2021; Khanagar et al. 2021a; Schwendicke et al. 2020b; Carrillo-Perez et al. 2022; Park and Park 2018; Hung et al. 2020b) (Fig. 4.1).

AI has been developed in three phases. In the 1980s and 1990s, the first generation of AI utilized predefined rules to process data and generate outputs. The second generation, in the 2000s, introduced the concept of "learning," where computers could autonomously establish rules based on human-provided input and data and apply those rules to produce outputs. Currently, we are in the third generation of AI, which focuses on "deep learning." Deep learning enables computers to automatically analyze new data, learn new rules, and generate outputs without the need for human interaction (https://www.impactfund.org/legal-practitioner-blog/ai-civilrights n.d.). The first chatbot computer program, ELIZA, was created in the

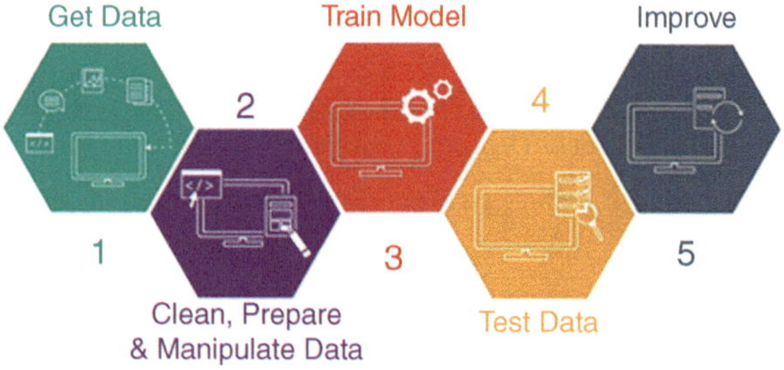

Fig. 4.1 Illustration showing the development of AI software

1960s, while in 1977, IBM's custom-built supercomputer, Deep Blue, made history by defeating a world chess champion. Apple's Siri, introduced as a feature in the iPhone 4S in October 2011, and Amazon's Alexa are examples of AI applications that have become part of our daily lives. Today, AI is pervasive across various industries, including self-driving cars, marketing chatbots, social media monitoring, manufacturing robots, healthcare management, and even dentistry. AI plays a significant role in the medical industry, including areas such as electronic health records, robotic surgery, and now, dentistry. According to Forbes, key AI areas in healthcare include administrative workflows, image analysis, robotic surgery, and clinical decision support (Marr 2018).

Although dentistry initially lagged behind in integrating AI, the advancements in dental technology have rapidly positioned AI as one of the essential tools in dental diagnosis and treatment. Dentistry heavily relies on digital workflows, and AI is increasingly being incorporated into the field. AI finds applications in dentistry such as diagnosis and treatment planning, image analysis, patient management, predictive analytics, and robotics. The potential impact of AI in dentistry is substantial, as it can improve diagnosis accuracy, reduce treatment time, and enhance patient care. This chapter focuses on the current use of AI in diagnosis and treatment planning in dentistry.

Applications of AI in Dentistry

Normal Anatomy

"Normal anatomy identification and segmentation are now possible with AI-generated algorithms. Today, AI successfully assists dentists in automatically detecting and segmenting anatomical structures in dental radiographs, particularly cone beam computed tomography (CBCT). In addition to the tooth and its structures, the successful segmentation of maxillofacial bones and other anatomical structures such as the maxillary sinus, pharyngeal airway, mandibular canal, and incisive canals provides dentists with significant advantages in making faster and more accurate decisions in the diagnosis and treatment planning processes (Fig. 4.2). With the help of AI-assisted software, both 2D radiographs and 3D CBCT volumes

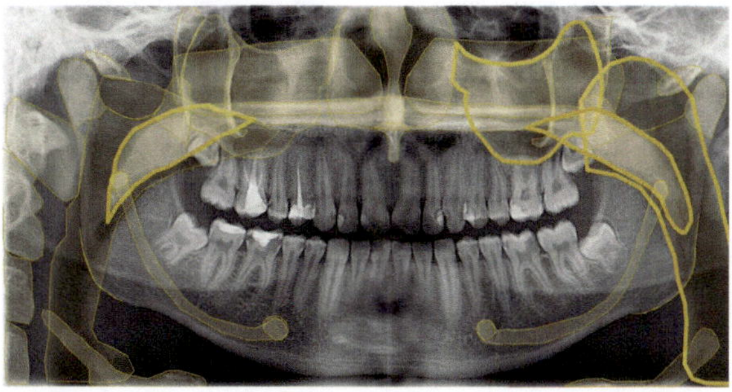

Fig. 4.2 AI-generated anatomic structure segmentation on panoramic radiograph. (Courtesy by CranioCatch AI software)

can now be segmented and separated for better viewing (Fig. 4.3). This allows clinicians to study the anatomy accurately and precisely (Lahoud et al. 2021; Hung et al. 2020a; Mohaideen et al. 2022; Hung et al. 2023; Orhan et al. 2022).

Reporting of Dental Status/Electronic Dental Record

AI can report the patient's status by performing tasks such as detecting and numbering teeth, identifying dental restorations, and detecting pathologies in dental radiographs and other images, including intraoral photographs and intraoral scanning images (Figs. 4.4, 4.5, and 4.6) (Bilgir et al. 2021; Görürgöz et al. 2022; Kilic et al. 2021; Yasa et al. 2021). This automation of determining the patient's current state before treatment greatly facilitates workflow and improves efficiency (Shan et al. 2021; Khanagar et al. 2021a; Schwendicke et al. 2020b; Carrillo-Perez et al. 2022; Park and Park 2018).

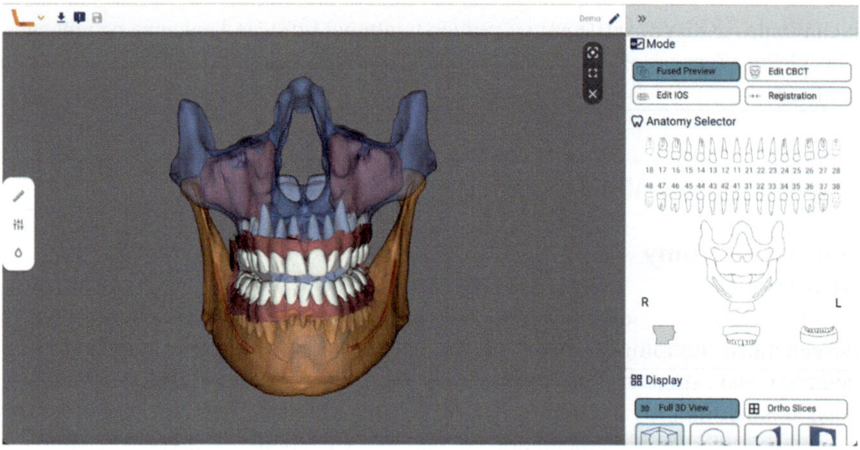

Fig. 4.3 AI-generated 3D Virtual Model. (Courtesy by Relu AI software)

Fig. 4.4 AI-generated teeth segmentation on panoramic radiograph. (Courtesy by CranioCatch AI software)

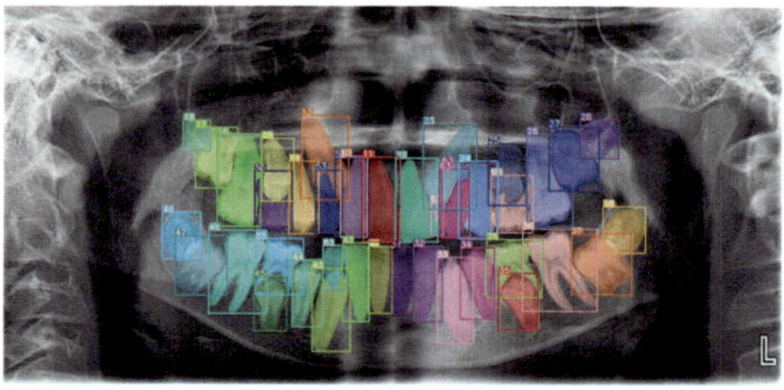

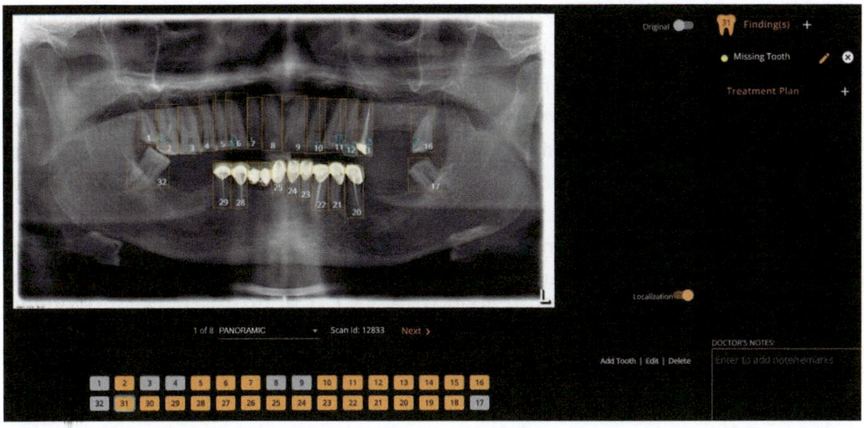

Fig. 4.5 AI system detecting teeth and caries on panoramic radiograph for dental status/record. (Courtesy by Velmeni AI software)

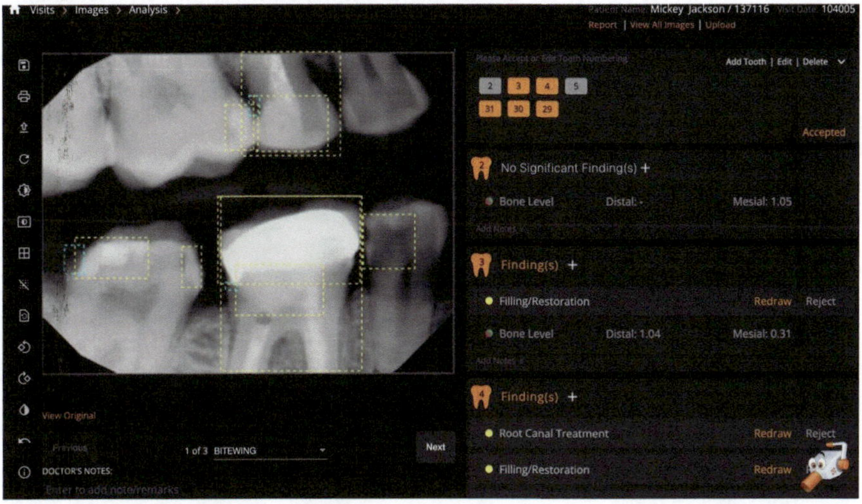

Fig. 4.6 Automatic segmentation of bitewing radiograph showing root canal treated teeth, restoration, and bone loss. (Courtesy by Velmeni AI software)

Cariology

Dental caries is one of the most common diseases in humans. Early and accurate detection of dental caries is crucial for appropriate treatment and prevention of further complications. Radiographic examination plays a vital role in identifying dental caries. Intraoral radiographs are particularly important for detecting early non-cavitated caries. While several diagnostic methods exist for dental caries detection, such as near-infrared-light transillumination (NILT), digital imaging fiber-optic transillumination (DIFOTI), quantitative light-induced fluorescence (QLF), and laser fluorescence, radiographic evaluation remains essential in caries detection. Numerous deep learning-based AI models have been developed to assist dentists in detecting and classifying dental caries in panoramic, periapical, bitewing, and CBCT images. Using AI for dental caries detection offers several potential benefits, including improved accuracy, faster diagnosis, and reduced reliance on human interpretation. The integration of AI in dental caries detection can enhance dental care and reduce the prevalence of dental diseases by enabling earlier and more accurate diagnoses (Shan et al. 2021; Khanagar et al. 2021a; Schwendicke et al. 2020b; Carrillo-Perez et al. 2022; Park and Park 2018; Hung et al. 2020b; Hung et al. 2023; Revilla-León et al. 2022; Schwendicke et al. 2023; Ezhov et al. 2021) (Figs. 4.7 and 4.8).

AI models have shown success in assessing the presence or absence of dental caries in radiographic images. According to various studies, AI models achieved caries diagnosis accuracy ranging from 76% to 88.3%, sensitivity ranging from 73% to 90%, and specificity ranging from 61.5% to 93%. For instance, Valizadeh et al. analyzed an AI model for diagnosing proximal caries from periapical radiographs, which achieved a 97% accuracy in diagnosing dentin caries but only 60% accuracy in diagnosing enamel caries (Valizadeh et al. 2015). Similarly, Devito et al. evaluated an AI model for diagnosing proximal caries from bitewing

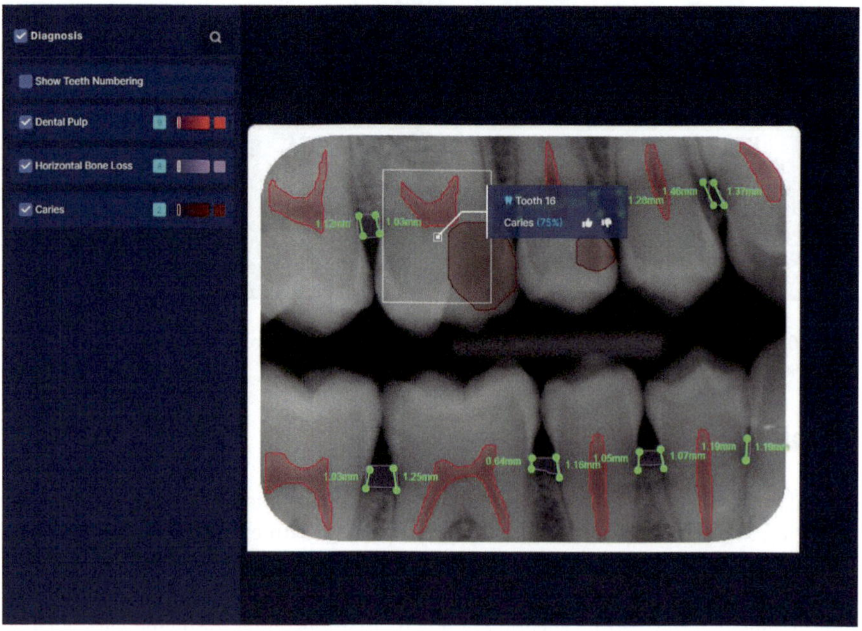

Fig. 4.7 AI-generated caries segmentation on dental bitewing radiograph. (Courtesy by CranioCatch AI software)

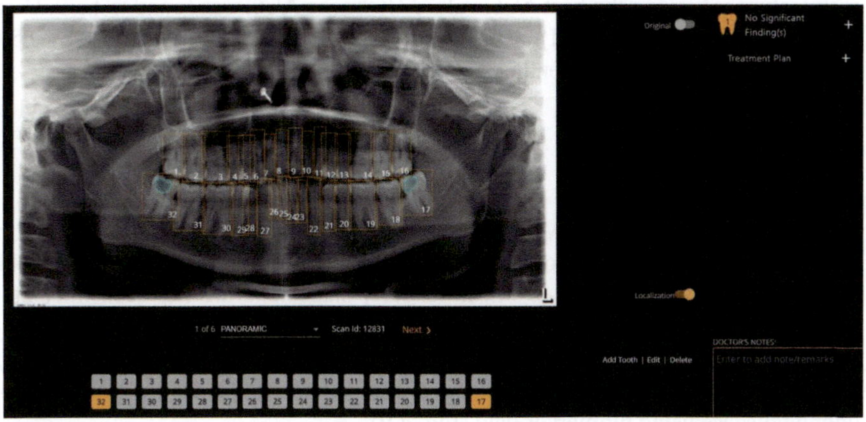

Fig. 4.8 Teeth identification and caries segmentation on panoramic radiograph. (Courtesy by Velmeni AI software)

radiographs, and AI showed better performance than the most accurate human examiner (Devito et al. 2008).

Lee et al. (2018a) evaluated the success of a pre-trained GoogleNet Inception v3 CNN model in detecting dental caries on periapical images. The accuracy rates for detecting dental caries in premolar, molar, and premolar-molar teeth were found to be 89.0%, 88.0%, and 82.0%, respectively. The premolar caries detection model achieved the highest AUC value and outperformed other caries detection models.

Srivastava et al. (2017) developed a CNN model for detecting dental caries on bitewing radiographs, which achieved a significantly higher sensitivity (81%) compared to three general dentists (34–48%) (Srivastava et al. 2017). Cantu et al. developed a deep learning-based AI model for segmenting dental caries on bitewing radiographs, achieving an accuracy, sensitivity, specificity, and F1 score of 0.80, 0.75, 0.83, and 0.73, respectively. The sensitivity rate of 0.75 surpassed that of the dentists (0.36) (Cantu et al. 2020).

Bayrakdar et al. developed AI models for dental caries, which demonstrated better performance than a 2-year-experienced resident of dento-maxillofacial radiology and a 3-year-experienced resident of restorative dentistry. Additionally, various AI models, including regression analysis, decision tree learning, and artificial neural networks, have been developed to diagnose dental caries using intraoral photographs. These AI models achieved diagnosis accuracy ranging from 80% to 86.3%, specificity ranging from 95.6% to 98.3%, and sensitivity ranging from 80% to 100% (Bayrakdar et al. 2022a).

Furthermore, Casalegno et al. developed a deep CNN model for the classification of dental caries as presence or absence using near-infrared-light transillumination (NILT) images, which achieved ROC (receiver operating characteristic) values of 83.6% and 85.6% for occlusal and interproximal dental caries, respectively (Casalegno et al. 2019). Schwendicke et al. employed deep CNN methods, including Resnet18 and Resnext50, to detect dental caries in NILT images, with Resnext50 architecture achieving the best AUC value. The mean AUC was found to be 0.74 at a 95% confidence interval (CI). Sensitivity and specificity were determined as 0.59 and 0.76, respectively (Schwendicke et al. 2020a).

Periodontics

Periodontal diseases are a prevalent group of diseases worldwide and can lead to the loss of alveolar bone and periodontal attachment, resulting in tooth loss. In the field of periodontal evaluation, AI is still in its early stages and has not been fully utilized. However, it has been employed in various areas such as detecting and evaluating alveolar bone loss and periodontally compromised teeth on dental radiographs, assessing gingivitis using intraoral images, and estimating the progression of periodontal disease using biomarker data (Fig. 4.9).

AI models have been utilized to detect alveolar bone loss, changes in bone density, and the classification of periodontitis stages on dental radiographs in periodontal evaluation (Fig. 4.10) (Scott et al. 2023). Studies that employed deep learning (DL) for detecting bone loss on radiographs in periodontics revealed F1 scores ranging from 0.75 to 0.93 on panoramic radiographs and 0.47 to 0.83 on periapical radiographs. The DL model developed by Chang et al. (2020) using the Mask R-CNN architecture achieved the best performance for diagnosing and staging periodontal disease on panoramic radiographs. Moran et al. (2021) employed an Inception transfer learning model to classify regions as either healthy or displaying periodontal bone loss on periapical radiographs. Lee et al. developed a CNN model that identified periodontally compromised posterior teeth on periapical images and estimated tooth prognosis, achieving an accuracy rate of 78.9%. The model showed a higher accuracy for premolars (>80%) than molars (Lee et al. 2018b).

Kurt Bayrakdar et al. developed a GoogleNet Inception v3-based CNN model to detect alveolar bone loss from dental panoramic radiographs, achieving an accuracy value of 0.9 for classifying panoramic radiographs as either showing alveolar bone loss or not (Kurt Bayrakdar et al. 2020). Thanathornwong and Suebnukarn developed a CNN model to identify periodontally compromised teeth on panoramic images (Thanathornwong and Suebnukarn 2020). Kim et al. and Krois et al. also

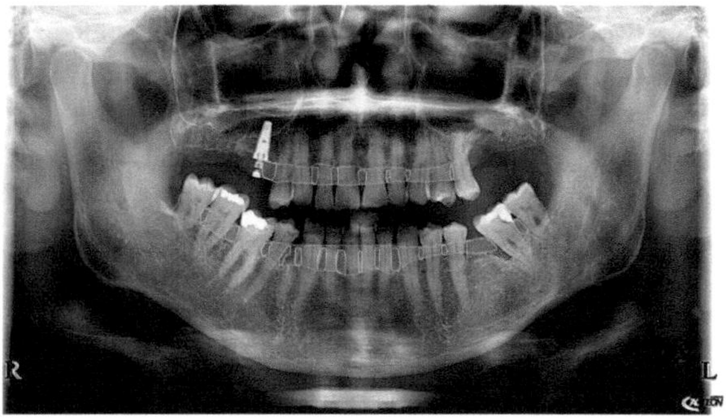

Fig. 4.9 AI-generated periodontal bone loss on panoramic radiograph. (Courtesy by CranioCatch AI software)

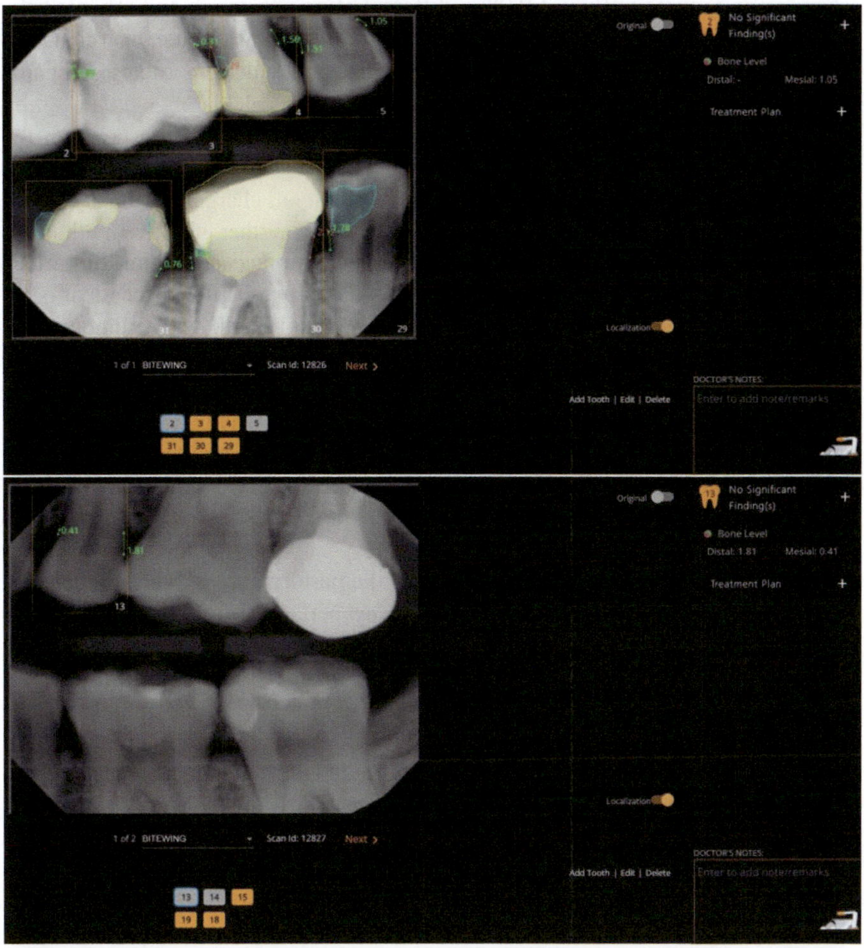

Fig. 4.10 Periodontal bone loss detection by AI software on bitewing radiographs. (Courtesy by Velmeni AI software)

developed CNN models that automatically detected periodontal bone loss on dental panoramic radiographs, with AUC values of 0.89–0.95, surpassing the performance of several general dentists (AUCs of 0.77–0.85). Furthermore, stages of alveolar bone loss were automatically classified using CNN models on periapical and panoramic radiographs (Kim et al. 2019; Krois et al. 2019).

Regarding intraoral photographs, DL models achieved accuracies ranging from 0.77 to 0.94 in detecting gingivitis, with the model developed by Liu et al. (2020) using Mask R-CNN as an object detector demonstrating the best performance. In terms of biomarker data, DL models achieved accuracies ranging from 0.73 to 0.98 in classifying periodontal disease. Papantonopoulos et al. (2014) employed a multilayer perceptron model based on immunological and clinical parameters, achieving an accuracy value of 0.98 in differentiating aggressive and chronic periodontitis. Additionally, Nakano et al. developed a multilayer perceptron that estimated oral malodors with an accuracy of 0.96 using saliva microbiota (Nakano et al. 2018).

Endodontics

AI has made significant advancements in the detection and prediction of various aspects in endodontics. In terms of detection, AI has been utilized for identifying periapical lesions, crown and root fractures, working length determination, and detecting root and canal morphology (Fig. 4.11). Prediction tasks include the estimation of retreatment need. Periapical lesions are common and pose challenges in diagnosis and treatment planning for dentists. Early identification of these lesions can improve treatment outcomes by preventing the spread of the disease to surrounding tissues (Shan et al. 2021; Khanagar et al. 2021a; Schwendicke et al. 2020b; Carrillo-Perez et al. 2022; Park and Park 2018; Hung et al. 2020b; Hung et al. 2023; Aminoshariae et al. 2021).

Endres et al. conducted a study comparing the performance of a DL model with 24 oral and maxillofacial surgeons in detecting periapical lesions on panoramic radiographs. The study concluded that DL-based AI algorithms outperformed some of the surgeons (Endres et al. 2020). Similarly, another study demonstrated that CNN models performed better than three oral and maxillofacial radiologists in detecting simulated periapical lesions on intraoral radiographs. Orhan et al. used 109 CBCT scans to test an AI system and reported high detection accuracy, with no significant differences in the lesion volumes measured by the software compared to a radiologist (Orhan et al. 2020). The integration of AI systems in clinical practice for detecting periapical lesions from dental radiographs can enhance reliability and

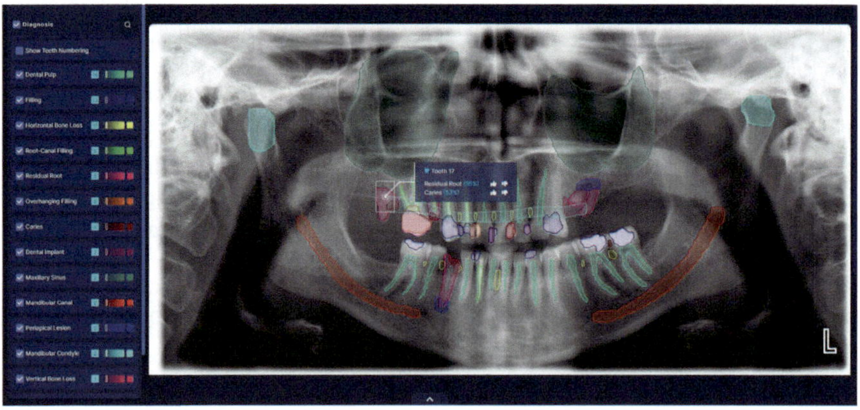

Fig. 4.11 AI-generated root canal morphology, anatomic structures, restorations, and pathologies on panoramic radiograph (courtesy by CranioCatch AI software)

accuracy, similar to experienced specialists. Additionally, it can save assessment time and assist in automated recording (Aminoshariae et al. 2021; Endres et al. 2020; Orhan et al. 2020; Bayrakdar et al. 2022b).

The diagnosis of horizontal and vertical root fractures is a challenging task that requires experience. CNN models have been developed to automatically detect root fractures on 2D and 3D dental radiographic images. Fukuda et al. demonstrated that CNNs can be a promising tool for diagnosing vertical root fractures on panoramic radiographs (Fukuda et al. 2020). Another study by Johari et al. used probabilistic neural network (PNN) for the detection of vertical root fractures and showed excellent performance with an accuracy rate of 96.6%. These evaluations indicate that AI algorithms can be highly effective in detecting vertical root fractures on CBCT images and panoramic radiographs (Johari et al. 2017).

Accurate determination of the working length is a critical step for successful root canal treatment. Studies have shown that artificial neural networks (ANNs) can be used for the accurate determination of the working length. Saghiri et al. reported that ANNs can be used as a supplementary tool for localizing the apical foramen on dental radiographs. They demonstrated no differences in root length measurements when comparing an ANN with actual measurements after extraction (Saghiri et al. 2012).

AI algorithms based on CNNs have shown high success rates in automatic tooth detection and segmentation on 2D and 3D dental radiographs. AI performs at a high level, comparable to human observers, but with much faster processing times. Determining root and canal morphology is crucial for the success of root canal treatment, and AI applications have the potential to contribute to these tasks. Hiraiwa et al. developed a DL system that exhibited high accuracy in detecting radix entomolaris in mandibular first molars (Hiraiwa et al. 2019).

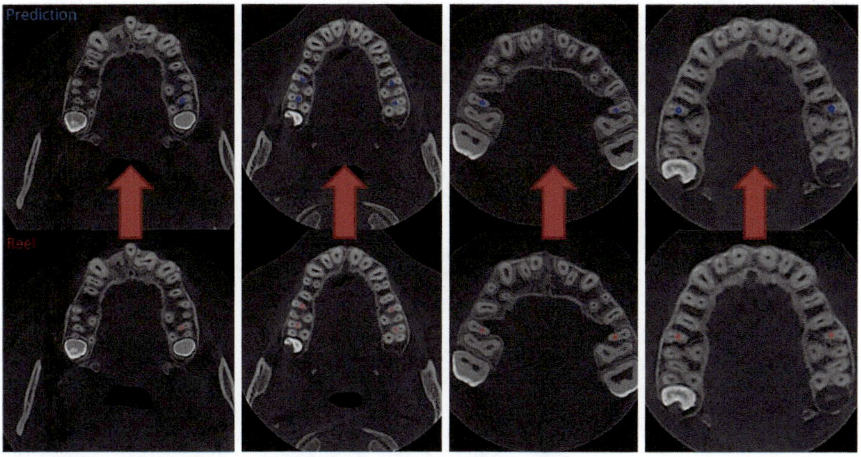

Fig. 4.12 Automatic MB2 segmentation on axial slices of CBCT images using the YOLOv5x based AI model. (Courtesy by CranioCatch AI software)

Automatic detection and classification of root canals, including the identification of canal numbers and variations such as C-shaped canals and mesio-buccal canals, have emerged as another area of AI application in endodontics (Fig. 4.12). Several CNN models have been developed for the automatic detection, segmentation, and classification of root canals on 2D and 3D dental radiographs. Additionally, AI has been applied for the detection of taurodont teeth. The success of these AI models has been demonstrated to be similar to or even superior to that of dentists (Lahoud et al. 2021; Leite et al. 2021; Hiraiwa et al. 2019; Zhang et al. 2022; Sherwood et al. 2021a; Jeon et al. 2021; Yang et al. 2022; Sherwood et al. 2021b; Duman et al. 2023). Regarding the estimation part, there have been studies highlighting the potential use of AI for retreatment predictions. However, further research is needed in this area (Aminoshariae et al. 2021).

Oral and Maxillofacial Surgery

In the field of oral and maxillofacial surgery, AI algorithms can be utilized for decision support in diagnosis, treatment, prediction of outcomes, and preoperative surgical planning. Impacted tooth detection and assessment of the relationship with surrounding anatomical structures such as the maxillary sinus, nasal fossa, and mandibular canal can be performed using AI algorithms with a high success rate (Fig. 4.13). AI technology has also been employed for predicting postoperative facial swelling following tooth extraction. Zhang et al. (2018) developed an AI model for predicting postoperative facial swelling after impacted mandibular third molar extraction, which demonstrated excellent predictive performance. In another study, the extraction difficulty of third molars was evaluated using a deep CNN model on panoramic radiographs with the Pederson Difficulty Score (PDS). The model achieved success rates of 82.03%, 90.23%, and 78.91% for determining the relationship with the ramus, angulation, and depth, respectively (Yoo et al. 2021).

Various AI tools have been developed to improve the diagnostic accuracy of dentists for different maxillofacial pathologies, thereby enhancing overall performance. CNN-based DL models for the detection and classification of ameloblastomas, odontogenic keratocysts, dentigerous cysts, and radicular cysts on panoramic radiographs have demonstrated high performance (Bispo et al. 2021; Yang et al. 2020).

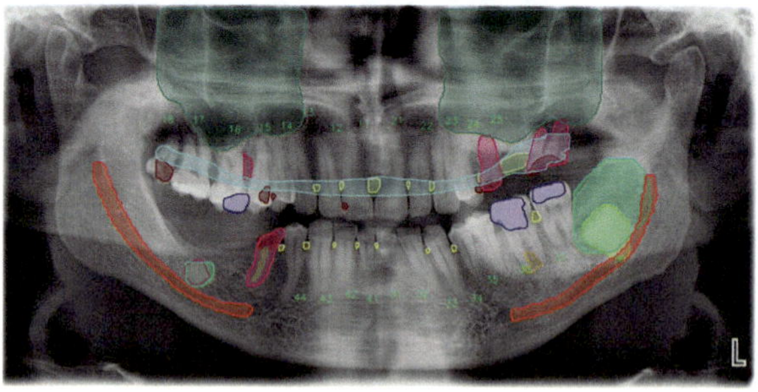

Fig. 4.13 AI-generated anatomic structures, restorations, and pathologies on panoramic radiograph. (Courtesy by CranioCatch AI software)

Additionally, Lee et al. developed CNN models for detecting, segmenting, and classifying odontogenic keratocysts, dentigerous cysts, and radicular cysts on panoramic and CBCT images, with the CBCT model showing better performance (Lee et al. 2020). A CNN-based AI model also exhibited superior performance compared to two radiologists in identifying metastatic cervical lymph nodes on contrast-enhanced CT images in patients with oral cancer (Ariji et al. 2022).

AI tools have proven effective in detecting and segmenting maxillofacial and dental fractures on panoramic and CBCT images as well as in automatically diagnosing TMJ osteoarthritis, measuring cortical thickness of the mandibular condyle head, and diagnosing mandibular condyle fractures (Fukuda et al. 2020; Johari et al. 2017; Rasteau et al. 2022; Eschert et al. 2022; Bianchi et al. 2021; Warin et al. 2023; Nishiyama et al. 2021).

Furthermore, automatic detection and segmentation tools for the maxillary sinus and pathologies using CNN-based AI models have been developed for panoramic and CBCT images. These AI tools have shown positive performance in aiding dentists in the diagnosis of maxillary sinus diseases, such as maxillary sinusitis, mucous retention cysts, and mucosal thickening (Hung et al. 2022a; Choi et al. 2022; Kuwana et al. 2021; Ha et al. 2023; Mori et al. 2021).

In the field of orthognathic surgery, the use of AI algorithms is rapidly expanding. Various AI models have been developed to assess facial asymmetry in patients and determine the need for orthognathic surgery using cephalometric radiographs and clinical photos (Fig. 4.14). CNN models have demonstrated clinically acceptable success rates in detecting cephalometric landmarks across different stages of orthognathic surgery, including initial, pre-surgery, post-surgery, and debonding phases. Additionally, neural network models have shown accurate estimation of postoperative infections following orthognathic surgery, achieving a success rate of

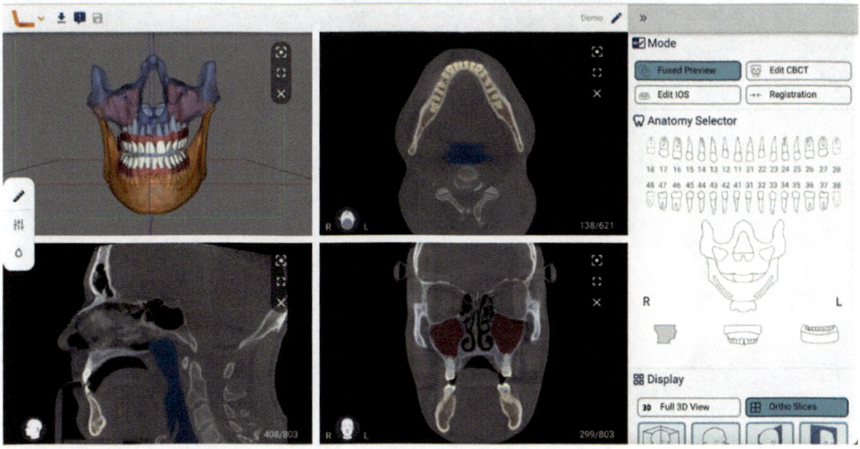

Fig. 4.14 AI-generated 3D virtual model + orthogonal CBCT slices. (Courtesy by Relu AI software)

98.7% (Mohaideen et al. 2022; Hung et al. 2023; Hung et al. 2022b; Shujaat et al. 2021; Rokhshad et al. 2023).

AI has proven to be valuable in the detection of oral cancers. CNN-based models have demonstrated the capability to automatically detect oral cancer in photographs and confocal laser microscopy images. These studies highlight the potential of AI models in facilitating early diagnosis of oral cancer, which can greatly improve patient outcomes (Mohaideen et al. 2022; Hung et al. 2023; Hung et al. 2022b; Khanagar et al. 2021b; Patil et al. 2022; Patcas et al. 2022).

Dental Implantology

CNN-based AI models have been utilized for the detection and analysis of various aspects related to dental implants. These models have shown high performance in detecting dental implants, implant fractures, and peri-implant bone loss on dental

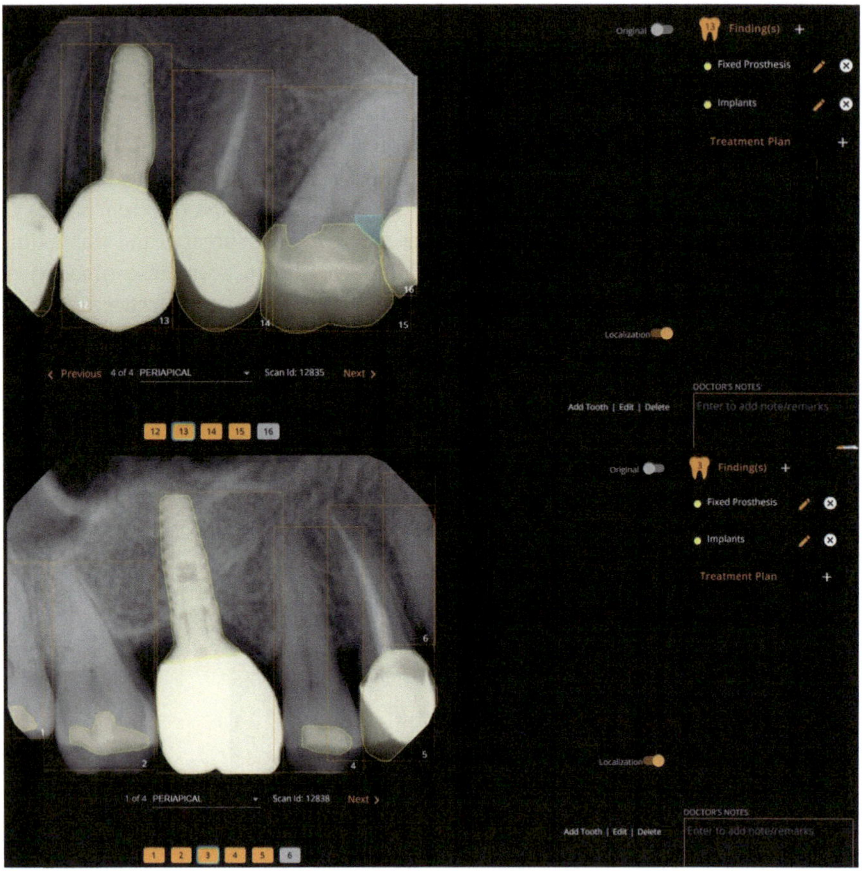

Fig. 4.15 Automatic implant detection on 2D imaging. (Courtesy by Velmeni AI software)

radiographs. They have also demonstrated proficiency in classifying dental implants based on various criteria (Revilla-León et al. 2023; Hadj Saïd et al. 2020; Liu et al. 2022; Cha et al. 2021; Lee et al. 2021; Kurt Bayrakdar et al. 2021; Mangano et al. 2023) (Fig. 4.15).

For instance, Liu et al. developed an AI algorithm that performed similarly to two general dentists in automatically detecting peri-implant bone loss on periapical images. Another CNN algorithm developed on dental periapical images exhibited high performance in measuring peri-implant bone loss and classifying its severity into categories such as normal, early, moderate, and severe (Liu et al. 2022; Cha et al. 2021).

CNN models have also been employed to detect implant fractures and classify them as horizontal or vertical fractures (Lee et al. 2021). In the realm of dental implant planning, CNN models have demonstrated the ability to automatically detect edentulous sites, nasal fossa, maxillary sinus, and mandibular canal as well as measure the heights and widths of residual alveolar bone at the edentulous sites using CBCT images (Kurt Bayrakdar et al. 2021).

Furthermore, a novel protocol combining AI and augmented reality (AR) was proposed for three-dimensional (3D) implant planning. The integration of AI and AR technologies has the potential to revolutionize modern guided implant surgery, potentially replacing conventional guided surgery software (Mangano et al. 2023).

Orthodontics

AI has tremendous potential in the field of orthodontics, with applications ranging from automated anatomical landmark detection and cephalometric analyses to diagnosis and treatment planning, growth and development assessment, and evaluation of treatment outcomes.

One of the most common areas of AI use in orthodontics is automatic cephalometric landmark detection and analysis, which holds great value for orthodontic diagnosis and treatment. AI-generated cephalometric tracings on both 2D and 3D radiographs are available, and the accuracy of these software tools is within an acceptable range, accurately predicting overall skeletal and dental growth in patients. CNN-based AI tools have been used with high accuracy rates compared to human observers. Studies in the literature have demonstrated that AI-generated measurements and angles in cephalometric analysis do not have statistically significant differences from manually traced analyses. This automation reduces human effort and time involved in the analysis process (Hung et al. 2020a; Hung et al. 2023; Bichu et al. 2021; Mohammad-Rahimi et al. 2021; Arsiwala-Scheppach et al. 2023; Uğurlu 2022).

Diagnosis and treatment planning are critical components of orthodontic treatments, and they involve subjectivity and complexity. AI-based clinical decision support systems help reduce these challenges by assisting clinicians. For example, the decision to extract teeth is an important one in orthodontics, and it can vary among physicians. Decision support systems based on artificial neural networks (ANNs) have demonstrated high accuracy in estimating tooth extraction decisions, achieving an accuracy rate of 94%. These tools can also be used to evaluate orthodontic treatment needs and estimate treatment outcomes. AI models have been developed for classifying skeletal patterns on radiographs and photographs, achieving excellent results with accuracy rates over 93% (Li et al. 2019; Lin et al. 2021).

Furthermore, AI models have been developed to assess facial symmetry before and after orthognathic surgery on CBCT images, reporting high accuracy rates of 90%. AI can also assist in predicting the location, orientation, and position of impacted teeth, such as canines, providing orthodontists with a 3D perspective of the clinical scenario and aiding in formulating a treatment plan (Chen et al. 2020) (Fig. 4.16).

The integration of AI in orthodontics holds great promise for improving diagnostic accuracy, treatment planning, and overall treatment outcomes, while also reducing the subjectivity and complexity associated with traditional approaches.

The advancements in intraoral scanners and aligner technology have paved the way for the development of AI-predicted software for orthodontic treatment. These digital treatment planning tools are intuitive and accurate, providing orthodontists with a more precise approach to treatment. AI-based software can accurately simulate and predict teeth movements during orthodontic treatment, allowing orthodontists to visualize the expected outcomes and plan treatment accordingly. This technology is also beneficial for patient education, as it provides a clear demonstration of the treatment process and potential results.

In addition to treatment planning, AI-assisted software plays a role in airway assessment in orthodontics. It can help determine airway patterns, identify anatomical variations, and calculate airway volume. The software utilizes color coding to provide easy visualization of the airspace and its structures (Figs. 4.17 and 4.18).

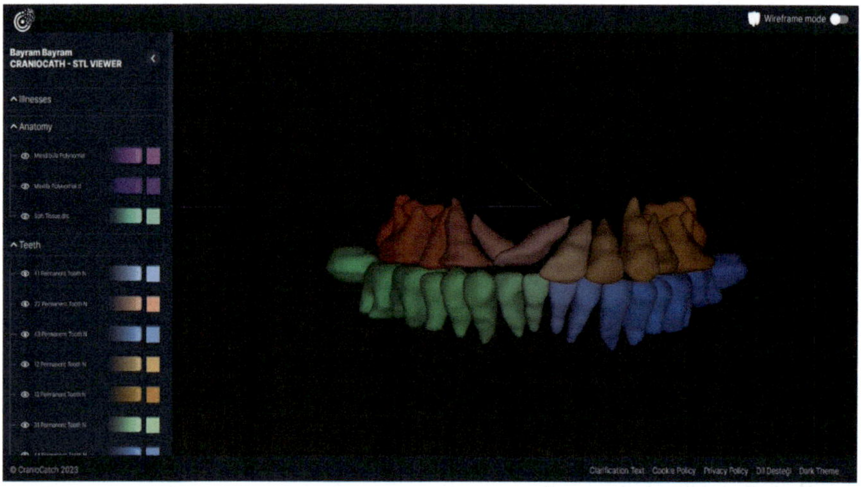

Fig. 4.16 AI-generated 3D perspective of teeth. (Courtesy by CranioCatch AI software)

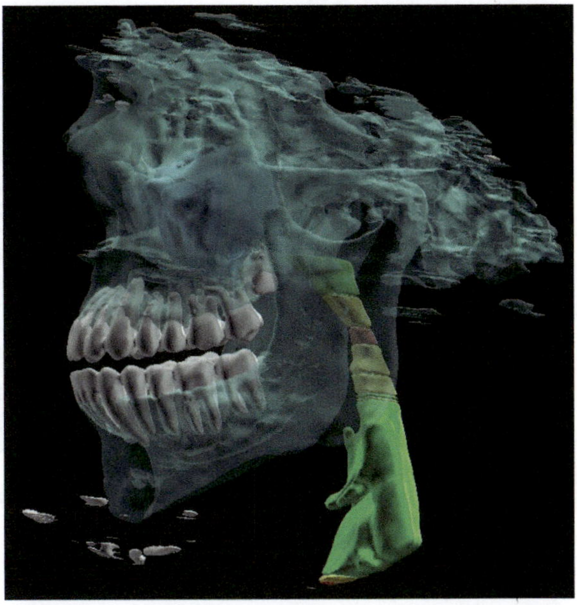

Fig. 4.17 3D airway assessment on cone beam computed tomography by an AI model. (Courtesy by Velmeni AI software)

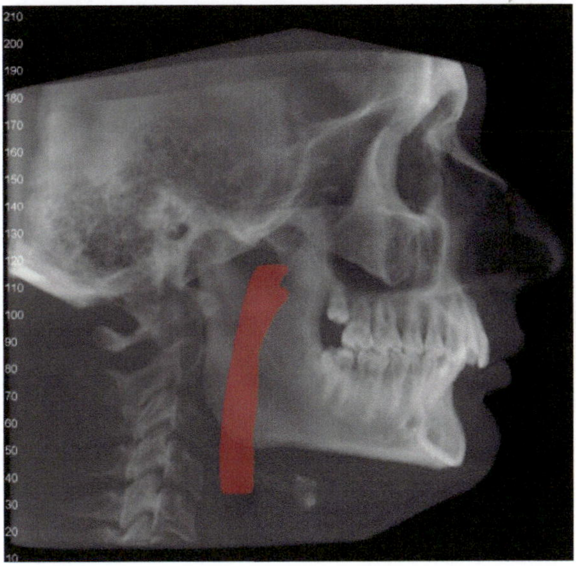

Fig. 4.18 AI-generated pharyngeal airway on CBCT-generated lateral cephalogram. (Courtesy by CranioCatch AI software)

This enables orthodontists to assess the airway more effectively and incorporate airway considerations into treatment planning (Fig. 4.19).

In the evaluation of growth and development and orthodontic treatment outcomes, AI algorithms have shown promising results in automated skeletal bone age assessment, cervical vertebrae maturation evaluation, classification of skeletal patterns, and assessing the effects of orthognathic surgery on facial appearance (Li

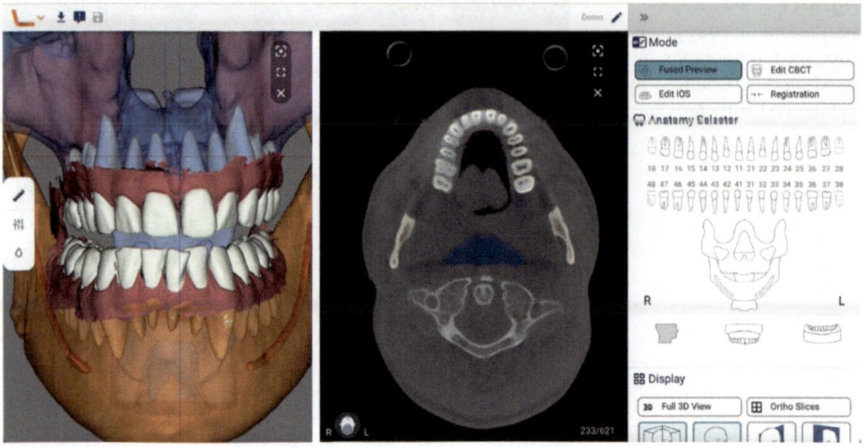

Fig. 4.19 AI-generated close-up of 3D teeth models + auto-segmentation on axial CBCT slice. (Courtesy by Relu AI software)

et al. 2019; Lin et al. 2021; Chen et al. 2020; Yu et al. 2020; Kök et al. 2019; Amasya et al. 2020b; Amasya et al. 2020a).

Prosthodontics

Prosthodontics is a specialized field of dentistry that focuses on treatments such as dentures, dental implants, crowns, and bridges. In recent years, AI has made significant contributions to various aspects of prosthodontics, including CAD/CAM technology, implant surgery template designing, esthetic dentistry, shade matching, and debonding predictions for CAD/CAM restorations. These AI technologies offer immense capabilities in producing occlusal surface designs for crowns, automatic setup designers for complete dentures, determining the emergence profile in dental implantology, and automatic framework designs for removable partial dentures (Figs. 4.20 and 4.21).

The integration of AI with intraoral scanners has revolutionized prosthodontics by enabling the prediction and design of prostheses within minutes with remarkable accuracy. This has greatly reduced the laboratory time required by dental technicians and has resulted in more predictable treatment outcomes (Bernauer et al. 2021; Lerner et al. 2020).

Pedodontics

AI has found applications in pedodontics, contributing to accurate diagnosis, clinical decision-making, preventive measures, and treatment planning, much like in other fields of dentistry. AI models have been developed for various clinical

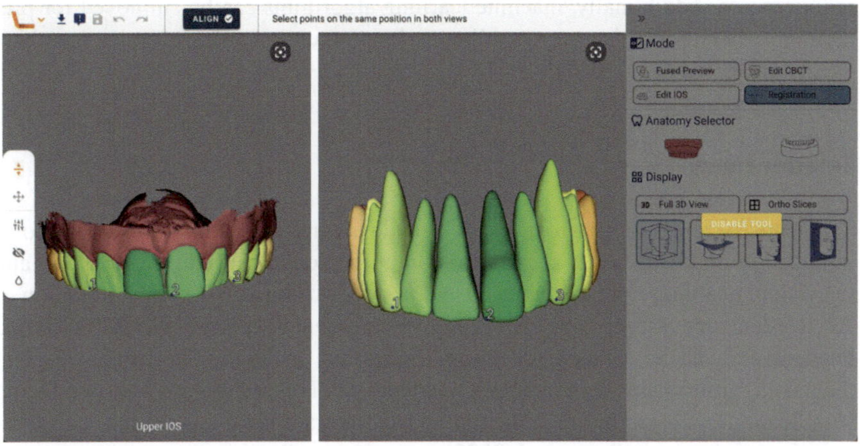

Fig. 4.20 Tool for registration of IOS crowns on CBCT roots. (Courtesy by Relu AI software)

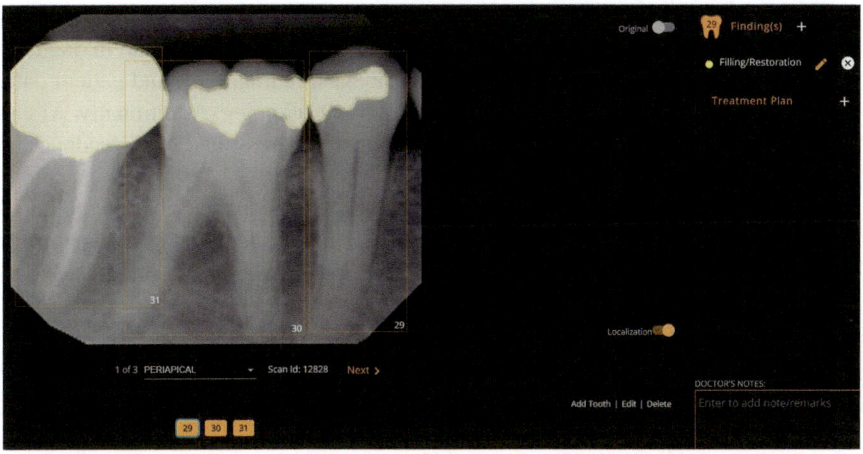

Fig. 4.21 Detection of crown and restoration by CNN-based AI model. (Courtesy by Velmeni AI software)

applications in pedodontics, including dental plaque detection on deciduous teeth and categorization of fissure sealants using intraoral photographs. Additionally, AI models have been used for the detection and numbering of deciduous and permanent teeth, identification of supernumerary teeth such as mesiodens, and assessment of ectopic eruption and submerged teeth in radiographs. Deep learning-based CNN models have been employed to classify tooth development stages and assess chronological age based on radiographs.

Furthermore, machine learning-based AI toolkits have been designed to evaluate children's oral health. These toolkits can aid dentists, parents, and even children themselves in understanding individual oral health needs and treatment requirements. Additionally, machine learning algorithms can be employed for predicting early childhood caries, enabling early intervention and preventive measures (Vishwanathaiah et al. 2023).

Teledentistry

Teledentistry refers to the provision of dental care and education through telecommunication platforms such as phones, computers, email, instant messengers, and television, enabling remote diagnosis and treatment advice. With the integration of AI, teledentistry is becoming increasingly intelligent and powerful. AI-supported teledentistry can be utilized for various purposes, including screening, triaging, diagnosing, follow-ups, and feedback mechanisms. This technology is experiencing significant growth and has the potential to replace traditional face-to-face consultations in certain cases (Batra et al. 2022).

The combination of teledentistry and AI offers numerous benefits, such as improved accessibility to dental care, especially in underserved areas or remote locations. AI algorithms can assist in remote screening and triaging, helping to prioritize patients and identify urgent cases. AI-based systems can also aid in diagnosing dental conditions remotely by analyzing images, radiographs, and patient data, providing valuable insights to dentists for treatment planning. Additionally, AI can support remote follow-up care, monitor treatment progress, and offer feedback to patients.

As technology continues to advance, AI-supported teledentistry has the potential to revolutionize the dental care landscape, providing efficient and effective remote dental services, reducing barriers to access, and improving overall oral health outcomes for patients.

Future of Artificial Intelligence in Dentistry

There is little doubt that AI has been a help in many industries, including dentistry. It acts as a link between patients and dentists. AI is being used in all dentistry disciplines, although it still has a wide range of scope.

Dentures, implant prostheses, and surgical templates are frequently fabricated using CBCT and 3D printing. However, in addition to CBCT and 3D printing, the use of AI to forecast bone quality and create surgical templates will significantly improve the accuracy of the templates and prostheses. Virtual smile designing and predictive esthetic outcomes will be the key areas of development in the AI world. Future training in the field of endodontics will be necessary for AI models to effectively predict the specificity of apical radiolucency and determine lamina dura widening. AI in orthodontics should aid in accurate diagnosis and the provision of the treatment plan. This would help reduce manual work, save patients time, provide proper care, and assist dentists in reducing human error. Future technology will enable dentists to educate their patients better and provide proper care by alleviating the discomfort associated with frequent dental appointments and assisting in the development of the best treatment strategy. Dental technology advancements are advantageous for patients and clinicians alike.

With the acceptance of AI-based technology, the question also arises: are humans being replaced by robots? But we must look at AI as our additional supportive colleague in the dental office, whose role is to simplify and efficiently predict the diagnosis and treatment planning, thereby improving the overall oral healthcare of the patients. There will always be the importance of human touch and emotions in dental treatment, which is irreplaceable. AI will play an important role in areas where there is a lack of accessibility to quality dentists or specialists. In the long term, AI and automation are going to be taking over so much of what gives humans a feeling of purpose" – Mat Bellamy.

In conclusion, AI is a valuable tool that simplifies diagnosis, treatment planning, oral health care, and overall well-being. It supports and enhances the capabilities of dentists and specialists, ultimately benefiting both patients and clinicians.

References

Amasya H, Cesur E, Yıldırım D, Orhan K. Validation of cervical vertebral maturation stages: artificial intelligence vs human observer visual analysis. Am J Orthod Dentofac Orthop. 2020a;158(6):e173–9.

Amasya H, Yildirim D, Aydogan T, Kemaloglu N, Orhan K. Cervical vertebral maturation assessment on lateral cephalometric radiographs using artificial intelligence: comparison of machine learning classifier models. Dentomaxillofac Radiol. 2020b;49(5):20190441.

Aminoshariae A, Kulild J, Nagendrababu V. Artificial intelligence in endodontics: current applications and future directions. J Endod. 2021;47(9):1352–7.

Ariji Y, Kise Y, Fukuda M, Kuwada C, Ariji E. Segmentation of metastatic cervical lymph nodes from CT images of oral cancers using deep-learning technology. Dentomaxillofac Radiol. 2022;51(4):20210515.

Arsiwala-Scheppach LT, Chaurasia A, Müller A, Krois J, Schwendicke F. Machine learning in dentistry: a scoping review. J Clin Med. 2023;12(3):937.

Batra P, Tagra H, Katyal S. Artificial intelligence in teledentistry. Discoveries (Craiova). 2022;10(3):153.

Bayrakdar IS, Orhan K, Akarsu S, Çelik Ö, Atasoy S, Pekince A, Yasa Y, Bilgir E, Sağlam H, Aslan AF, Odabaş A. Deep-learning approach for caries detection and segmentation on dental bitewing radiographs. Oral Radiol. 2022a;38(4):468–79.

Bayrakdar IS, Orhan K, Çelik Ö, Bilgir E, Sağlam H, Kaplan FA, Görür SA, Odabaş A, Aslan AF, Różyło-Kalinowska I. A U-net approach to apical lesion segmentation on panoramic radiographs. Biomed Res Int. 2022b;2022:7035367.

Bernauer SA, Zitzmann NU, Joda T. The use and performance of artificial intelligence in prosthodontics: a systematic review. Sensors (Basel). 2021;21(19):6628.

Bianchi J, Ruellas A, Prieto JC, Li T, Soroushmehr R, Najarian K, Gryak J, Deleat-Besson R, Le C, Yatabe M, Gurgel M, Turkestani NA, Paniagua B, Cevidanes L. Decision support systems in temporomandibular joint osteoarthritis: a review of data science and artificial intelligence applications. Semin Orthod. 2021;27(2):78–86.

Bichu YM, Hansa I, Bichu AY, Premjani P, Flores-Mir C, Vaid NR. Applications of artificial intelligence and machine learning in orthodontics: a scoping review. Prog Orthod. 2021;22(1):18.

Bilgir E, Bayrakdar İŞ, Çelik Ö, Orhan K, Akkoca F, Sağlam H, Odabaş A, Aslan AF, Ozcetin C, Kıllı M, Rozylo-Kalinowska I. An artificial ıntelligence approach to automatic tooth detection and numbering in panoramic radiographs. BMC Med Imaging. 2021;21(1):124.

Bispo MS, de Queiroz Pierre MLG, Apolinario AL, Dos Santos JN, Junior BC, Neves FS, et al. Computer tomographic differential diagnosis of ameloblastoma and odontogenic keratocyst: classification using a convolutional neural network. Dentomaxillofac Radiol. 2021;20210002

Cantu AG, Gehrung S, Krois J, Chaurasia A, Rossi JG, Gaudin R, et al. Detecting caries lesions of different radiographic extension on bitewings using deep learning. J Dent. 2020;100:103425.

Carrillo-Perez F, Pecho OE, Morales JC, Paravina RD, Della Bona A, Ghinea R, Pulgar R, Pérez MDM, Herrera LJ. Applications of artificial intelligence in dentistry: a comprehensive review. J Esthet Restor Dent. 2022;34(1):259–80.

Casalegno F, Newton T, Daher R, et al. Caries detection with near-infrared transillumination using deep learning. J Dent Res. 2019;98:1227e33.

Cha JY, Yoon HI, Yeo IS, Huh KH, Han JS. Peri-implant bone loss measurement using a region-based convolutional neural network on dental periapical radiographs. J Clin Med. 2021;10(5):1009.

Chang HJ, Lee SJ, Yong TH, et al. Deep learning hybrid method to automatically diagnose periodontal bone loss and stage periodontitis. Sci Rep. 2020;10(1):7531.

Chen S, Wang L, Li G, Wu TH, Diachina S, Tejera B, et al. Machine learning in orthodontics: introducing a 3D auto-segmentation and auto-landmark finder of CBCT images to assess maxillary constriction in unilateral impacted canine patients. Angle Orthod. 2020;90(1):77–84.

Choi H, Jeon KJ, Kim YH, Ha EG, Lee C, Han SS. Deep learning-based fully automatic segmentation of the maxillary sinus on cone-beam computed tomographic images. Sci Rep. 2022;12(1):14009.

Devito KL, de Souza BF, Felippe Filho WN. An artificial multilayer perceptron neural network for diagnosis of proximal dental caries. Oral Surg Oral Med Oral Pathol Oral Radiol Endod. 2008;106(6):879–84.

Duman S, Yılmaz EF, Eşer G, Çelik Ö, Bayrakdar IS, Bilgir E, Costa ALF, Jagtap R, Orhan K. Detecting the presence of taurodont teeth on panoramic radiographs using a deep learning-based convolutional neural network algorithm. Oral Radiol. 2023;39(1):207–14.

Endres MG, Hillen F, Salloumis M, Sedaghat AR, Niehues SM, Quatela O, Hanken H, Smeets R, Beck-Broichsitter B, Rendenbach C, Lakhani K, Heiland M, Gaudin RA. Development of a deep learning algorithm for periapical disease detection in dental radiographs. Diagnostics. 2020;10(6):430.

Eschert T, Schwendicke F, Krois J, Bohner L, Vinayahalingam S, Hanisch M. A survey on the use of artificial intelligence by clinicians in dentistry and oral and maxillofacial surgery. Medicina (Kaunas). 2022;58(8):1059.

Ezhov M, Gusarev M, Golitsyna M, Yates JM, Kushnerev E, Tamimi D, Aksoy S, Shumilov E, Sanders A, Orhan K. Clinically applicable artificial intelligence system for dental diagnosis with CBCT. Sci Rep. 2021;11(1):15006. https://doi.org/10.1038/s41598-021-94093-9. Erratum in: Sci Rep. 2021;11(1):22217

Fukuda M, Inamoto K, Shibata N, et al. Evaluation of an artificial intelligence system for detecting vertical root fracture on panoramic radiography. Oral Radiol. 2020;36:337–43.

Görürgöz C, Orhan K, Bayrakdar IS, Çelik Ö, Bilgir E, Odabaş A, Aslan AF, Jagtap R. Performance of a convolutional neural network algorithm for tooth detection and numbering on periapical radiographs. Dentomaxillofac Radiol. 2022;51(3):20210246.

Ha EG, Jeon KJ, Choi H, Lee C, Choi YJ, Han SS. Automatic diagnosis of retention pseudocyst in the maxillary sinus on panoramic radiographs using a convolutional neural network algorithm. Sci Rep. 2023;13(1):2734.

Hadj Saïd M, Le Roux MK, Catherine JH, Lan R. Development of an artificial intelligence model to identify a dental implant from a radiograph. Int J Oral Maxillofac Implants. 2020;36(6):1077–82.

Hiraiwa T, Ariji Y, Fukuda M, Kise Y, Nakata K, Katsumata A, Fujita H, Ariji E. A deep-learning artificial intelligence system for assessment of root morphology of the mandibular first molar on panoramic radiography. Dentomaxillofac Radiol. 2019;48(3):20180218.

https://www.impactfund.org/legal-practitioner-blog/ai-civilrights

Hung K, Montalvao C, Tanaka R, Kawai T, Bornstein MM. The use and performance of artificial intelligence applications in dental and maxillofacial radiology: a systematic review. Dentomaxillofac Radiol. 2020a;49(1):20190107.

Hung K, Yeung AWK, Tanaka R, Bornstein MM. Current applications, opportunities, and limitations of AI for 3D imaging in dental research and practice. Int J Environ Res Public Health. 2020b;17(12):4424.

Hung KF, Ai QYH, King AD, Bornstein MM, Wong LM, Leung YY. Automatic detection and segmentation of morphological changes of the maxillary sinus mucosa on cone-beam computed tomography images using a three-dimensional convolutional neural network. Clin Oral Investig. 2022a;26(5):3987–98.

Hung KF, Ai QYH, Wong LM, Yeung AWK, Li DTS, Leung YY. Current applications of deep learning and radiomics on CT and CBCT for maxillofacial diseases. Diagnostics (Basel). 2022b;13(1):110.

Hung KF, Yeung AWK, Bornstein MM, Schwendicke F. Personalized dental medicine, artificial intelligence, and their relevance for dentomaxillofacial imaging. Dentomaxillofac Radiol. 2023;52(1):20220335.

Jeon SJ, Yun JP, Yeom HG, Shin WS, Lee JH, Jeong SH, Seo MS. Deep-learning for predicting C-shaped canals in mandibular second molars on panoramic radiographs. Dentomaxillofac Radiol. 2021;50(5):20200513.

Johari M, Esmaeili F, Andalib A, Garjani S, Saberkari H. Detection of vertical root fractures in intact and endodontically treated premolar teeth by designing a probabilistic neural network: an ex vivo study. Dentomaxillofac Radiol. 2017;46(2):20160107.

Khanagar SB, Al-Ehaideb A, Maganur PC, Vishwanathaiah S, Patil S, Baeshen HA, Sarode SC, Bhandi S. Developments, application, and performance of artificial intelligence in dentistry - a systematic review. J Dent Sci. 2021a;16(1):508–22.

Khanagar SB, Naik S, Al Kheraif AA, Vishwanathaiah S, Maganur PC, Alhazmi Y, Mushtaq S, Sarode SC, Sarode GS, Zanza A, Testarelli L, Patil S. Application and performance of artificial intelligence technology in oral cancer diagnosis and prediction of prognosis: a systematic review. Diagnostics (Basel). 2021b;11(6):1004.

Kılıc MC, Bayrakdar IS, Çelik Ö, Bilgir E, Orhan K, Aydın OB, Kaplan FA, Sağlam H, Odabaş A, Aslan AF, Yılmaz AB. Artificial intelligence system for automatic deciduous tooth detection and numbering in panoramic radiographs. Dentomaxillofac Radiol. 2021;50(6):20200172.

Kim J, Lee HS, Song IS, Jung KH. DeNTNet: deep neural transfer network for the detection of periodontal bone loss using panoramic dental radiographs. Sci Rep. 2019;9:17615.

Kök H, Acilar AM, İzgi MS. Usage and comparison of artificial intelligence algorithms for determination of growth and development by cervical vertebrae stages in orthodontics. Prog Orthod. 2019;20(1):41.

Krois J, Ekert T, Meinhold L, Golla T, Kharbot B, Wittemeier A, et al. Deep learning for the radiographic detection of periodontal bone loss. Sci Rep. 2019;9:8495.

Kurt Bayrakdar S, Celik O, Bayrakdar IS, Orhan K, Bilgir E, Odabas A, Aslan AF. Success of artificial intelligence system in determining alveolar bone loss from dental panoramic radiography images. Cumhuriyet Den J. 2020;23(4):318–24.

Kurt Bayrakdar S, Orhan K, Bayrakdar IS, Bilgir E, Ezhov M, Gusarev M, Shumilov E. A deep learning approach for dental implant planning in cone-beam computed tomography images. BMC Med Imaging. 2021;21(1):86.

Kuwana R, Ariji Y, Fukuda M, Kise Y, Nozawa M, Kuwada C, Muramatsu C, Katsumata A, Fujita H, Ariji E. Performance of deep learning object detection technology in the detection and diagnosis of maxillary sinus lesions on panoramic radiographs. Dentomaxillofac Radiol. 2021;50(1):20200171.

Lahoud P, EzEldeen M, Beznik T, Willems H, Leite A, Van Gerven A, Jacobs R. Artificial intelligence for fast and accurate 3-dimensional tooth segmentation on cone-beam computed tomography. J Endod. 2021;47(5):827–35.

Lee JH, Kim DH, Jeong SN, Choi SH. Detection and diagnosis of dental caries using a deep learning-based convolutional neural network algorithm. J Dent. 2018a;77:106–11.

Lee JH, Kim DH, Jeong SN, Choi SH. Diagnosis and prediction of periodontally compromised teeth using a deep learning-based convolutional neural network algorithm. J Periodontal Implant Sci. 2018b;48(2):114–23.
Lee JH, Kim DH, Jeong SN. Diagnosis of cystic lesions using panoramic and cone beam computed tomographic images based on deep learning neural network. Oral Dis. 2020;26:152–8.
Lee DW, Kim SY, Jeong SN, Lee JH. Artificial intelligence in fractured dental implant detection and classification: evaluation using dataset from two dental hospitals. Diagnostics (Basel). 2021;11(2):233.
Leite AF, Gerven AV, Willems H, Beznik T, Lahoud P, Gaêta-Araujo H, Vranckx M, Jacobs R. Artificial intelligence-driven novel tool for tooth detection and segmentation on panoramic radiographs. Clin Oral Investig. 2021;25(4):2257–67.
Lerner H, Mouhyi J, Admakin O, Mangano F. Artificial intelligence in fixed implant prosthodontics: a retrospective study of 106 implant-supported monolithic zirconia crowns inserted in the posterior jaws of 90 patients. BMC Oral Health. 2020;20(1):80.
Li P, Kong D, Tang T, Su D, Yang P, Wang H, et al. Orthodontic treatment planning based on artificial neural networks. Sci Rep. 2019;9(1):2037.
Lin H-H, Chiang W-C, Yang C-T, Cheng C-T, Zhang T, Lo L-J. On construction of transfer learning for facial symmetry assessment before and after orthognathic surgery. Comput Methods Programs Biomed Mar. 2021;200:105928.
Liu L, Xu J, Huan Y, Zou Z, Yeh SC, Zheng LR. A smart dental health IoT platform based on intelligent hardware, deep learning, and mobile terminal. IEEE J Biomed Health Inform. 2020;24(3):898–906.
Liu M, Wang S, Chen H, Liu Y. A pilot study of a deep learning approach to detect marginal bone loss around implants. BMC Oral Health. 2022;22(1):11.
Mangano FG, Admakin O, Lerner H, Mangano C. Artificial intelligence and augmented reality for guided implant surgery planning: a proof of concept. J Dent. 2023;104485
Marr B. How is AI used in healthcare—5 powerful real-world examples that show the latest advances. Forbes. 2018.
Mohaideen K, Negi A, Verma DK, Kumar N, Sennimalai K, Negi A. Applications of artificial intelligence and machine learning in orthognathic surgery: a scoping review. J Stomatol Oral Maxillofac Surg. 2022;123(6):e962–72.
Mohammad-Rahimi H, Nadimi M, Rohban MH, Shamsoddin E, Lee VY, Motamedian SR. Machine learning and orthodontics, current trends and the future opportunities: a scoping review. Am J Orthod Dentofac Orthop. 2021;160(2):170–192.e4.
Moran M, Faria M, Giraldi G, Bastos L, Conci A. Do radiographic assessments of periodontal bone loss improve with deep learning methods for enhanced image resolution? Sensors. 2021;21(6):2013.
Mori M, Ariji Y, Katsumata A, Kawai T, Araki K, Kobayashi K, Ariji E. A deep transfer learning approach for the detection and diagnosis of maxillary sinusitis on panoramic radiographs. Odontology. 2021;109(4):941–8.
Nakano Y, Suzuki N, Kuwata F. Predicting oral malodour based on the microbiota in saliva samples using a deep learning approach. BMC Oral Health. 2018;18(1):1–7.
Nishiyama M, Ishibashi K, Ariji Y, Fukuda M, Nishiyama W, Umemura M, Katsumata A, Fujita H, Ariji E. Performance of deep learning models constructed using panoramic radiographs from two hospitals to diagnose fractures of the mandibular condyle. Dentomaxillofac Radiol. 2021;50(7):20200611.
Orhan K, Bayrakdar IS, Ezhov M, Kravtsov A, Özyürek T. Evaluation of artificial intelligence for detecting periapical pathosis on cone-beam computed tomography scans. Int Endod J. 2020;53(5):680–9.
Orhan K, Shamshiev M, Ezhov M, Plaksin A, Kurbanova A, Ünsal G, Gusarev M, Golitsyna M, Aksoy S, Mısırlı M, Rasmussen F, Shumilov E, Sanders A. AI-based automatic segmentation of craniomaxillofacial anatomy from CBCT scans for automatic detection of pharyngeal airway evaluations in OSA patients. Sci Rep. 2022;12(1):11863.

Papantonopoulos G, Takahashi K, Bountis T, Loos BG. Artificial neural networks for the diagnosis of aggressive periodontitis trained by immunologic parameters. PLoS One. 2014;9(3):e89757.
Park WJ, Park JB. History and application of artificial neural networks in dentistry. Eur J Dent. 2018;12(4):594–601.
Patcas R, Bornstein MM, Schätzle MA, Timofte R. Artificial intelligence in medico-dental diagnostics of the face: a narrative review of opportunities and challenges. Clin Oral Investig. 2022;26(12):6871–9.
Patil S, Albogami S, Hosmani J, Mujoo S, Kamil MA, Mansour MA, Abdul HN, Bhandi S, Ahmed SSSJ. Artificial intelligence in the diagnosis of oral diseases: applications and pitfalls. Diagnostics (Basel). 2022;12(5):1029.
Rasteau S, Ernenwein D, Savoldelli C, Bouletreau P. Artificial intelligence for oral and maxillofacial surgery: a narrative review. J Stomatol Oral Maxillofac Surg. 2022;123(3):276–82.
Revilla-León M, Gómez-Polo M, Vyas S, Barmak AB, Özcan M, Att W, Krishnamurthy VR. Artificial intelligence applications in restorative dentistry: a systematic review. J Prosthet Dent. 2022;128(5):867–75.
Revilla-León M, Gómez-Polo M, Vyas S, Barmak BA, Galluci GO, Att W, Krishnamurthy VR. Artificial intelligence applications in implant dentistry: a systematic review. J Prosthet Dent. 2023;129(2):293–300.
Rokhshad R, Keyhan SO, Yousefi P. Artificial intelligence applications and ethical challenges in oral and maxillo-facial cosmetic surgery: a narrative review. Maxillofac Plast Reconstr Surg. 2023;45(1):14.
Saghiri MA, Asgar K, Boukani KK, Lotfi M, Aghili H, Delvarani A, Karamifar K, Saghiri AM, Mehrvarzfar P, Garcia-Godoy F. A new approach for locating the minor apical foramen using an artificial neural network. Int Endod J. 2012;45(3):257–65.
Schwendicke F, Elhennawy K, Paris S, Friebertshäuser P, Krois J. Deep learning for caries lesion detection in near-infrared light transillumination images: a pilot study. J Dent. 2020a;92:103260.
Schwendicke F, Samek W, Krois J. Artificial intelligence in dentistry: chances and challenges. J Dent Res. 2020b;99(7):769–74.
Schwendicke F, Chaurasia A, Wiegand T, Uribe SE, Fontana M, Akota I, Tryfonos O, Krois J. IADR e-oral health network and the ITU/WHO focus group AI for health. Artificial intelligence for oral and dental healthcare: Core education curriculum. J Dent. 2023;128:104363.
Scott J, Biancardi AM, Jones O, Andrew D. Artificial intelligence in periodontology: a scoping review. Dent J (Basel). 2023;11(2):43.
Shan T, Tay FR, Gu L. Application of artificial intelligence in dentistry. J Dent Res. 2021;100(3):232–44.
Sherwood AA, Sherwood AI, Setzer FC, Shella Devi K, Shamili JV, John C, Schwendicke F. A deep learning approach to segment and classify C-shaped canal morphologies in mandibular second molars using cone-beam computed tomography. J Endod. 2021a;47(12):1907–16.
Sherwood AA, Sherwood AI, Setzer FC, et al. A deep learning approach to segment and classify C-shaped canal morphologies in mandibular second molars using cone-beam computed tomography. J Endod. 2021b;47(12):1907–16.
Shujaat S, Bornstein MM, Price JB, Jacobs R. Integration of imaging modalities in digital dental workflows - possibilities, limitations, and potential future developments. Dentomaxillofac Radiol. 2021;50(7):20210268.
Srivastava MM, Kumar P, Pradhan L, Varadarajan S. Detection of tooth caries in bitewing radiographs using deep learning. arXiv. 2017.
Thanathornwong B, Suebnukarn S. Automatic detection of periodontal compromised teeth in digital panoramic radiographs using faster regional convolutional neural networks. Imaging Sci Dent. 2020;50:169–74.
Uğurlu M. Performance of a convolutional neural network- based artificial intelligence algorithm for automatic cephalometric landmark detection. Turk J Orthod. 2022;35(2):94–100.
Valizadeh S, Goodini M, Ehsani S, Mohseni H, Azimi F, Bakhshandeh H. Designing of a computer software for detection of approximal caries in posterior teeth. Iran J Radiol. 2015;12(4):e16242.

Vishwanathaiah S, Fageeh HN, Khanagar SB, Maganur PC. Artificial intelligence its uses and application in pediatric dentistry: a review. Biomedicine. 2023;11(3):788.

Warin K, Limprasert W, Suebnukarn S, Paipongna T, Jantana P, Vicharueang S. Maxillofacial fracture detection and classification in computed tomography images using convolutional neural network-based models. Sci Rep. 2023;13(1):3434.

Yang H, Jo E, Kim HJ, Cha IH, Jung YS, Nam W, et al. Deep learning for automated detection of cyst and tumors of the jaw in panoramic radiographs. J Clin Med. 2020;9:1–14.

Yang S, Lee H, Jang B, Kim KD, Kim J, Kim H, Park W. Development and validation of a visually explainable deep learning model for classification of C-shaped canals of the mandibular second molars in periapical and panoramic dental radiographs. J Endod. 2022;48(7):914–21.

Yasa Y, Çelik Ö, Bayrakdar IS, Pekince A, Orhan K, Akarsu S, Atasoy S, Bilgir E, Odabaş A, Aslan AF. An artificial intelligence proposal to automatic teeth detection and numbering in dental bite-wing radiographs. Acta Odontol Scand. 2021;79(4):275–81.

Yoo JH, Yeom HG, Shin W, Yun JP, Lee JH, Jeong SH, et al. Deep learning based prediction of extraction difficulty for mandibular third molars. Sci Rep. 2021;11:1954.

Yu HJ, Cho SR, Kim MJ, Kim WH, Kim JW, Choi J. Automated skeletal classification with lateral cephalometry based on artificial intelligence. J Dent Res. 2020;99(3):249–56.

Zhang W, Li J, Li ZB, Li Z. Predicting postoperative facial swelling following impacted mandibular third molars extraction by using artificial neural networks evaluation. Sci Rep. 2018;8:12281.

Zhang L, Xu F, Li Y, Zhang H, Xi Z, Xiang J, Wang B. A lightweight convolutional neural network model with receptive field block for C-shaped root canal detection in mandibular second molars. Sci Rep. 2022;12(1):17373.

Applications of AI in Endodontics and Restorative Dentistry

5

Kaan Orhan, Umut Aksoy, and Seçil Aksoy

Introduction

The landscape of healthcare, characterized by its continuous evolution, has been significantly shaped by innovation and technological advancements. Of these, artificial intelligence (AI), with its various manifestations such as machine learning algorithms and deep learning networks, has emerged as a transformative force. The potential of AI to revolutionize healthcare delivery is vast, with dentistry representing one of the many fields impacted by this technological evolution.

Endodontics and restorative dentistry, two fundamental domains within dental care, have experienced substantial influence from AI technologies. Endodontics, which concentrates on the study and treatment of dental pulp and periradicular tissues, and restorative dentistry, which focuses on the restoration and maintenance of oral functionality and aesthetics, have both witnessed significant enhancements through the integration of AI.

The objective of this chapter is to illuminate the diverse applications of AI within these critical fields of dentistry. Initially, we provide a foundational understanding of AI, tracing its evolution and explaining its relevance within the dental profession. This forms the basis for subsequent detailed exploration of AI's specific applications within endodontics and restorative dentistry.

K. Orhan
Faculty of Dentistry, Department of Dentomaxillofacial Radiology, Ankara University, Ankara, Turkey

U. Aksoy (✉)
Faculty of Dentistry, Department of Endodontics, Near East University, Nicosia, Cyprus
e-mail: umut.aksoy@neu.edu.tr

S. Aksoy
Faculty of Dentistry, Department of Dentomaxillofacial Radiology, Near East University, Nicosia, Cyprus
e-mail: secil.aksoy@neu.edu.tr

K. Orhan, R. Jagtap (eds.), *Artificial Intelligence in Dentistry*,
https://doi.org/10.1007/978-3-031-43827-1_5

We then examine the role of AI in endodontics, discussing its utility in diagnostic processes, treatment planning, and procedural aspects. Similarly, the influence of AI in restorative dentistry is explored, including its application in diagnosing dental conditions, planning restorative treatments, and facilitating restorative procedures.

In acknowledging the transformative potential of AI, we also evaluate its broader impact on dental practice. This includes a discussion of the benefits, limitations, and ethical considerations associated with integrating AI in dental care, as well as potential legal implications. The chapter concludes with a forward-looking perspective, discussing emerging trends, potential new applications, and the possible future trajectory of AI within endodontics and restorative dentistry.

Our aspiration is that this chapter contributes substantively to the current discourse on AI in dentistry, offering a comprehensive understanding of its role within the fields of endodontics and restorative dentistry, and grounding the discussion in contemporary research and professional practice.

Background

The advent of AI dates back to the mid-twentieth century—a period marked by the inception of the idea of machine-based humanlike intelligence. This concept evolved over subsequent decades, weathering periods of skepticism and progressing through moments of significant advancement. AI has transformed from its rudimentary beginnings with rule-based systems to its current state, characterized by sophisticated machine learning and deep learning algorithms.

As AI matured, its applications proliferated across numerous fields, with dentistry being one of them. Initially, AI was employed in dentistry to perform simple tasks such as data analysis and image recognition. However, as the technology evolved, its role within dental practice expanded to encompass diagnostics, treatment planning, procedural assistance, and patient management.

The impact of AI has been particularly notable within the fields of endodontics and restorative dentistry. In endodontics, AI has enhanced diagnostic processes traditionally dependent on radiographic interpretation, a task often affected by subjectivity and variability. AI algorithms have improved the accuracy and consistency of these processes. Additionally, AI has facilitated the identification of root canal anomalies and improved treatment planning through its predictive capabilities (Figs. 5.1 and 5.2).

In restorative dentistry, AI has revolutionized caries detection by transforming it from a subjective process into an objective and reliable one. AI has also transformed the design and fabrication of restorations, leading to personalized, accurate, and efficient restorative outcomes. Furthermore, AI aids in the selection of restorative materials and techniques, enhancing the quality of treatment outcomes.

In essence, the significance of AI within endodontics and restorative dentistry lies in its ability to improve accuracy, efficiency, and personalization of dental care. AI has initiated a new era—an era marked by precision, predictability, and

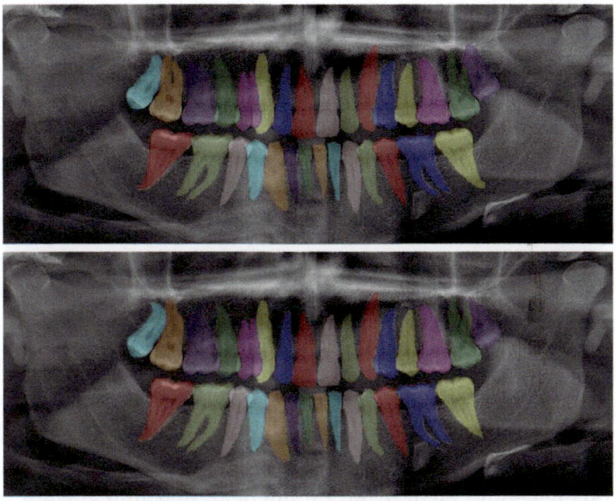

Fig. 5.1 Automatic segmentation of the teeth. Manual segmentation (upper image) and automatic segmentation (lower image) can be seen above. Each tooth has a unique label according to the FDI World Dental Federation notation

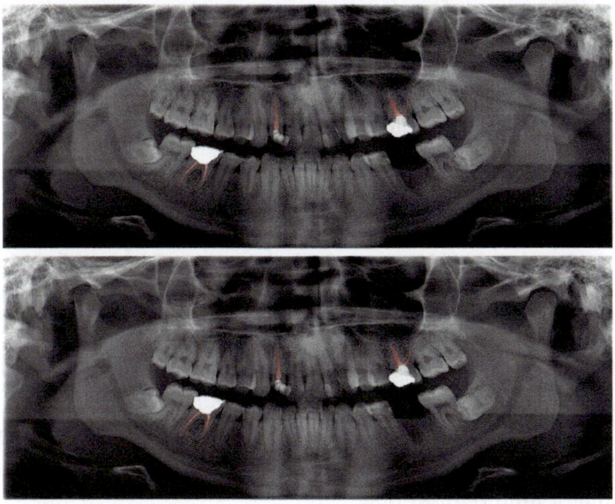

Fig. 5.2 Automatic segmentation of root-canal fillings. Manual segmentation (upper image), automatic segmentation (lower image) can be seen above

personalization. As we stand on the threshold of this exciting epoch, it is evident that the influence of AI will continue to grow.

AI in Endodontics

AI Models for Assessing Root Morphology

In the realm of endodontics and restorative dentistry, the assessment of root morphology plays a pivotal role in diagnosis, treatment planning, and prognosis determination. The complexity of root canal anatomy, particularly in cases of variations like C-shaped canals, poses significant challenges to clinicians. Traditionally, the evaluation of root morphology has relied on two-dimensional radiographic images, which often fall short in accurately representing the three-dimensional intricacies of root canal systems. This limitation can lead to suboptimal treatment outcomes, highlighting the need for more advanced, reliable, and precise assessment tools. Artificial intelligence (AI), with its ability to analyze complex data and identify patterns, offers a promising solution to this challenge.

One notable study, conducted by Hiraiwa et al. (2019), focused on evaluating the diagnostic performance of a deep learning system in classifying the root morphology of mandibular first molars using panoramic radiographs. To establish a reliable gold standard, dental cone-beam CT (CBCT) images were utilized for comparison. The results showed that a diagnostic accuracy of 86.9% was achieved by the deep learning system in determining whether distal roots were single or had extra roots. The conclusion was drawn by the authors that high accuracy was shown by the deep learning system in the differential diagnosis of a single or extra root in the distal roots of mandibular first molars. It was also suggested that the interpretation of images could be assisted by the deep learning system for inexperienced doctors.

Another study by Sherwood et al. (2021) presents a study that aims to develop a deep learning model to classify C-shaped canal anatomy in mandibular second molars from cone-beam computed tomographic (CBCT) volumes (Sherwood et al. 2021). The conclusion drawn from the study was that the detection and classification of C-shaped canal anatomy could potentially be aided by deep learning. It was suggested that an understanding of C-shaped canal morphologies could be enhanced by an automated segmentation tool for CBCT images, thereby improving the safety and efficiency of patient treatment.

Jeon et al. (2021) conducted a study (Jeon et al. 2021) to assess the effectiveness of a convolutional neural network (CNN) system in predicting C-shaped canals in panoramic radiographs of mandibular second molars. The findings indicated that the CNN model achieved impressive performance metrics, with accuracy, sensitivity, specificity, and precision values of 95.1%, 92.7%, 97.0%, and 95.9%, respectively. As a result, the authors concluded that the deep-learning system exhibited significant accuracy in predicting C-shaped canals in mandibular second molars on panoramic radiographs.

Yang et al. (2022) recently conducted a study (Yang et al. 2022) where they created and validated a visually interpretable deep learning model to classify C-shaped canals in periapical and panoramic radiographs of mandibular second molars. The study aimed to assess the diagnostic capabilities of the deep learning system in determining whether the second mandibular molar exhibited a C-shaped canal configuration, using CBCT as the reference standard. The findings revealed that the deep convolutional neural network algorithm model demonstrated excellent accuracy in predicting the presence of C-shaped canal variations in mandibular second molars, regardless of whether periapical or panoramic images were used.

These studies collectively suggest that AI models can significantly aid in the assessment of root morphology, specifically C-shaped canals in mandibular molars, potentially improving clinical practice and education in endodontics. However, they also highlight the need for further research and development to fully realize the potential of AI in this field.

AI in Predicting Case Difficulty

The application of artificial intelligence (AI) in endodontics has shown promising results, particularly in predicting case difficulty. This is a crucial aspect of endodontic treatment planning, as it allows for more accurate diagnosis, better patient communication, and more effective treatment outcomes.

One of the innovative approaches in this area is the use of machine learning algorithms to predict the difficulty level of endodontic cases. A study by Mallishery et al. (2020) demonstrated the potential of such an approach. The researchers used the standard American Society of Endodontists Endodontic Case Difficulty Assessment Form (American Association of Endodontists n.d.) to diagnose 500 potential root canal patients. Two pre-calibrated endodontists evaluated the completed forms, seeking a third endodontist's input in the event of differing opinions. Utilizing an artificial neural network, an algorithm was generated.

The results of the study were encouraging, with the machine learning algorithm achieving a sensitivity of 94.96%. This high sensitivity indicates the potential of machine learning algorithms in accurately predicting case difficulty in endodontics. In their conclusion, the authors found that the machine learning algorithm offers an alternative to the traditional approach of predicting case complexity. This innovation enables faster decision-making and potential referrals, introducing automation into the process.

Qu et al. (2023) endeavored to construct and authenticate machine learning models with the objective of forecasting the complexity of cases in endodontic microsurgery, thereby providing a tool for clinicians to conduct preoperative evaluations.

The investigators gathered cone-beam computed tomographic images from a sample of 261 patients, encompassing 341 teeth, which were subjected to radiographic examination and measurement. Four distinct models were established, utilizing a variety of machine learning algorithms, namely, linear regression (LR), support vector regression (SVR), and extreme gradient boosting (XGBoost). These models underwent validation through a process of five-fold cross-validation.

The efficacy of the models was assessed through a range of metrics, which included the mean absolute error (MAE), coefficient of determination (R2), explained variance score (EVS), mean squared error (MSE), and median absolute error (MedAE). The XGBoost model demonstrated superior performance across all evaluation metrics, thereby indicating its potential utility in assisting clinicians in preoperative analysis.

The research also identified a number of factors that could serve as predictors of case difficulty in endodontic microsurgery. These factors, arranged in the order of their relative importance, encompassed lesion size, the distance between the apex and adjacent important anatomical structures, tooth type, root canal curvature, root apex diameter, root filling density, root resorption, tooth length, root filling length, and the number of root canals.

In their conclusion, the authors posited that the XGBoost model surpassed the LR and SVR models in its ability to predict case difficulty in endodontic microsurgery. They proposed that the relative importance of features could serve as a reference for the development of a scoring system for case difficulty assessment in endodontic microsurgery. They further recommended the execution of a larger-scale multicenter study involving experienced endodontists who were not part of the algorithm development team for the purpose of further optimization of the models.

While the results are promising, the application of AI in predicting case difficulty in endodontics is not without challenges. The algorithm's performance can vary depending on the complexity of the case and the quality of the input data. Therefore, further research and development are needed to improve the accuracy and reliability of these AI models.

In conclusion, AI models, particularly machine learning algorithms, have shown significant potential in predicting case difficulty in endodontics. These models can enhance the speed and accuracy of decision-making, potentially improving patient outcomes. However, further research and development are needed to fully realize the potential of AI in this field.

AI in Detecting Pulpal Diseases

Artificial intelligence (AI) has shown promising results in the field of the detection of pulpal diseases. Deep learning models, specifically convolutional neural networks (CNNs), have been used to diagnose deep caries and pulpitis with high accuracy.

Tumbelaka et al. (2014) demonstrated the potential of AI in diagnosing pulpitis. The researchers utilized ten tooth radiographs and applied edge detection, texture description, and artificial neural networks (ANNs) to identify pulpitis. The model was particularly efficient in diagnosing reversible and irreversible pulpitis, providing valuable insights for pulp interpretation. However, the authors suggested that direct reading radiography should be digitized for better diagnosis validation.

A recent study conducted by Zheng et al. (2021) embarked on an exploration of deep learning, a subset of artificial intelligence, to detect and diagnose deep caries and pulpitis. They employed a specific type of deep learning model known as a convolutional neural network (CNN), which has shown remarkable success in image recognition tasks. To test the performance of their models, Zheng and his team used a total of 844 radiographs. They allocated 85% of these images for training the models and reserved the remaining 15% for testing. The results were impressive. Their model outperformed its counterparts and even the experienced clinicians. However, it's important to note that this study had its limitations. The focus was solely on teeth with single carious lesions, leaving out cases with multiple carious lesions. This suggests that while the study provides a promising direction, there is still a need for further research.

AI in Detecting Periapical Lesions

In the rapidly evolving field of AI application in detecting periapical lesions, several promising strides have been made to improve the accuracy and efficiency of diagnoses. Periapical lesions, which are often a consequence of pulpal diseases, can be challenging to detect accurately using traditional methods. However, the advent of AI has brought forward models that can assist in this task.

As an example of such advancements, the study by Ekert et al. (2019) developed a deep learning model for detecting apical lesions using panoramic radiographs. While the model showed promise with an AUC of 0.85, the authors pointed out room for improvement, particularly in sensitivity. Moving from this point, it is clear that while the potential for AI in lesion detection is high, there is still a need for further fine-tuning in model performance.

Taking a different approach, another study (Endres et al. 2020) used a deep learning model to aid oral and maxillofacial (OMF) surgeons in detecting periapical radiolucencies on panoramic radiographs. Highlighting the variability in dental professionals' abilities to read panoramic radiographs, the study pointed to the potential of AI to reduce the rate of misdiagnosis and improve patient outcomes.

Next, in the realm of CBCT images, Orhan et al. (2020) used an artificial intelligence system based on deep convolutional neural network methods to detect periapical pathosis. Their AI system showed a high reliability of 92.8% in correctly detecting a periapical lesion, hinting at the usefulness of AI in the diagnosis and treatment of periapical diseases.

Building upon the application of AI in CBCT images, Setzer et al. (2020) used a deep learning (DL) algorithm for the automated segmentation of CBCT images and the detection of periapical lesions. Their findings underscored the potential for AI to improve the accuracy of periapical lesion detection in CBCT images.

On the other hand, Li et al. (2021) employed a convolutional neural network (CNN) to detect dental apical lesions using periapical radiographs. While they found that their model performed better than other methods, they also recognized the need for future development in the field.

In a comparative study by Pauwels et al. (2021), the diagnostic performance of convolutional neural networks (CNNs) was compared with human observers for the detection of simulated periapical lesions. With CNNs showing diagnostic performance comparable to or better than human observers, the potential for AI in clinical applications becomes more apparent.

Transitioning from detection to segmentation of lesions, Bayrakdar et al. (2022) used a deep-convolutional neural network (D-CNN) model to segment apical lesions on dental panoramic radiographs. The results suggested that AI systems might overcome certain clinical challenges, facilitating the assessment of periapical pathology based on panoramic radiographs.

Making significant strides in the field, Calazans et al. (2022) developed an automatic classification system for the detection of endodontic lesions in pairs of cone-beam computed tomography sections. The success of the system highlighted the potential for AI as a useful tool in lesion detection, albeit with noted challenges in detecting very small lesions.

In a unique two-step approach, Kirnbauer et al. (2022) developed a deep convolutional neuronal network for the automated detection of osteolytic periapical lesions in CBCT data sets. The success of this approach showcased the potential of AI, even in the face of variability in lesion appearance, size, and shape.

Finally, a study by Moidu et al. (2022) demonstrated the potential for AI in scoring periapical lesions. Their CNN model trained to score periapical lesions based on the periapical index (PAI) scoring system showed promising results. This suggests the potential application of AI not only in detection but also in the severity assessment of periapical lesions.

To summarize, these studies represent the tremendous strides made in the application of AI for the detection of periapical lesions. However, they also highlight the ongoing need for improvements in model performance, as well as the potential for future development in the field.

AI in Segmentation of the Pulp Cavity

The utilization of artificial intelligence (AI) in segmenting the pulp cavity has garnered increasing attention within the field of endodontics. In a study conducted by Lin et al. (2021), a fresh data pipeline was introduced, utilizing micro-computed tomographic (micro-CT) data to train the U-Net network. The aim was to achieve automatic and precise segmentation of the pulp cavity and tooth structures in cone-beam computed tomographic (CBCT) images. This groundbreaking approach has paved the way for exciting possibilities in applying AI to the field of endodontics.

In order to carry out this process, the scientists gathered data from 30 teeth, including both CBCT and micro-CT scans. The CBCT data underwent processing and were converted into high-resolution, small field-of-view images for each tooth. Out of the 30 sets, 25 were randomly chosen for the training set, while the remaining five sets were designated as the test set. This collection and processing of data formed the foundation of the study, establishing the groundwork for the subsequent stages.

Building on this, two data pipelines were used for U-Net network training: one manually labeled by an endodontic specialist as the control group and one processed from the micro-CT data as the experimental group. This dual approach allowed for a comprehensive comparison of the effectiveness of manual labeling versus AI-based segmentation.

The 3-dimensional models constructed using micro-CT data in the test set were taken as the ground truth. The Dice similarity coefficient, Hausdorff distance, recall rate, precision rate, average symmetric surface distance, and morphologic analysis were used for performance evaluation. The results of this evaluation were pivotal in determining the effectiveness of the AI-based approach.

The segmentation accuracy of the experimental group measured by these metrics were significantly better than the control group. These findings underscored the potential of AI in enhancing the accuracy of pulp cavity segmentation.

To conclude, this study suggests that the proposed approach for segmenting teeth and pulp cavities in CBCT images has potential applications in both research and clinical settings. It offers precise training samples for neural networks, enabling accurate labeling even for small root canals that may pose challenges for specialists when interpreting CBCT images. This method mitigates differences in individual image recognition and ensures reliable training samples for neural networks.

However, the study also emphasizes the need for further research in this domain of dental research. With the advent of AI, researchers are striving to develop increasingly advanced models for tooth segmentation to achieve precise results. Nevertheless, the focus on providing high-quality training samples for AI segmentation models has been comparatively limited. This serves as a reminder that despite the promising prospects of AI in endodontics, there are still unresolved challenges that must be addressed to fully harness its potential.

AI in Determining Working Length

The determination of working length in endodontics is a critical step in ensuring successful root canal treatment. Accurate working length determination is essential to avoid over-instrumentation, which can lead to posttreatment complications such as pain and infection, or under-instrumentation, which can leave residual bacteria and debris in the canal. Traditionally, working length determination has been achieved through a combination of tactile sensation, radiographic interpretation, and electronic apex locators. However, these methods have their limitations, including operator subjectivity, radiation exposure, and inaccuracies due to anatomical variations or the presence of electrolytes in the canal.

In this context, the application of artificial intelligence (AI) in determining the working length has emerged as a promising avenue of research. AI, with its ability to learn from data and make predictions, has the potential to overcome the limitations of traditional methods and improve the accuracy and consistency of working length determination. A study by Qiao et al. (2020) explored this potential, specifically focusing on a multifrequency impedance method based on a neural network for root canal length measurement. This method combines the principles of electronic length determination with the power of AI to provide a more accurate and reliable method for working length determination. The study proposed that the neural network-based multifrequency method can be used to determine the working length in endodontics. It provides a more accurate and robust method compared to the traditional dual-impedance ratio method. However, the study also highlighted that further improvements in accuracy can be considered, such as improving the neural network structure, using different judgment strategies, using different optimization methods, and most importantly, expanding the data set.

AI in Diagnosing Vertical Root Fracture

Vertical root fracture (VRF) is a challenging diagnosis in endodontics and restorative dentistry. Traditional diagnostic methods, such as clinical examination and radiographic imaging, have limitations in detecting VRFs. However, recent advances in artificial intelligence (AI) have shown promise in improving the accuracy of VRF diagnosis.

In a recent study by Fukuda et al. (2020), a convolutional neural network (CNN) system was developed to detect VRFs on panoramic radiography. The CNN model was trained on a dataset of 1000 panoramic radiographs and achieved a recall of 0.75, precision of 0.93, and an F measure of 0.83. These results suggest that AI-based systems have the potential to improve the accuracy of VRF diagnosis on panoramic radiography.

While this study focused on panoramic radiography, other imaging modalities such as cone-beam computed tomography (CBCT) have also been investigated for VRF diagnosis using AI. A systematic review and meta-analysis by Ma et al. (2016) found that CBCT had high detection accuracy for root fractures, with a sensitivity of 0.91 and specificity of 0.98. AI-based systems could potentially improve the accuracy of VRF diagnosis on CBCT as well.

In conclusion, AI-based systems have shown promise in improving the accuracy of VRF diagnosis in endodontics and restorative dentistry. While further research is needed to validate these findings and optimize the performance of AI models, the potential benefits of AI in VRF diagnosis are promising.

AI in Restorative Dentistry

Artificial intelligence (AI) has been making significant strides in various fields, including dentistry. In the realm of restorative dentistry, AI has shown promising potential in enhancing diagnosis, treatment planning, and prediction of treatment outcomes.

AI models have been increasingly used to diagnose dental caries, detect tooth preparation margins, and predict restoration failure. The use of these models has grown substantially since 2019, indicating a rising trend in the integration of AI in restorative dentistry (Revilla-León et al. 2022).

AI models can provide a powerful tool to assist in the diagnosis of dental caries (Fig. 5.3). These models can analyze complex patterns in dental images, enabling more accurate and early detection of these conditions. This can lead to timely interventions and improved patient outcomes.

Furthermore, AI can be used to detect the tooth finishing line, an essential step in restorative procedures such as crown placement. This can improve the precision of restorations, leading to better fit and longevity of the dental prosthesis.

AI models can also predict the failure of dental restorations. By analyzing various factors such as the type of restoration, patient characteristics, and oral health status, these models can provide valuable insights into the likelihood of restoration

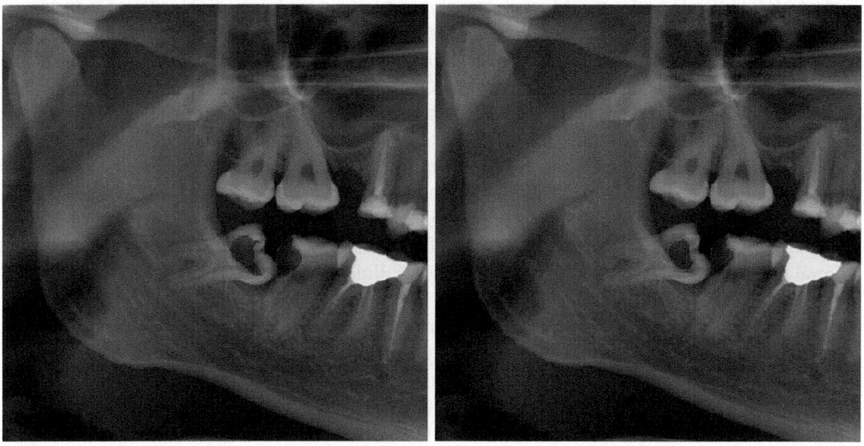

Fig. 5.3 Automatic segmentation of the carious lesions at the lower-right second and third molar. Manual segmentation (left) as well as automatic segmentation (right) can be seen above

failure. This can guide dentists in choosing the most suitable restorative materials and techniques for each patient, potentially reducing the need for future re-treatments.

However, it's important to note that the dental applications of AI models are still under development. Further studies are required to assess the clinical performance of AI models in restorative dentistry. The standardization and benchmarking of datasets might increase the accuracy of AI models in diagnosing dental conditions and predicting failures of dental restorations. The availability of open datasets will facilitate the development of AI models.

In conclusion, AI has the potential to revolutionize restorative dentistry by enhancing diagnostic accuracy, improving treatment planning, and predicting treatment outcomes. As AI models continue to evolve and improve, they are expected to play an increasingly important role in restorative dentistry.

References

American Association of Endodontists. Endodontic Case Difficulty Assessment Form and Guidelines. https://www.aae.org

Bayrakdar IS, Orhan K, Çelik Ö, et al. A U-Net approach to apical lesion segmentation on panoramic radiographs. Biomed Res Int. 2022;2022:7035367. Published 2022 Jan 15. https://doi.org/10.1155/2022/7035367.

Calazans MAA, Ferreira FABS, Alcoforado MLMG, Santos AD, Pontual ADA, Madeiro F. Automatic classification system for periapical lesions in cone-beam computed tomography. Sensors (Basel). 2022;22(17):6481. Published 2022 Aug 28. https://doi.org/10.3390/s22176481.

Ekert T, Krois J, Meinhold L, et al. Deep learning for the radiographic detection of apical lesions. J Endod. 2019;45(7):917–922.e5. https://doi.org/10.1016/j.joen.2019.03.016.

Endres MG, Hillen F, Salloumis M, et al. Development of a deep learning algorithm for periapical disease detection in dental radiographs. Diagnostics (Basel). 2020;10(6):430. Published 2020 Jun 24. https://doi.org/10.3390/diagnostics10060430.

Fukuda M, Inamoto K, Shibata N, et al. Evaluation of an artificial intelligence system for detecting vertical root fracture on panoramic radiography. Oral Radiol. 2020;36(4):337–43. https://doi.org/10.1007/s11282-019-00409-x.

Hiraiwa T, Ariji Y, Fukuda M, et al. A deep-learning artificial intelligence system for assessment of root morphology of the mandibular first molar on panoramic radiography. Dentomaxillofac Radiol. 2019;48(3):20180218. https://doi.org/10.1259/dmfr.20180218.

Jeon SJ, Yun JP, Yeom HG, et al. Deep-learning for predicting C-shaped canals in mandibular second molars on panoramic radiographs. Dentomaxillofac Radiol. 2021;50(5):20200513. https://doi.org/10.1259/dmfr.20200513.

Kirnbauer B, Hadzic A, Jakse N, Bischof H, Stern D. Automatic detection of periapical osteolytic lesions on cone-beam computed tomography using deep convolutional neuronal networks. J Endod. 2022;48(11):1434–40. https://doi.org/10.1016/j.joen.2022.07.013.

Li CW, Lin SY, Chou HS, et al. Detection of dental apical lesions using CNNs on periapical radiograph. Sensors (Basel). 2021;21(21):7049. Published 2021 Oct 24. https://doi.org/10.3390/s21217049.

Lin X, Fu Y, Ren G, et al. Micro-computed tomography-guided artificial intelligence for pulp cavity and tooth segmentation on cone-beam computed tomography. J Endod. 2021;47(12):1933–41. https://doi.org/10.1016/j.joen.2021.09.001.

Ma RH, Ge ZP, Li G. Detection accuracy of root fractures in cone-beam computed tomography images: a systematic review and meta-analysis. Int Endod J. 2016;49(7):646–54. https://doi.org/10.1111/iej.12490.

Mallishery S, Chhatpar P, Banga KS, Shah T, Gupta P. The precision of case difficulty and referral decisions: an innovative automated approach. Clin Oral Investig. 2020;24(6):1909–15. https://doi.org/10.1007/s00784-019-03050-4.

Moidu NP, Sharma S, Chawla A, Kumar V, Logani A. Deep learning for categorization of endodontic lesion based on radiographic periapical index scoring system. Clin Oral Investig. 2022;26(1):651–8. https://doi.org/10.1007/s00784-021-04043-y.

Orhan K, Bayrakdar IS, Ezhov M, Kravtsov A, Özyürek T. Evaluation of artificial intelligence for detecting periapical pathosis on cone-beam computed tomography scans. Int Endod J. 2020;53(5):680–9. https://doi.org/10.1111/iej.13265.

Pauwels R, Brasil DM, Yamasaki MC, et al. Artificial intelligence for detection of periapical lesions on intraoral radiographs: comparison between convolutional neural networks and human observers. Oral Surg Oral Med Oral Pathol Oral Radiol. 2021;131(5):610–6. https://doi.org/10.1016/j.oooo.2021.01.018.

Qiao X, Zhang Z, Chen X. Multifrequency impedance method based on neural network for root canal length measurement. Appl Sci. 2020;10(21):7430. https://doi.org/10.3390/app10217430.

Qu Y, Wen Y, Chen M, Guo K, Huang X, Gu L. Predicting case difficulty in endodontic microsurgery using machine learning algorithms. J Dent. 2023;133:104522. https://doi.org/10.1016/j.jdent.2023.104522.

Revilla-León M, Gómez-Polo M, Vyas S, et al. Artificial intelligence applications in restorative dentistry: a systematic review. J Prosthet Dent. 2022;128(5):867–75. https://doi.org/10.1016/j.prosdent.2021.02.010.

Setzer FC, Shi KJ, Zhang Z, et al. Artificial intelligence for the computer-aided detection of periapical lesions in cone-beam computed tomographic images. J Endod. 2020;46(7):987–93. https://doi.org/10.1016/j.joen.2020.03.025.

Sherwood AA, Sherwood AI, Setzer FC, et al. A deep learning approach to segment and classify C-shaped canal morphologies in mandibular second molars using cone-beam computed tomography. J Endod. 2021;47(12):1907–16. https://doi.org/10.1016/j.joen.2021.09.009.

Tumbelaka B, Baihaki F, Oscandar F, Rukmo M, Sitam S. Identification of pulpitis at dental X-ray periapical radiography based on edge detection, texture description and artificial neural networks. Saudi Endod J. 2014;4:115.

Yang S, Lee H, Jang B, et al. Development and validation of a visually explainable deep learning model for classification of C-shaped canals of the mandibular second molars in periapical and panoramic dental radiographs. J Endod. 2022;48(7):914–21. https://doi.org/10.1016/j.joen.2022.04.007.
Zheng L, Wang H, Mei L, Chen Q, Zhang Y, Zhang H. Artificial intelligence in digital cariology: a new tool for the diagnosis of deep caries and pulpitis using convolutional neural networks. Ann Transl Med. 2021;9(9):763. https://doi.org/10.21037/atm-21-119.

Artificial Neural Networks for the Design Optimization of Implants

6

Jason A. Griggs

Challenges of AI Use in Engineering Design

AI is commonly used in the health sciences for object recognition (Vujanovic and Jagtap 2023) or diagnosis (Yamaguchi et al. 2019) because it lends itself to easy use for those applications. The portion of the protocol that the AI takes over is the majority of the total protocol, leaving little remaining work for the operator to do. However, engineering design presents some additional challenges because the operator is required to define design parameters and constraints in advance of the AI contribution. This includes determining which measurements or design features can be varied, over what range each of them can be varied, and how to best define design parameters so they are independent of each other and do not impinge on each other as a result of variation. These definitions require substantial effort on the part of the operator without the aid of AI. The AI is then trained to predict a numerical performance metric, and it saves a lot of time following training because it is capable of predicting the performance of a design in a fraction of a second. In engineering design, the data for training are not existing images paired with expert human interpretation. The training and validation data are either from physical testing of prototypes (requiring days for the operator to acquire each data point) or more commonly from finite element analysis software (requiring hours for each data point). In either case, acquiring the data to create the AI is effort-intensive. After training and validation, the operator is often required to guide the AI or use a genetic algorithm because the performance predictions output by the AI often form a complex response surface that contains many local maxima and minima. The gratuitous number of designs corresponding to these points in the design space thwarts many algorithms from finding the globally optimum design. Thus, current AI technology saves a smaller

J. A. Griggs (✉)
Department of Biomedical Materials Science, School of Dentistry, University of Mississippi Medical Center, Jackson, MS, USA
e-mail: jgriggs@umc.edu

K. Orhan, R. Jagtap (eds.), *Artificial Intelligence in Dentistry*,
https://doi.org/10.1007/978-3-031-43827-1_6

proportion of human effort for engineering design problems compared to the effort that it saves in object recognition and medical diagnosis. Nevertheless, AI has been a valuable tool for engineers both inside and outside the health sciences as illustrated by the examples below. Before describing the projects that successfully used AI for design optimization, it will be useful to provide an overview of the design optimization process.

Process of Design Optimization

Figure 6.1 summarizes the steps of the engineering design optimization process.

Step 1 is to define the design factors and their limits. A design factor is an aspect of the implant that can be controlled and that is expected to have an effect on the performance of the implant. Examples include implant length, implant outer diameter, and implant inner diameter. However, it is best to define geometrical factors in terms of distances between landmarks on the product. Otherwise, the factors may come into conflict when they are varied. For example, when the outer diameter is decreased and the inner diameter is increased, it may result in an implant with no wall thickness. Inner diameter and wall thickness would never come into conflict with each other though. In addition, one should be careful to identify factors that are not truly independent of each other and combine them into a single factor.

Step 2 is to define the design objectives. Design objectives are the performance metrics for which the goal is either to maximize their value (strength, lifetime, fatigue limit), minimize their value (variability in strength, cost, deflection), or target a moderate value (strain on bone within a healthy range without atrophy and without microfracture). A desirability function may be constructed for each objective, which provides a quantitative and nonsubjective means for comparing competing product designs (Fig. 6.2). The desirability function ranges from $d = 0$ (undesirable) to $d = 1$ (desirable). If the design objective is to be maximized, then $d = 0$ until the objective reaches the lower limit (L). From the lower limit to the target value (T), d increases from 0 to 1. Above the target value, $d = 1$ because there is no reward for increasing the objective higher than the target value. On the other hand, if the objective is something that we wish to minimize, then $d = 0$ above the

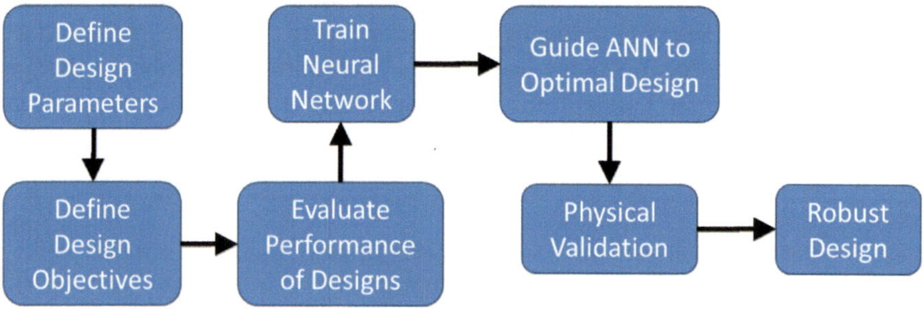

Fig. 6.1 Flowchart for the engineering design optimization process

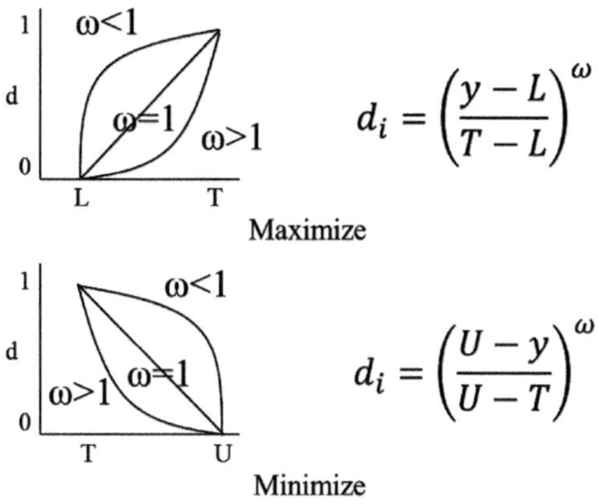

$$D = \left(d_1^{r_1} d_2^{r_2} \cdots d_n^{r_n}\right)^{1/(r_1+r_2+\cdots+r_n)}$$

Fig. 6.2 Desirability functions for maximizing and minimizing the design objective

upper limit (U), and $d = 1$ below the target value. If an intermediate level is most valuable for the objective, then the desirability function will contain both upper and lower limits, and d will be penalized in either direction from the target value. In cases where there is more than one design objective, it is unlikely that the same combination of design factors will result in maximum d for every objective, and the factors must be chosen to compromise between the various objectives to produce the highest overall desirability (D). *D* is calculated as the harmonic mean of the individual d values (Fig. 6.2).

Step 3 is to determine what level of desirability or objective results from each combination of design factors. This could be done by milling or 3D-printing a prototype for each design and physically testing them, but engineers usually employ finite element analysis (FEA) software to save time in predicting the performance of each design. A virtual "solid" model is created in the computer using a combination of computed tomography (CT) scans and CAD software. Then, material properties (Young's modulus, Poisson's ratio, etc.) are assigned to each component, and virtual forces and supports are applied at appropriate locations on the device. FEA can predict the direction and magnitude of stress and strain in an implant, stress and strain in the adjacent bone, amount of deflection or micromotion, natural harmonic frequency, fluid flow, and changes in temperature.

However, it is usually too labor intensive to test or predict the performance of every possible combination of design factors. For an implant with 16 different factors, even if only three settings are considered for each factor the burden would be $3^{16} = 43{,}046{,}721$ different designs! A common strategy is to use only two settings per factor, but that is not advisable because the experiment will not be able to notice nonlinear behavior and would overlook optimal designs that may exist at intermediate settings (Fig. 6.3). A better solution is to use fractional factorial experiments. A half-factorial experiment cuts the number of designs by half (Fig. 6.4), and the only

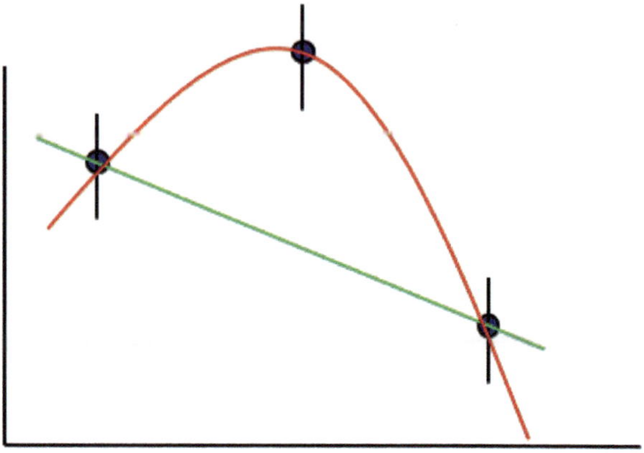

Fig. 6.3 Illustration of the way in which a two-level design (green) fails to register a nonlinear behavior, thereby missing optimal designs (red)

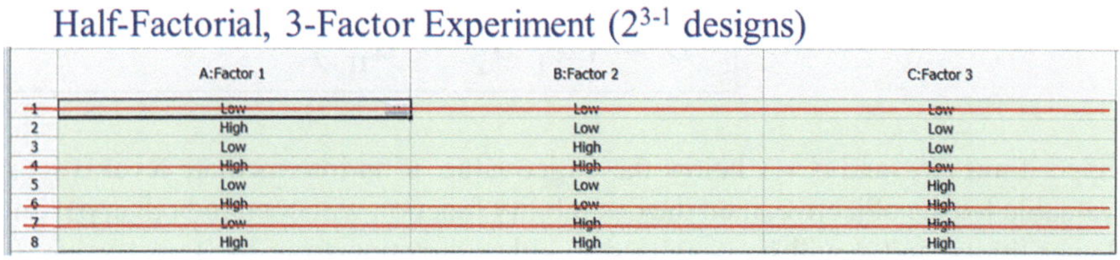

	A:Factor 1	B:Factor 2	C:Factor 3
1	Low	Low	Low
2	High	Low	Low
3	Low	High	Low
4	High	High	Low
5	Low	Low	High
6	High	Low	High
7	Low	High	High
8	High	High	High

Fig. 6.4 Illustration of how fractional factorial experiments reduce the number designs to be evaluated

loss is the ability to detect the highest-order interaction. For example, for three design factors a half-factorial experiment would be able to detect the main effects of the factors and their two-way interactions but not the possible three-way interactions. According to the Pareto principle (also known as the sparsity of effects principle or the 80/20 rule), 80% of the effects are controlled by 20% of the factors and their low-order interactions. Experiments may be cut in half multiple times, and they only lose one order of interaction with each halving. This leads to highly fractional designs such as the popular Taguchi orthogonal arrays. By varying more than one factor at a time in a strategic manner, orthogonal arrays allow later analysis with either multiple regression or ANN to isolate the effect of each factor based on the performance of only 8–27 designs for 7–16 factors (Fig. 6.5). A wide variety of design of experiments (DOE) software packages are available to plan fractional factorial experiments and create orthogonal arrays (Burnham 1998).

Step 4 is to fit a statistical model to the data or train an ANN on the data so that the performance of additional hypothetical designs can be predicted without spending additional time on FEA or manufacturing prototypes. This is where ANNs excel. A simple ANN with one hidden layer and two neurons (Fig. 6.6) is capable of learning the effects of a large number of design factors and their interactions. It is inadvisable to use a single neuron because there are classes of problems that a single neuron cannot solve, but a few neurons suffice for most engineering design problems. The ANN multiplies each design factor by a weighting factor (w) and sums all

	A:Factor 1	B:Factor 2	C:Factor 3	D:Factor 4	E:Factor 5	F:Factor 6	G:Factor 7
1	Low	Low	Low	Low	Low	Low	Low
2	Low	Low	High	High	Low	High	High
3	Low	High	Low	High	High	Low	High
4	Low	High	High	Low	High	High	Low
5	High	Low	Low	High	High	High	Low
6	High	Low	High	Low	High	Low	High
7	High	High	Low	Low	Low	High	High
8	High	High	High	High	Low	Low	Low

Fig. 6.5 Taguchi orthogonal array for measuring the main effects of seven design factors using only eight designs

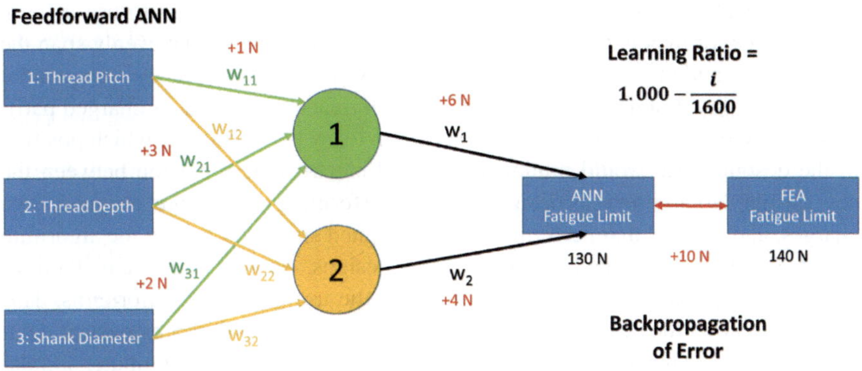

Fig. 6.6 The structure and training of a simple artificial neural network with one hidden layer containing two neurons

of the products to calculate the membrane potential of a neuron. For example, in Fig. 6.6, thread pitch (TP), thread depth (TD), and shank diameter (SD) all contribute to the membrane potential (MP) or input of Neuron 1 in the hidden layer: TP • w_{11} + TD • w_{21} + SD • w_{31} = MP_1. The output or action potential (AP) of a neuron can be any function based on its input. It is common to use a sigmoidal (S-shaped) function where little action occurs up to a threshold input level (θ) and the action rapidly climbs after that threshold in reached.

$$AP_1 = \frac{1}{1 - \exp\left(\theta - MP_{1.}\right)}.$$

The sigmoidal function aids in modeling nonlinear effects, and it also mimics the action of biological neurons. The ANN is trained by the backpropagation of error. For each design, the ANN's prediction of performance or desirability is compared to the data from prototype testing or the prediction of FEA. The discrepancy is divided among the neurons according to the proportion of each neuron's contribution, and the weighting factors are adjusted to reduce the discrepancy. Only a portion of the error is corrected so that the ANN remembers all of its past training, and the portion of error corrected is usually decreased over time to avoid the ANN from trying to learn minute fluctuations in product performance. These fluctuations are probably caused by stochastic variation instead of design effects. In lieu of using an

ANN, multiple regression can be used to fit polynomials to the data. However, ANNs consistently outperform multiple regression.

Step 5 is to identify the combination of design factors that corresponds to maximum performance (maximum overall desirability, D). This step can be surprisingly difficult. Although the trained ANN can predict the performance of any given design in a fraction of a second, it lacks the ability to guide itself regarding which designs to evaluate. The excellent ability of ANNs to fit data sets often results in a complex response surface that contains many local maxima and minima. The gratuitous number of designs corresponding to these points thwarts many algorithms from finding the globally optimum design. A common starting point is to use a Latin square, cube, or hypercube generator to create a list of designs that evenly span the design space and then to submit that list to the ANN. Another strategy is sequential minimal energy design (Dasgupta 2007), which treats the designs as charged particles and chooses the location of the next design to try by calculating which position in the design space would minimize the total electrostatic repulsion between the new design and all previous designs. Poorly performing designs are assigned large charges, and designs that perform well are assigned small charges, so the algorithm spends more time near the better performing designs. Another effective method for locating the global performance maximum is the use of genetic algorithms. This involves treating the designs as if they are genomes competing in a process of natural selection. The desirability function is the measure of fitness. A computer simulation automatically queries the ANN about the predicted fitness of each design in the population and breeds new generations of designs that inherit some design factors from the superior designs in the previous generation while also including the occasional design factor setting that occurs by mutation. MATLAB software can be used both to construct ANNs and genetic algorithms, and the two features work together well (MATLAB 2015, 2020).

Steps 6 and 7 are often neglected. They are, respectively, to validate the predicted performance of the optimal design by physical tests on prototypes and optimization for decreased variability using Taguchi robust design (Taguchi 1986). Robust design traditionally adds an outer orthogonal array that consists of extraneous (nuisance) factors. It locates the design that has close to optimal performance and also has similar performance under all conditions (low technique sensitivity). A modern approach to robust design is to include the standard deviation of the performance among the objectives, assigning a separate desirability function to minimize the standard deviation. The overall desirability will be the harmonic mean of the performance with its standard deviation. Maximizing the overall desirability will identify a design that reaches a compromise between performance and robustness.

Examples of Using AI for Design Optimization

Simple backpropagation artificial neural networks have been successfully used for designing fluid impellers, radio antennae, and variable cross-section structural beams among many other engineering applications outside the health sciences

(Babiker et al. 2012; Kim et al. 2009; Mahouti 2019). However, there are only seven cases of using ANN for medical implant design to date.

Dental Implants

Dental implant components. At first glance, a dental implant may appear similar in design and function to an orthopedic screw. Dental implants do have external screw threads, and those screw threads help dental implants to penetrate bone and maintain stability within bone. However, the need for delayed loading and for angulation require a much more complex design for dental implants than for bone screws. The human jawbone will not tolerate even microscopic motion of the implant relative to the bone. Any such motion results in the formation of a fibrous capsule around the implant and subsequent failure to osseointegrate. In order to avoid this type of failure, dental implants usually consist of two segments: the implant body, which is screwed into the bone and allowed sufficient time (sometimes months) to fully osseointegrate, and the implant abutment that is installed onto the implant body later (after osseointegration is complete). Another reason that this modular design is used in most dental implants is there may be insufficient bone to anchor the implant along the long-axis of the tooth that is being replaced. In that case, the implant body is placed at an angle in the jaw to ensure contact with sufficient bone, and it is necessary to install an implant abutment that is angled to the same degree (and in the opposite direction) so that the prosthetic tooth that sits on the abutment will be properly aligned with the other teeth in the mouth. The implant abutment either slides into the implant body (internal connection) or sits atop the platform of the implant body (external connection). Regardless of the connection type, a tiny connector screw is required to penetrate and transfix both the implant abutment and the implant body. These three components may experience micromotion between them that creates a risk of loosening the connection, leading to fatigue fracture. Connection loosening is currently the most common complication in dental implants (Griggs 2017). Anti-rotation features such as a hexagonal or octagonal socket, cone-shaped (Morse taper) socket, or a combination of these are implemented to decrease loosening. The connector screw is also designed to take a heavy preload, which protects the other two components and decreases the incidence of loosening. The functions of the three components are so varied that it is increasingly common for them to be made from different materials (grade 4 CP Ti for the implant body, Ti-6Al-4 V alloy for the implant abutment, and 316 L stainless steel for the connector screw).

Fatigue fracture resistance. Reduced-diameter implants are used to replace mandibular incisors and lateral maxillary incisors. Although fatigue fracture is rare for standard diameter implants, reduced-diameter implants suffer from a greater incidence of connector screw loosening and fatigue fracture (Griggs 2017). A project was conducted to maximize the fatigue limit of reduced-diameter implants without increasing the overall implant dimensions (Satpathy 2022). Fatigue testing of physical specimens was conducted to develop more rapid methods of gathering fatigue resistance data from prototypes (Duan and Griggs 2018) and to validate the accuracy of FEA to predict the fatigue lifetime of reduced-diameter implants (Duan et al. 2018). In a preliminary study, four different commercially available implant systems were subjected to physical accelerated lifetime testing (Gonzalez 2010). The implant system with the best performance (3.25 × 15 mm parallel walled with external hex connection, 3i T3, Biomet 3i Dental) was chosen as the reference model for the subsequent design optimization study. Initially 26 design factors were identified. It was later determined that several of the factors could not be varied independently from each other, so a reduced set of 16 design factors was defined (Table 6.1). Each design factor was varied by ±20% from the reference setting, creating three settings for each factor. A Taguchi orthogonal array permitted exploring the three settings for all 16 factors with only 27 implant designs. SOLIDWORKS was used to construct a virtual solid model for each of the 27 designs, and the models were meshed and solved in ABAQUS. The fe-safe post-processor was used to determine the fatigue limit for each design (Fig. 6.7). The fatigue limit was defined as the maximum bite force that could be withstood for an infinite number of cycles. The geometry of the holder material and the load application were defined according to ISO 14801. Preliminary studies were conducted to determine the most accurate methods for simulating the preload on the connector screw and the effect of osseointegration on implant fatigue limit (Satpathy et al. 2022a,b). A simple ANN with one hidden layer and two neurons was trained on the fatigue limit data with a learning ratio that decreased from 100% to 0% over 1600 iterations. The ANN was better at fitting the data ($R^2 = 0.99$) compared to a multiple regression model with

Table 6.1 Definition of 16 design parameters for a reduced-diameter dental implant

	Design parameters	20% lower (mm)	Reference (mm)	20% higher (mm)
1	Degree of coronal taper (A)	0.192	0.240	0.288
2	Implant body total length (B)	12.096	15.120	18.144
3	Implant Body Screw Pitch (C)	0.48	0.60	0.72
4	Thread height (coronal) (D)	0.12	0.15	0.18
5	Body screw diameter without threads (coronal) (Z)	2.28	2.85	3.42
6	Degree of apical taper (E)	0.264	0.330	0.396
7	Distance from bone level to top of implant body (F)	0.512	0.640	0.768
8	Body screw diameter without threads (coronal) - Internal cavity diameter (with threads) (G)	0.56	0.70	0.84
9	Abutment screw total length (H)	5.872	7.340	8.808
10	Abutment screw head diameter - abutment screw diameter with threads (I)	0.36	0.45	0.54
11	Bone level to top of abutment screw (J)	2.496	3.120	3.744
12	Distance between bottom of abutment screw and bottom of internal cavity (K)	1.048	1.310	1.572
13	Internal cavity diameter with threads - abutment screw diameter with threads (L)	0.04	0.05	0.06
14	Abutment screw thread height - internal cavity thread height (M)	0.008	0.010	0.012
15	Abutment screw pitch (N)	0.336	0.420	0.504
16	Bone level to most coronal abutment screw thread (O)	0.536	0.670	0.804

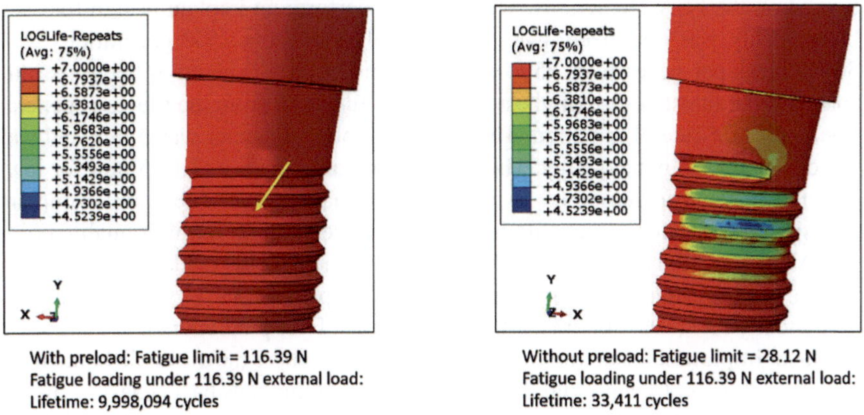

Fig. 6.7 Effect of connector screw preload on fatigue lifetime as predicted by the FEA post-processor (fe-safe). The heat shows the expected failure time for each location on the implant with cool colors (blue) indicating short lifetime and hot colors (red) indicating long lifetime. With permission from (Satpathy et al. 2022a,b)

quadratic and interaction terms ($R^2 = 0.95$). A Latin hypercube generator was used to create a list of 1000 implant designs that were spread across the 16-dimensional design space. Manual searching of the response surface was also conducted. Both the manual search and the multiple regression model predicted optimal designs in the corner of the design space, and FEA models were constructed to validate the fatigue limit at these locations. However, both the ANN and the multiple regression model overestimated the fatigue limit of these designs because of a sparsity of training data in the corners of the design space. The ANN was retrained using the validation data, and new optimal designs were identified in an iterative loop. Ultimately, the ANN identified a design that had 8.6% higher fatigue limit than the reference model, whereas the best design identified by multiple regression had only 0.7% higher fatigue limit than the reference model.

Bone microstrain. A combination of ANN and genetic algorithm was used to optimize an endosseous dental implant with the goal of maintaining 2500 microstrain in the bone adjacent to the implant (Roy et al. 2018). Since 1500–3000 microstrain is the windows for healthy bone in Frost's mechanostat (Frost 1987) with both lower strains and higher strains leading to bone deterioration, a desirability function was constructed with 1500 and 3000 microstrain as the limits. The desirability increased from 0 to 1 as microstrain increased from 1500 to 2500, and the desirability decreased from 1 to 0 as the microstrain increased from 2500 to 3000. FEA was used to predict the microstrain in the adjacent bone. FE models were constructed for 180 cases in a full-factorial design. The design parameters were implant porosity (0%, 10%, and 20%), implant length (9, 10, 11, and 12 mm), and implant diameter (4, 5, and 6 mm). The extraneous factor was bone quality (Young's modulus = 1.872, 2.497, 3.121, and 3.745 GPa). Bite force was assumed to be 120 N applied along the long axis of the implant. A simple ANN with one hidden layer and 12 neurons was trained on the FEA predictions. Then, the top performing implant design for each bone quality was optimized using a genetic algorithm over 500 generations with 500 designs per generation, 95% of the designs in each generation being the offspring of the fittest design (highest desirability function) from the previous generation, and a 1% rate of mutation. The optimal implant diameter was 5 mm and was not dependent on bone quality. The optimal implant length was 10.5 mm for low-quality bone and increased to 12 mm for high quality bone. The optimal implant porosity was 16% for low-quality bone and increased to 20% for high-quality bone. The ANN predicted that all optimal designs would achieve 100% desirability (being within 1 microstrain of 2500). However, the ANN predictions for microstrain were consistently low (199–400 microstrains lower than FEA predictions).

Basal implants. Basal implants are used in cases where the available bone in the jaw is insufficient for a normal dental implant. Basal implants have a design similar to that of a lag bolt, and the screw threads find purchase in the cortical bone farthest from the occlusal surface. One study optimized the designs of basal implants in an attempt to keep the strain in the adjacent bone within the adapted window of Frost's mechanostat (Choudhury et al. 2022). A Taguchi robust design was used to explore five different levels for each of the three design factors (screw thread depth, screw thread length, and screw thread pitch) and two extraneous factors (bone height and bone width). The implants were assumed to be subjected to a 200 N axial load applied to coronal aspect of the implant, which was shaped as if to mate with an overdenture. FEA was used to predict the microstrain in the bone for each implant design in each shape of bone, and a fitness function was calculated for each case as the square of the difference between the desired and achieved bone microstrain. The design objective was to minimize the fitness parameter. After the ANN was trained the design space was explored using genetic algorithms to breed the best performing designs while introducing a controlled amount of variation from mutations in each generation of offspring. The optimal setting for each of the three design parameters was dependent on the shape of the bone – with the optimal screw thread length ranging from 4 mm to 6 mm, the optimal screw thread depth ranging from 3 mm to 5 mm, and the optimal screw thread pitch ranging from 0.5 mm to 1.5 mm.

Orthopedic Implants

Spinal fusion. ANN was successfully used to optimize the design of bone cages for use in anterior lumbar interbody fusion (Nassau et al. 2012). The goal was to minimize the von Mises stress on the bone adjacent to the implant because a common mode of failure for this application is subsidence, where implant penetration induces failure of the adjacent vertebral body. Six design factors were varied (the height, width, and obliqueness of ridges on the surface of the implant; the surface area covered by ridges; the surface area of the implant; and the stiffness of the material). A Taguchi orthogonal array was used to plan the minimum number of designs necessary to elucidate the importance of each of the six design factors. The maximum stress on the bone for each design was predicted using finite element analysis (FEA).

A simple ANN having one hidden layer with three neurons was trained on the data and achieved good accuracy, having 1% or lower error in predicting the maximum von Mises stress as judged by the FEA predictions for the 18 original designs in the orthogonal array. However, the optimal design was located in one corner of the six-dimensional design space, which raises the question of whether a design with better performance might be located outside of the boundaries of the design space. It also raises the question of whether the ANN error would be low for predicting the performance of this design if it were included in the validation set.

Femoral implant primary stability. Similarly to dental implants, it is desirable to minimize micromotion at the bone-implant interface for femoral implants. A combination of ANN and genetic algorithms was able to decrease the primary mobility by 37% compared to that of a commercially available femoral implant (Chanda et al. 2016). The training data for micromotion were provided by FEA. The solid model was constructed from the medical records of one specific patient. Young's modulus, Poisson's ratio, and density of bone were varied by location according to radiolucency. The elastic constants for the implant were held constant at the values commonly used for Ti-6Al-4 V alloy. The FE model was loaded with forces that seven muscles are known to exert on the femur during normal walking and during the climbing of stairs (Bergmann et al. 2001). The micromotion along the bone-implant interface was integrated to provide an overall normalized Index of Instability (IoI). The design objective was to minimize IoI by varying the design parameters that control the cross-sectional shape of the implant at four locations along its length. At each cross-section, the major axis, minor axis, and the degree of chamfer were varied. A series of simple ANNs having one hidden layer and from two to eight neurons in the hidden layer were trained on the IoI data, and it was determined that four neurons along with a learning rate of 20% and a momentum constant of 0.4 resulted in the best accuracy ($R^2 = 0.82$). Once the ANN was trained on 160 implant designs and validated using 26 more implant designs, its predictions were used to save time by eliminating the need for further use of FEA to predict IoI for candidate designs. The 12-dimensional design space was explored using genetic algorithms. The most rapid decrease in IoI was produced when the population size (number of designs per generation) was 125 and 80% of the design factors were inherited from the fittest design in the previous generation. The results converged after only 40 generations on an implant design that was predicted to have 37% lower IoI compared to the stock commercially available implant.

Tibial locking screws. Multiple regression models (linear, quadratic, and quadratic with interactions) were compared with ANN for ability to minimize the stress in tibial locking screws (Hsu et al. 2011). It was assumed that the screws would be embedded in an equal amount of bone on either end and loaded laterally at the midpoint. This would generate maximum tensile stress at the midpoint of the screw length on the surface opposite the point of loading. The design objective was to minimize the tensile stress as predicted by FEA at the location where it is greatest. The design parameters that could be varied included the diameter including screw threads (crest-to-crest), the diameter of the screw shank (root-to-root), screw thread pitch, screw thread width, and the angle between the screw threads and the normal to the screw (angle to the long axis of the screw minus 90 °). A Taguchi orthogonal array was prepared that contained five different levels for each design factor. This provided 22 designs for training the ANN, and five designs were randomly selected for validation. Three simple ANNs having one hidden layer with either one, two, or three neurons were trained on the FEA predictions. The ANN with one neuron had similar error (0.4%–14.0%, $R^2 = 0.980$) as the multiple linear regression (0.2%–9.5%, $R^2 = 0.980$), the multiple quadratic regression (0.3%–11.5%, $R^2 = 0.988$), and the regression with interaction terms (0.2%–8.8%, $R^2 = 0.990$). The performances of the ANN with two neurons (0.0%–8.9%, $R^2 = 0.992$) and the ANN with three neurons (0.0%–4.0%, $R^2 = 0.998$) were both superior to all regression models. The optimal design was one of the training designs and was close to a corner of the design space, having either the maximum or minimum allowed value for every design parameter other than screw thread angle. The fact that a search of the design space beyond the original orthogonal array and validation points was not conducted raises the question of whether another nearby design could have superior performance. Given the location of the optimal design near the corner of the design space, it seems likely that there could be better designs outside the allowed design space.

Spinal pedical screws. ANN was used to minimize the stress in spinal pedicle screws (Hsu et al. 2011). These screws were modeled as being embedded in bone along the complete length of the threaded portion with a lateral load applied to the bone near the tip of the screw. The head of the screw was considered to be fixed in location. The design objective was to minimize the tensile stress as predicted by FEA at the location where it is greatest (the surface of the screw shank adjacent to the screw head). The design parameters that could be varied included the diameter of the screw shank, the screw thread width, the thread pitch, the angle of the thread on the proximal side (screw head side), the radius of curvature at the root of the screw thread, and the distance on the distal side between one screw thread and the beginning of curvature for the next screw thread. A Taguchi orthogonal array was prepared that contained five different levels for each design factor. This provided 22 designs for training the ANN, and five designs were randomly selected for validation. Three simple ANNs having one hidden layer with either one, two, or three neurons were trained on the FEA predictions. The error for the ANN with one neuron (0.2%–11.1%, $R^2 = 0.979$), the ANN with two neurons (0.0%–7.1%, $R^2 = 0.997$), and the ANN with three neurons (0.0%–5.6%, $R^2 = 0.998$) were all superior compared to the multiple linear regression (2.0%–27.2%, $R^2 = 0.857$), the multiple quadratic regression (1.3%–16.9%, $R^2 = 0.955$), and the regression with interaction terms (0.1%–17.5%, $R^2 = 0.968$).

Summary

Simple artificial neural networks having one hidden layer and only a few neurons were able to achieve a good accuracy after training on the results of finite element analysis for a variety of implant applications in dentistry and orthopedics. Taguchi orthogonal arrays are frequently used to efficiently explore a large number of design factors. Genetic algorithms are useful in guiding a neural network toward the optimal design.

Acknowledgment This work was sponsored by NIH grants DE017991 and DE026144.

References

Babiker S, Adam F, Mohamed A. Design optimization of reinforced concrete beams using artificial neural network. Int J Eng Invent. 2012;1(8):07–13.

Bergmann G, Deuretzbacher G, Heller M, Graichen F, Rohlmann A, Strauss J, et al. Hip contact forces and gait patterns from routine activities. J Biomech. 2001;34(7):859–71.

Burnham R. How to select design of experiments software. Quality Digest. 1998;18:32–6.

Chanda S, Gupta S, Pratihar DK. A combined neural network and genetic algorithm based approach for optimally designed femoral implant having improved primary stability. Appl Soft Comput. 2016;38:296–307.

Choudhury S, Rana M, Chakraborty A, Majumder S, Roy S, RoyChowdhury A, et al. Design of patient specific basal dental implant using finite element method and artificial neural network technique. Proc Inst Mech Eng Part H. 2022;236(9):1375–87.

Dasgupta T. Robust parameter design for automatically controlled systems and nanostructure synthesis. Georgia Institute of Technology; 2007.

Duan Y, Griggs JA. Effect of loading frequency on cyclic fatigue lifetime of a standard-diameter implant with an internal abutment connection. Dent Mater. 2018;34(12):1711–6.

Duan Y, Gonzalez JA, Kulkarni PA, Nagy WW, Griggs JA. Fatigue lifetime prediction of a reduced-diameter dental implant system: Numerical and experimental study. Dent Mater. 2018;34(9):1299–309.

Frost HM. Bone "mass" and the "mechanostat": A proposal. Anat Rec. 1987;219:1–9.

Gonzalez J. Fatigue load resistance in reduced diameter implants: The Texas A&M. University System Health Science Center; 2010.

Griggs JA. Dental implants. In: Ferracane J, Bertassoni LE, Pfeifer CS, editors. Dental biomaterials, an issue of dental clinics of North America, vol. 61. Elsevier Health Sciences; 2017.

Hsu C-C, Lin J, Chao C-K. Comparison of multiple linear regression and artificial neural network in developing the objective functions of the orthopaedic screws. Comput Methods Programs in Biomedi. 2011;104(3):341–8.

Kim J-H, Choi J-H, Kim K-Y, editors. Design optimization of a centrifugal compressor impeller using radial basis neural network method. Turbo Expo Power Land Sea Air. 2009;48883:443–51.

Mahouti P. Design optimization of a pattern reconfigurable microstrip antenna using differential evolution and 3D EM simulation-based neural network model. Int J RF Microwave Comput Aided Eng. 2019;29(8):e21796.

MATLAB. What Is a Genetic Algorithm? 2015. https://youtu.be/1i8muvzZkPw.

MATLAB. Getting Started with Neural Networks Using MATLAB. 2020. https://youtu.be/6T2yYTSw8z0.

Nassau CJ, Litofsky NS, Lin Y. Analysis of spinal lumbar interbody fusion cage subsidence using Taguchi method, finite element analysis, and artificial neural network. Front Mech Eng. 2012;7:247–55.

Roy S, Dey S, Khutia N, Chowdhury AR, Datta S. Design of patient specific dental implant using FE analysis and computational intelligence techniques. Appl Soft Comput. 2018;65:272–9.

Satpathy M. Optimizing the design of reduced-diameter dental implants to increase their fatigue lifetime. The University of Mississippi Medical Center; 2022.

Satpathy M, Duan Y, Betts L, Priddy M, Griggs JA. Effect of Bone Remodeling on dental implant fatigue limit predicted using 3D finite element analysis. J Dent Oral Epidemiol. 2022a:2.

Satpathy M, Jose RM, Duan Y, Griggs JA. Effects of abutment screw preload and preload simulation techniques on dental implant lifetime. JADA Found Sci. 2022b;1:100010.

Taguchi G. Introduction to quality engineering: designing quality into products and processes; 1986.

Vujanovic T, Jagtap R. Evaluation of artificial intelligence for automatic tooth and periapical pathosis detection on panoramic radiography. Oral Surg Oral Med Oral Pathol Oral Radiol. 2023;135(2):e51.

Yamaguchi S, Lee C, Karaer O, Ban S, Mine A, Imazato S. Predicting the debonding of CAD/CAM composite resin crowns with AI. J Dent Res. 2019;98(11):1234–8.

Outlook for AI in Oral Surgery and Periodontics

7

Sevda Kurt-Bayrakdar, Kaan Orhan, and Rohan Jagtap

Introduction

Today, artificial intelligence (AI) refers to computer or machine systems that imitate human intelligence, enabling them to think, learn, and evaluate like humans (Khanagar et al. 2021). The term "AI" was officially coined and defined as "the science and engineering of making intelligent machines" at a conference in 1956 (Ossowska et al. 2022; Hamet and Tremblay 2017). In the 1970s, concerns were raised about how this technology could potentially harm the careers of professional groups such as medicine and dentistry (Scott et al. 2023). However, despite these initial apprehensions, AI has emerged as one of the most innovative technologies, offering solutions to problems across various areas of healthcare today (Alami et al. 2020).

AI has proven to be highly capable of handling the rapid increase in data and data complexity within the medical field (Schwendicke et al. 2020). It can efficiently analyze and interpret this data, providing a valuable decision-support mechanism to

S. Kurt-Bayrakdar (✉)
Division of Oral and Maxillofacial Radiology, Department of Care Planning and Restorative Sciences, University of Mississippi Medical Center, Jackson, MS, USA

Department of Periodontology, School of Dentistry Eskisehir Osmangazi University, Eskisehir, Turkey

K. Orhan
Department of Dentomaxillofacial Radiology, School of Dentistry Ankara University, Ankara, Turkey

R. Jagtap
Division of Oral and Maxillofacial Radiology, Department of Care Planning and Restorative Sciences, University of Mississippi Medical Center, Jackson, MS, USA

K. Orhan, R. Jagtap (eds.), *Artificial Intelligence in Dentistry*,
https://doi.org/10.1007/978-3-031-43827-1_7

physicians (Amann et al. 2020). Due to these and similar benefits, AI-based research in dentistry has grown in parallel with medicine (Mohammad-Rahimi et al. 2022), leading to its adoption in numerous subfields of dentistry, including periodontics, oral surgery, oral implantology, endodontics, orthodontics, and restorative dentistry (Fatima et al. 2022). This study aims to explore the applications of AI in periodontics and oral surgery, based on the current information available.

AI in Oral Surgery

In surgical branches, accurate diagnosis and treatment planning are crucial to ensure patient safety during the operation and to implement the most optimal solution when faced with multiple options (Miladinović et al. 2017). Surgeons are required to make complex decisions rapidly, considering various factors simultaneously (Rasteau et al. 2022). However, factors such as fatigue, workload, mood, and differences in experience among physicians can hinder the idealization of these stages (Rasteau et al. 2022; Park et al. 2020; Schwalbe and Wahl 2020; Kurt Bayrakdar et al. 2021). To address these challenges and minimize errors, AI has emerged as an innovative technology that provides decision-support mechanisms to healthcare professionals (Miladinović et al. 2017; Vikram and Karjodkar 2009). Consequently, AI systems and computer-assisted technologies have gained significant attention across all areas of dentistry. Despite the increasing academic interest in AI technologies in oral and maxillofacial surgery, it is observed that oral surgeons have not fully maximized the use of this technology yet (Rasteau et al. 2022).

The complex anatomical structure of the oral region makes radiographic diagnosis critical for surgical planning (Yan et al. 2021; Weiss 2nd and Read-Fuller 2019). Successful execution of the process requires a detailed interpretation of patient records, dental/medical histories, and other diagnostic images (Langdon et al. 2017). AI can utilize radiographic images, patient photos, medical histories, and various health records as inputs and generate evaluations as outputs. This characteristic makes it promising for automating processes such as diagnosis, treatment planning, estimation, and gene analysis in oral and maxillofacial surgery (Agrawal and Nikhade 2022). Studies have indicated that the use of AI technologies in surgery can achieve performance levels comparable to experts (Yan et al. 2021).

Currently, there are numerous AI studies in various aspects of oral surgery, including routine protocols, orthognathic surgery, dental implantology, oral diseases, and oral cancers (Yan et al. 2021). These studies have been systematically categorized and summarized under different headings.

General Oral Surgery

AI has proven to be highly effective in the radiographic evaluation of critical anatomical structures in oral surgical procedures, such as sinuses, fossae, nerve canals, and vascular bundles (Shujaat et al. 2023; Minnema et al. 2022). It has also demonstrated

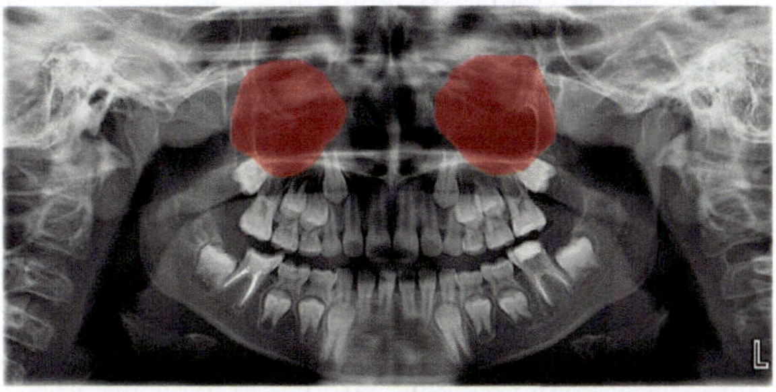

Fig. 7.1 Automatic detection of maxillary sinuses on panoramic radiography. (Courtesy of CranioCatch AI software)

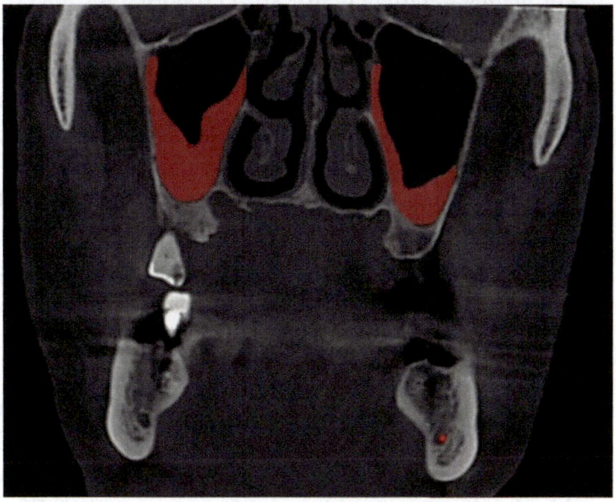

Fig. 7.2 Detection of maxillary sinus membrane mucosal thickening with artificial intelligence software on CBCT image section. (Courtesy of CranioCatch AI software)

success in detecting variations, pathologies, and diseases in these anatomical regions (Kim et al. 2019b; Agbaje et al. 2017; Lahoud et al. 2022) (Figs. 7.1 and 7.2).

For instance, Cha et al. (2021a) utilized the semantic segmentation method on panoramic radiographs commonly used in dental clinics for their research. They demonstrated that AI systems can easily detect anatomical formations, including the sinus, maxilla, mandible, and mandibular canal. The segmentation performance of their developed system achieved precision values ranging from 0.802 to 0.959 (Cha et al. 2021a).

In another study, Morgan et al. (2022) focused on an AI model designed for the automatic detection of maxillary sinuses using cone-beam computed tomography (CBCT) images. Their model achieved a high Dice similarity coefficient value of 98.4%, indicating the model's accuracy in detecting maxillary sinuses (Morgan et al. 2022).

Additionally, several studies have reported the successful performance of AI systems in mandibular canal detection (Kurt Bayrakdar et al. 2021; Lahoud et al. 2022; Jaskari et al. 2020). Existing research has demonstrated that these AI systems can effectively detect canal variations, such as bifid mandibular canal, as well as certain pathologies and variations in the sinuses. These variations include mucosal thickening, arterial localizations, the presence of maxillary sinusitis, mucous retention cysts, fungal ball presence, and concha bullosa, which can be easily detected and segmented with the help of these AI systems (Lahoud et al. 2022; Huang et al. 2020a; Kim et al. 2022; Parmar et al. 2020; Hung et al. 2022a,b).

As it is widely recognized, impacted third molar tooth problems are among the most commonly encountered situations by oral surgeons (Friedland et al. 2008; Yan et al. 2021). Deciding whether extraction of these teeth is necessary and predicting potential complications related to the extraction can be challenging for physicians. However, AI systems offer a solution by automatically detecting the localizations and positions of impacted teeth (Fig. 7.3).

For instance, Orhan et al. (2021) reported the successful development of a deep-convolutional neural network (CNN) algorithm that accurately detected impacted third molars in CBCT images (Orhan et al. 2021). Additionally, these AI technologies can be used to examine the relationship of the impacted tooth with the inferior alveolar canal or other surrounding anatomical structures, thereby minimizing potential complications associated with the extraction. Studies conducted by Choi et al. (2022) and Zhu et al. (2021) demonstrated the application of AI in determining the position of the third molar and its relationship with the mandibular canal (Choi et al. 2022; Zhu et al. 2021). Likewise, these algorithms can be utilized to detect the presence of impacted teeth, supernumerary teeth, residual roots, or ankylosed teeth (Orhan et al. 2021; Mladenovic et al. 2023; Mine et al. 2022; Kuwada et al. 2020; Başaran et al. 2022) (Figs. 7.3 and 7.4). There have been successful performances reported in cases such as jaw fractures and tooth root fractures as well (Fukuda et al. 2020; Schramm et al. 2009; Hashem and Hassanein 2019). Fukuda et al. (2020) confirmed that their CNN algorithm, based on 300 panoramic radiography images, could identify teeth with root fractures with 0.75 recall, 0.93 precision, and 0.83 F-measure (Fukuda et al. 2020).

Machine learning technology enables the estimation of prognosis for teeth and the prediction of potential complications (Vollmer et al. 2022; Kim et al. 2018; Etemad et al. 2021). Real et al. (2022) demonstrated the creation of automatic orthodontic tooth extraction prediction models using a machine learning system (Real

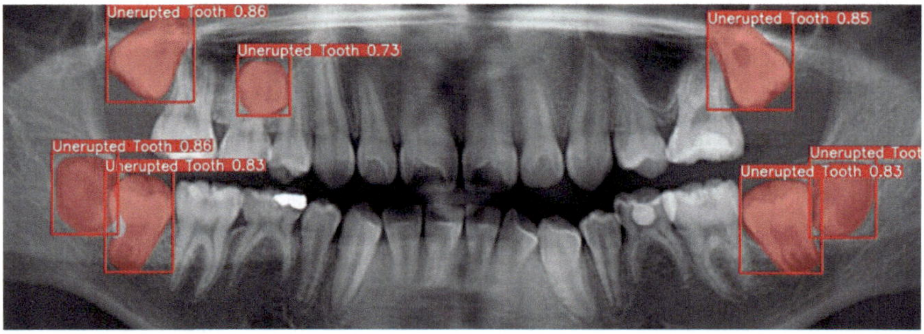

Fig. 7.3 Impacted tooth detection on panoramic radiography by CNN algorithm. (Courtesy of CranioCatch AI software)

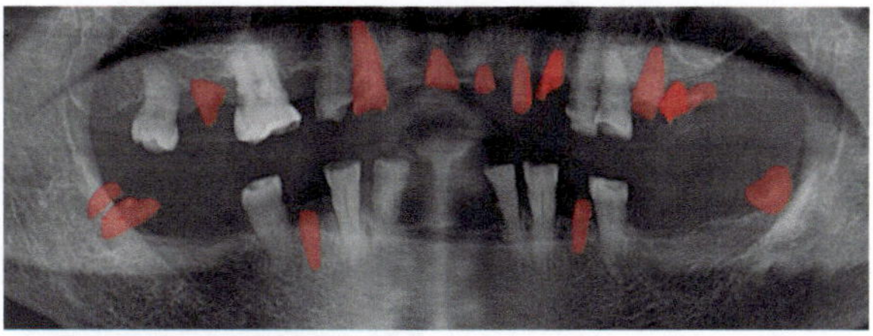

Fig. 7.4 Automatic detection of residual roots that need to be extracted. (Courtesy of CranioCatch AI software)

et al. 2022). Furthermore, Lee et al. (2022) reported that AI systems can aid in estimating the prognosis of teeth with periodontal damage (Lee et al. 2022). This enhanced estimation facilitates more accurate extraction decisions and surgical planning in oral surgery practice. Additionally, the literature contains studies in which AI is used for purposes such as estimating tooth extraction difficulty (Yoo et al. 2021) and predicting post-extraction swelling (Zhang et al. 2018). Another study reported that panoramic radiographs can be analyzed, and oroantral fistula that may occur after tooth extraction can be predicted using AI systems (Vollmer et al. 2022).

Oral Diseases and Pathologies

New computer-assisted technologies and AI systems are proving to be valuable tools in the diagnosis of oral lesions, cysts, and both benign and malignant tumors (Keser et al. 2023; Poedjiastoeti and Suebnukarn 2018; Yang et al. 2020; Yilmaz et al. 2017; Ariji et al. 2019, 2022; Kwon et al. 2020; Bispo et al. 2021; Lee et al. 2020). Early diagnosis of premalignant conditions is especially critical in oral surgery practice, but it can be challenging for nonspecialists to identify such situations (Rasteau et al. 2022). AI algorithms that can automatically determine oral diseases offer promising solutions to aid practitioners in this aspect (Figs. 7.5 and 7.6).

A wide range of diagnostic materials can be utilized with AI for detecting oral diseases. For instance, Keser et al. (2023) conducted a study on the automatic detection of oral lichen planus lesions using intraoral photographs. They employed a classification method and reported that the developed algorithm achieved 100% success in detecting the lesioned photographs (Keser et al. 2023). In various other studies, AI technologies have been proven effective in detecting various oral cancers, such as carcinoma, using oral photographs (Fu et al. 2020; Warin et al. 2021; Tanriver et al. 2021; Shamim et al. 2022; Jubair et al. 2022).

In another study, artificial neural networks (ANN) were utilized for the automatic classification of autofluorescence spectra instead of intraoral photographs. These algorithms demonstrated great success in interpreting autofluorescent spectra and determining the tissue dysplasia level of oral leukoplakia (van Staveren et al. 2000). The related algorithm exhibited 86% sensitivity and 100% specificity in detecting abnormal tissue, while also accurately analyzing homogeneous and nonhomogeneous tissues (van Staveren et al. 2000).

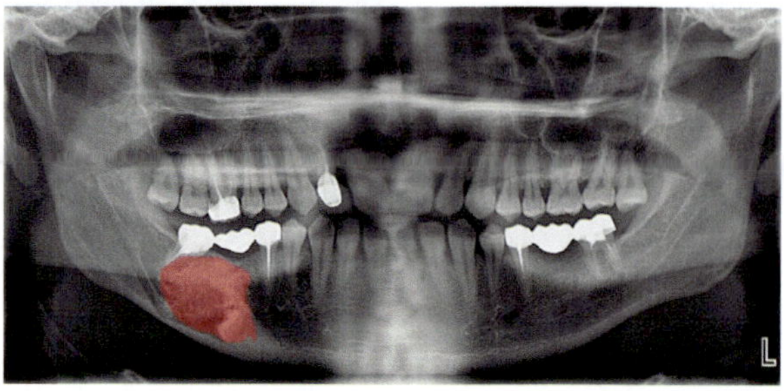

Fig. 7.5 Automatic detection of mandibular pathology. (Courtesy of CranioCatch AI software)

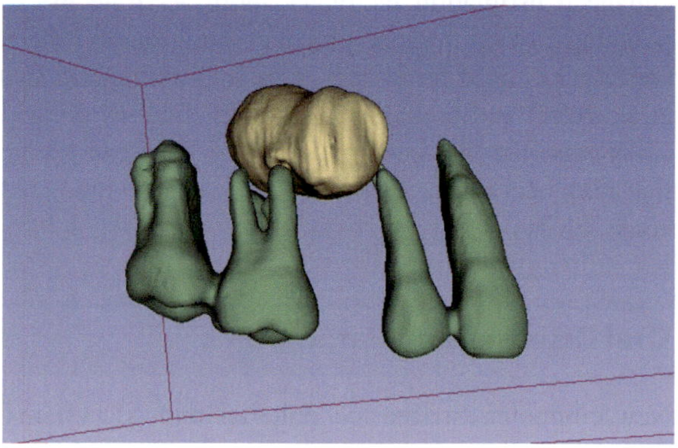

Fig. 7.6 Automatic 3D segmentation of cystic lesion. (Courtesy of Velmeni AI software)

It is known that oral diseases and oral cancers can be detected using AI systems to analyze biological materials such as saliva (Kouznetsova et al. 2021; Romm et al. 2021). In a study, Kouznetsova et al. (2021) used an algorithm that automatically examines salivary metabolites to evaluate the presence of cancer. They reported that this system could detect oral cancer using saliva samples with an accuracy of 79.54% (Kouznetsova et al. 2021). Additionally, Romm et al. (2021) carried out a similar study and demonstrated successful results of the system (Romm et al. 2021).

Several studies have shown that artificial intelligence systems could be utilized in the detection and segmentation of ameloblastomas, odontogenic keratocyst, dentigerous cysts, radicular cysts, follicular cysts, and various oral tumors from radiographs (Poedjiastoeti and Suebnukarn 2018; Yang et al. 2020; Yilmaz et al. 2017; Ariji et al. 2019, 2022; Kwon et al. 2020; Bispo et al. 2021; Lee et al. 2020; Mikulka et al. 2013; Nurtanio et al. 2013; Rana et al. 2015; Abdolali et al. 2016, 2017). Some of these studies used two-dimensional (2D) radiography images, such as panoramic radiography (Yang et al. 2020; Ariji et al. 2019; Mikulka et al. 2013; Nurtanio et al. 2013), while others employed three-dimensional (3D) radiography images, such as computed tomography (CT) and CBCT (Yilmaz et al. 2017; Lee et al. 2020; Abdolali et al. 2016, 2017).

Poedjiastoeti and Suebnukarn (2018) used 500 panoramic radiography images in their study and developed a CNN system that automatically detects ameloblastomas.

The accuracy rate of the system was found to be 83.09%, higher than that of the oral and maxillofacial surgeon. The authors emphasized that artificial intelligence can detect such pathologies in a shorter time and more effectively (Poedjiastoeti and Suebnukarn 2018). Yilmaz et al. (2017), on the other hand, proposed an artificial intelligence system that provides a decision support mechanism to the physician for the classification of dental periapical cysts and keratocystic odontogenic tumors from CBCT images. They demonstrated that this system, trained with 50 CBCT images, classifies lesions with high accuracy (Yilmaz et al. 2017).

Ariji et al. (2022) studied a deep learning (DL) model aiming at lymph node segmentation of oral cancer patients and analyzing possible metastases. In this study, 158 metastatic and 514 nonmetastatic lymph nodes were segmented using CT images, and artificial intelligence training was performed on this dataset. The algorithm outperformed the radiologist, achieving a 0.950 AUC (Ariji et al. 2022).

As shown, tools developed using intraoral photographs, autofluorescence spectra, radiographs, and biological materials have been studied to determine oral diseases. The use of these systems in the detection of diseases, where physicians face real difficulty in diagnosis and where early diagnosis plays an essential role in patient prognosis, has promising results for the coming years.

Overall, AI systems offer promising potential in improving the diagnostic capabilities of practitioners and facilitating the early detection of oral diseases, leading to better patient outcomes in oral surgery practice.

Orthognathic Surgery

Orthognathic surgery is the repositioning of the jaws for improved function and aesthetics (Khechoyan 2013). Usually, this process is carried out in cooperation with both a surgeon and an orthodontist (Luther et al. 2003). The use of artificial intelligence systems for purposes such as diagnosis, treatment planning, and prognosis estimation in cases requiring orthognathic surgery is increasing day by day. Physicians must carefully examine clinical records, cephalometric radiographs, and CBCT images throughout all stages of orthognathic surgery (Chaiprasittikul et al. 2023). Artificial intelligence systems allow clinicians to conduct a more efficient treatment process by reducing the workload during these multiple analysis phases (Chaiprasittikul et al. 2023; Mohaideen et al. 2022). However, studies in this area are still in their early stages, and system efficiencies can be enhanced through more comprehensive research, leading to modernized processes (Mohaideen et al. 2022).

When examining studies conducted in this field, it is evident that the majority focus on diagnosis. These studies utilize datasets such as lateral/frontal cephalograms (Choi et al. 2019; Kim et al. 2021; Shin et al. 2021), facial photography/imaging (Jeong et al. 2020; Knoops et al. 2019), and CBCT and CT images (Seo et al. 2021; Chung et al. 2020).

Choi et al. (2019) developed an artificial intelligence model to determine the decision for orthognathic surgery and tooth extraction, and they evaluated its performance. In this study, they trained their model using 12 measurements from lateral cephalograms and 6 additional indexes, based on data from 316 patients. The reported success rate of the model was 96% for surgery decisions and 91% for tooth extraction decisions (Choi et al. 2019).

Similarly, Kim et al. (2021) conducted a study on the same purpose and developed an artificial intelligence model. When evaluating the model's performance, they found that CNN models achieved a success rate ranging from 91.13% to 93.80% (Kim et al. 2021).

Jeong et al. (2020) assessed the detectability of facial models that would require orthognathic surgery using artificial intelligence with facial photos. Their study, which included data from 822 individuals, revealed that the CNN algorithm worked with an accuracy rate of 89.3% (Jeong et al. 2020).

Seo et al. (2021) demonstrated that artificial intelligence systems can be utilized to calculate soft tissue changes after surgery in patients with cleft lip and palate (Seo et al. 2021). In a study by Chung et al. (2020), it was reported that artificial intelligence can be employed to evaluate CBCT images for orthognathic surgery planning (Chung et al. 2020). Shujaat et al. (2021) developed a CNN model using 103 CBCT images and reported that the model could automatically detect the pharyngeal airway space, a critical aspect of orthognathic surgery, with high success rates (with 0.97 precision and 0.96 recall) (Shujaat et al. 2021).

Stehrer et al. (2019) evaluated the success of an AI system they developed in calculating perioperative blood loss instead of directly diagnosing orthognathic surgery. The study involved scanning a total of 1472 patients, and model training was conducted with data from 950 patients. The researchers found a statistically significant correlation between actual blood losses and the system's calculations ($p < 0.001$). This study highlights the potential to create estimation sets using AI for surgical planning and to make preliminary estimations of different parameters (Stehrer et al. 2019). In another study attempting to estimate the blood transfusion needed during surgery using 1243 patient data, the system achieved an f1 score value of 0.91 when its performance was evaluated (Jalali et al. 2021).

As evident from the mentioned studies, there are numerous possibilities for employing these technologies for various purposes at different stages of orthognathic surgery practice. The number of such studies is expected to increase even further in the coming years. Utilizing these models as assistive systems for physicians in clinics can accelerate the orthognathic surgery workflow and potentially improve success rates in surgeries (Fig. 7.7).

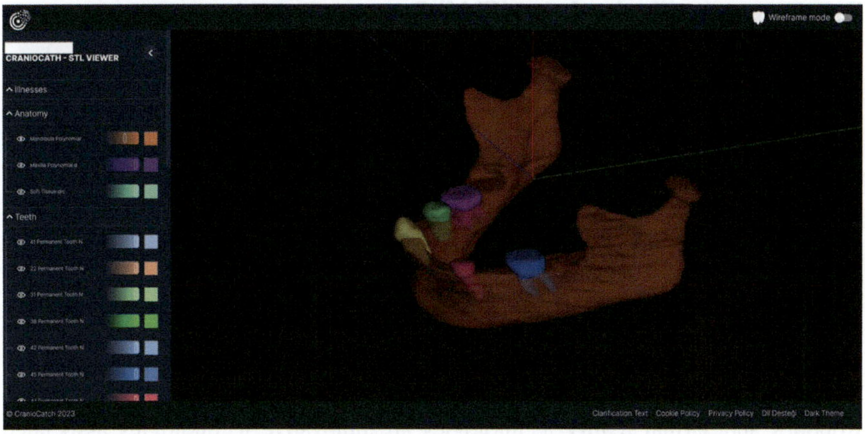

Fig. 7.7 Automatic 3D model creation. (Courtesy of CranioCatch AI software)

Implant Surgery

AI holds a wide potential for use in the diagnosis, treatment planning, and patient follow-up stages associated with oral implantology. Studies have shown that AI models can automatically detect many conditions related to dental implants, such as peri-implantitis and implant fracture, from dental radiographs (Liu et al. 2022; Cha et al. 2021b; Lee et al. 2021).

Kurt Bayrakdar et al. (2021) evaluated the success of an AI model in determining alveolar bone height and thickness. They reported that the system recognizes surrounding anatomical structures, such as the mandibular canal, sinus, and nasal fossa, which are crucial for implant planning in CBCT images. This finding shows a promising potential for the automatic measurement of bone thickness/width (Kurt Bayrakdar et al. 2021). The development of these systems can lead to reduced complications related to implant surgery and enable more detailed surgical planning. In another study, Mangano et al. (2023) demonstrated that these systems can perform implant planning with minimal deviations and achieve highly successful results (Mangano et al. 2023).

In addition to these, studies have been conducted to automatically detect implant brands from radiographic images (Sukegawa et al. 2021, 2022; Lee and Jeong 2020). These studies offer an opportunity to prevent radical surgical decisions in cases such as abutment fractures. Furthermore, there are studies on AI tools for measuring implant site bone density, which can significantly enhance the success of implant surgery (Xiao et al. 2022; Chen et al. 2022).

On the other hand, Sakai et al. (2022) developed an AI model that automatically determines the drilling protocol during implant surgery using CBCT images obtained from 60 patients. They reported that the AI model demonstrated high success in decision-making at this critical stage, which is essential for establishing primary stability (Sakai et al. 2022).

Temporomandibular Joint (TMJ) Surgery

AI models have shown successful results in the automatic detection of TMJ-related diseases and the radiographic examination of joint-related anatomical structures (Bianchi et al. 2021; Nishiyama et al. 2021; Warin et al. 2023; Almăşan et al. 2023). These studies primarily focus on diagnostic applications and can assist surgeons in making accurate diagnoses. However, further comprehensive research is required in this area to expand the potential applications and enhance the efficacy of AI in TMJ-related disease detection and evaluation.

Robotics and Virtual Reality

Robotics and virtual reality technologies are innovative technologies associated with AI (Khanna and Dhaimade 2017) (Fig. 7.8). Robotic surgery applications were first introduced in oral and maxillofacial surgery practice in 1999, and interest in this field has been steadily increasing in recent years (De Ceulaer et al. 2012). This technology holds revolutionary potential for the future of oral surgery.

Walvekar et al. (2011) demonstrated in their studies that robotic systems can be used successfully in the excision of bilateral ranula. It has been reported that anatomical structures such as nerves and canals are better preserved in robotic surgery, leading to more successful outcomes compared to traditional surgery (Walvekar et al. 2011). Additionally, studies have shown that robotic systems can be employed in surgeries for tongue-related pathologies and diseases (Sayin et al. 2015; Vicini et al. 2012). In a study related to a surgical robot system used in zygomatic implant placement, it was stated that the use of surgical robot systems increased the accuracy of the operation (Cao et al. 2020). Although there have been only a limited number of studies on the use of robotic technologies in dental implantology surgery, ongoing research in this area continues (Wu et al. 2019).

Virtual and augmented reality can be utilized in the training stages of oral surgery procedures and have the potential to significantly enhance the quality of education (Ayoub and Pulijala 2019). Moreover, these technologies provide the possibility of performing virtual planning in orthognathic surgery (Jandali and Barrera 2020).

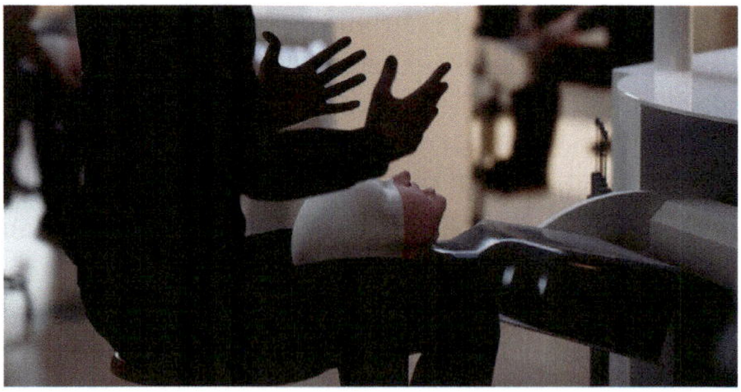

Fig. 7.8 Virtual reality and robotic technology in dentistry. (Courtesy of Dentaverse Company)

AI in Periodontics

Periodontal diseases are inflammatory diseases that affect the tissues supporting the teeth (Di Benedetto et al. 2013; Papapanou et al. 2018). Gingivitis is a mild form of periodontal disease characterized by limited reversible soft tissue inflammation (Papapanou et al. 2018; Gasner and Schure 2023). On the other hand, periodontitis is an irreversible disease where inflammation progresses and leads to the loss of alveolar bone supporting the teeth (Papapanou et al. 2018; Gasner and Schure 2023). If left untreated, periodontal disease can result in tooth loss, tooth mobility, and a decline in chewing and speech functions (Sroussi et al. 2017; Kuze et al. 2023).

Moreover, periodontal diseases are associated with various general health conditions, such as heart disease, diabetes, pneumonia, and preeclampsia (Nazir 2017; Bui et al. 2019). These associations can lead to the onset or exacerbation of diseases and undesirable situations (Nazir 2017). Therefore, early diagnosis and correct treatment planning are critical in managing periodontal diseases, which are among the most common diseases worldwide (Scott et al. 2023).

During routine dental examinations, the first step involves questioning the patient's systemic and dental history (Vuorjoki-Ranta et al. 2016). Subsequently, a detailed intraoral and extraoral examination should be conducted to ensure no condition is overlooked (Al-Helou 2021). The periodontal examination comprises the clinical and radiographic assessment of all teeth and supporting tissues, including the gingiva, cementum, periodontal ligament, and alveolar bone, with the recording of all findings (Tugnait et al. 2004). Clinical examination involves measurements such as attachment loss, pocket depth, plaque index, gingival index, and bleeding index during probing (Tugnait et al. 2004; Beltrán-Aguilar et al. 2012). Furthermore, a comprehensive periodontal assessment is essential to evaluate conditions such as frenulum attachment, amount of attached gingiva, gingival enlargement, gingival recession, tooth mobility, and furcation involvement (Beltrán-Aguilar et al. 2012; Miller Jr and Allen 1996; Lang and Bartold 2018). Radiographic evaluation includes taking 2D radiographic images such as panoramic, bitewing, periapical, and 3D radiographic images like CBCT, which are then meticulously examined (Mol 2004; Xiang et al. 2010). The accurate execution of these steps is vital for a correct diagnosis.

In 2017, a new periodontal disease classification system was introduced, based on criteria set by the American Academy of Periodontology and the European Federation of Periodontology (Papapanou et al. 2018). This system defines the severity of periodontitis by stages and the rate of disease progression by grades (Papapanou et al. 2018). To classify periodontal disease, various factors like clinical attachment levels, existing bone loss, number of teeth lost, smoking habits, diabetes, or other systemic diseases must be considered together (Papapanou et al. 2018).

Periodontal examination and determining the periodontal disease/condition are multistage, time-consuming, and repetitive processes for dentists (Armitage 2004). Density, fatigue, lack of experience, and patient compliance issues may lead to overlooked details. Consequently, in recent years, focus has shifted toward decision-support software and digitalized systems to assist dentists in some of these stages.

These technologies can automatically determine patient information from diagnostic images (Scott et al. 2023).

Deep learning, an AI technology, enables the recording and easy processing of large patient data by using artificial neurons (Scott et al. 2023; Jiang et al. 2010). Convolutional neural networks (CNN), a subset of DL, can discern patterns in images and examine each pixel in detail (Scott et al. 2023; Le Cun et al. 1990). These technologies facilitate automated radiographic and histopathological diagnoses and can identify anatomical structures from diagnostic images (Garland et al. 2021). Consequently, they have become a prominent topic in processing and interpreting diagnostic images in the healthcare field today (Zhang et al. 2021).

It can be observed that dentistry has entered a digitalization period with the emergence of technologies like CAD-CAM systems, implant guide systems, and intraoral scanners (Joda et al. 2019; Joda and Zitzmann 2022). However, some traditional practices have not been completely abandoned in certain dental specialties. The use of some traditional methods in the diagnosis of periodontal diseases can result in a serious lack of standardization and compliance (Scott et al. 2023). For instance, variations in applied probe pressure and angulation can lead to inconsistent and contradictory pocket depth measurements, which are crucial for clinical evaluation (Scott et al. 2023; Leroy et al. 2010). Similarly, differences in radiation dose and cone angulation during radiographic evaluations may hinder achieving ideal results (Scott et al. 2023).

Fortunately, AI systems offer solutions to these challenges by enabling the digitization of patient registration processes and achieving standardization with the aid of computer systems (Cui and Zhang 2021; Wang et al. 2020). This reduces or eliminates human errors, provides decision-support to physicians during diagnosis, and facilitates more regular and efficient record-keeping of patient diagnostic data (Scott et al. 2023; Park et al. 2020; Schwalbe and Wahl 2020; Kurt Bayrakdar et al. 2021; Cui and Zhang 2021; Wang et al. 2020).

Periodontal diseases are complex conditions, and various factors play a role in their etiology (Cekici et al. 2014; Baelum and López 2013; Scannapieco and Gershovich 2020). AI systems are known for their success in analyzing and solving complex and multivariate problems (Scott et al. 2023; Antonov 2011). This raises the question of the usability of these technologies in conducting etiological studies in the field of periodontics. It is well-established that dental bacterial plaque accumulating on the tooth surface is the main etiological factor for this disease, and the main inflammatory changes occur due to the host's immune response (Preshaw 2008; Saini et al. 2009; Mallikarjun et al. 2014).

Academic studies have demonstrated that the healthy periodontal sulcus primarily contains Gram-positive bacteria (Kesic et al. 2008). Conversely, the presence and increase in the number of Gram-negative periopathogens have been linked to periodontal disease (Ivanov and Webster 2017; Monterubbianesi et al. 2022). Some bacteria already proven to cause the disease include *Porphyromonas gingivalis* (*P. gingivalis*), *Aggregatibacter actinomycetemcomitans* (*A. actinomycetemcomitans*), *Tannerella forsythia* (*T. forsythia*), and *Treponema denticola* (*T. denticola*) (Kesic et al. 2008; Silva et al. 2015). However, research in the field of periodontics continues to explore the bacterial composition that is effective in the etiology (Kesic et al. 2008; Belibasakis et al. 2023) since the oral flora contains a vast variety of different bacterial species (Parahitiyawa et al. 2010). Consequently, microbiological examinations in periodontology can be challenging and time-consuming. To address these knowledge gaps, an increasing number of studies are utilizing new technologies supported by computer and machine systems (Wang et al. 2021; Aberin and de Goma 2018).

These innovative systems can also be employed to determine the immune response profiles of patients and investigate the role of different molecules, such as cytokines, chemokines, and growth factors, in the disease (Kouznetsova et al. 2021; Romm et al. 2021; Kim et al. 2020; Bezruk et al. 2017). This enables the analysis and interpretation of numerous variables directly or indirectly involved in the periodontal disease process and helps create risk profiles for patients (Kouznetsova et al. 2021; Kim et al. 2020; Chapple 1997; Valko et al. 2007; Troiano et al. 2023; Yoon et al. 2018; Sunmoo et al. 2018).

Despite the mentioned diagnostic advantages, the advancements related to artificial intelligence systems in periodontics are still in their early stages and have not yet reached their full potential.

Radiography-Based Studies

Intraoral and extraoral dental radiographs play a significant role in determining periodontal disease (Figs. 7.9, 7.10, and 7.11). Among the most preferred radiographs in dentistry workflow are periapical, bitewing, and panoramic radiographs, which provide 2D images (Feijo et al. 2012; Songa et al. 2014). Although these radiographs offer general information to the physician, they have limitations and disadvantages since they depict 3D structures as 2D images (Songa et al. 2014; Theilade 1965). In contrast, cone beam computed tomography (CBCT) is a 3D

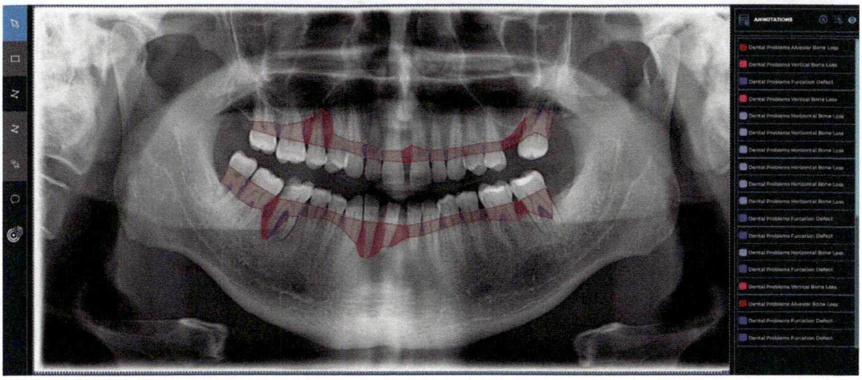

Fig. 7.9 Periodontal bone loss segmentation on panoramic radiograph using an AI software. (Courtesy of CranioCatch AI software)

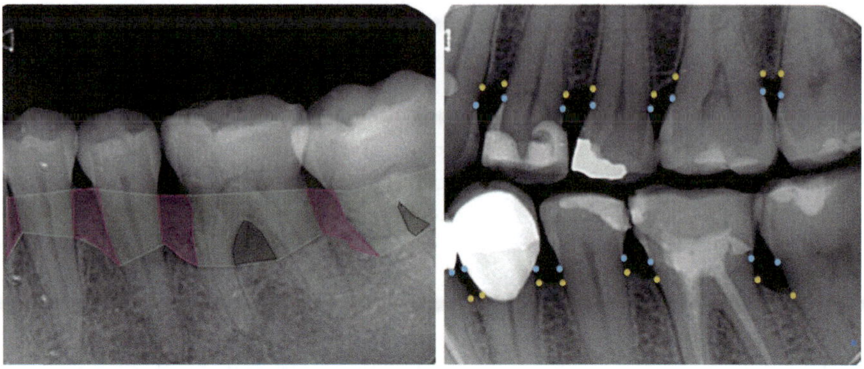

Fig. 7.10 Periodontal bone loss-related conditions' segmentation on periapical and bitewing radiographs. (Courtesy of CranioCatch AI software)

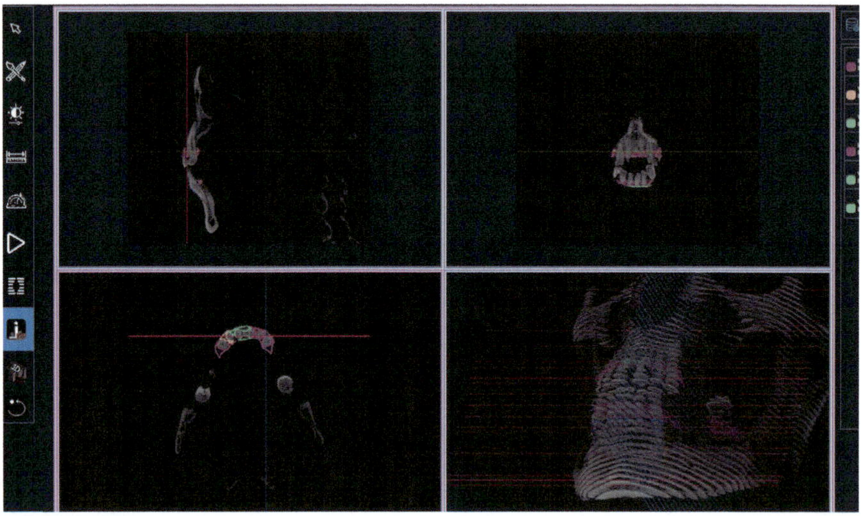

Fig. 7.11 Periodontal status labeling in CBCT images for use in an AI model training. (Courtesy of CranioCatch AI software)

imaging method that provides more detailed information (Vandenberghe et al. 2007). All these radiographs are valuable for disease diagnosis, bone density assessment, identifying periodontal defect types, patient follow-up, evaluating treatment success, and assessing other periodontal conditions, such as periodontal space widening (Corbet et al. 2009).

Currently, over half of the AI-based studies conducted to facilitate diagnosis in periodontics focus on image processing and automatic periodontal diagnosis from dental radiographs (Scott et al. 2023). These studies aim to detect the periodontal status from radiographs using AI systems and can be summarized as follows:

Panoramic Radiograph-Based Studies

Kong et al. (2020) conducted a study in China to evaluate the performance of detecting bone destruction using the segmentation method of the AI algorithm with 2602 panoramic radiography images. Their custom CNN demonstrated a high success rate of 98%, outperforming the U-net and FCN-8 architectures (Kong et al. 2020).

Kim et al. (2019a) utilized the deep-CNN method and developed an AI system with 12,179 panoramic radiographs to determine periodontal bone loss. The study revealed that the AI system achieved a higher F1 score performance (75%) compared to the average F1 score of the five participating clinicians (69%). The researchers suggested that future studies with more patient data could offer significant benefits for clinical applications (Kim et al. 2019a).

In a study by Krois et al. in 2019, they used the CNN method to determine periodontal bone resorption with 2001 panoramic radiographs. The results were compared with those of 6 dentists, and the AI system achieved accuracy, sensitivity, and specificity values of approximately 81%. The authors emphasized that the use of AI systems for radiographic diagnosis could lead to more effective results and time-saving benefits (Krois et al. 2019).

Chang et al. (2020) developed an algorithm based on the Feature Pyramid Network (FPN) architecture using 340 panoramic radiographs to perform staging according to the new periodontal disease classification. The study reported a 73% correlation between the AI results and radiologists' diagnosis of the periodontitis stage. The authors suggested that such algorithms could be employed by dentists to aid in making disease decisions and facilitate the implementation of the new classification (Chang et al. 2020).

Kurt Bayrakdar et al. (2020) conducted a study with 2276 panoramic radiographs and developed an algorithm to automatically detect panoramic radiographs with bone destruction. The AI system achieved a success rate of 94% sensitivity and 91% accuracy in this regard (Kurt Bayrakdar et al. 2020).

Thanathornwong and Suebnukarn (2020) worked on an AI algorithm capable of detecting periodontally damaged teeth in panoramic radiographs. Utilizing the Faster R-CNN architecture, the study reported a successful detection rate of over 81% for damaged teeth. The authors highlighted the advantages of the system, such as its speed, and suggested its use for diagnosis purposes (Thanathornwong and Suebnukarn 2020).

Jiang et al. (2022) conducted an AI-based study in China using 640 panoramic radiographs. The U-net and YOLOv4 architectures were used to determine the percentage of periodontal bone loss and furcation defects, following the 2017 periodontal disease classification standards. The accuracy rate of the system was reported to be 0.77 (Jiang et al. 2022).

Periapical Radiograph-Based Studies

Lee et al. (2018) conducted a study to evaluate the success of a CNN algorithm (VGG-19 architecture-based) they developed to detect periodontally compromised teeth from periapical radiographs, rather than periodontal bone loss. The algorithm achieved a success rate of 81% for premolars and 76.7% for molars in determining periodontally compromised teeth (Lee et al. 2018).

Danks et al. (2021) reported that they analyzed the bone loss of single-, double-, and triple-rooted teeth using an AI algorithm they developed, which utilized dental landmarks on periapical radiographs ($n = 340$). They emphasized that the detection of anatomical landmarks was automatic with a success rate of 73.9% or higher, and the stage of periodontitis was estimated with a success rate of 68.3%. The researchers also suggested that much more successful algorithms could be developed with larger datasets (Danks et al. 2021).

Moran et al. (2020) evaluated the success of an AI algorithm capable of detecting bone resorption from periapical radiography in their study. They utilized ResNet and inception architectures in training the system. In the study, which examined 467 periapical radiographs and 1079 periodontal spaces, the diagnostic accuracy and specificity values of the system were reported as 0.817 and 0.762, respectively (Moran et al. 2020).

Khan et al. (2021) developed a DL algorithm using 206 digital periapical radiographs, based on the diagnosis and image labeling provided by three specialists (2 oral pathologists and 1 endodontist). They found that using radiographic images of varying qualities reduced the success of the system. The authors emphasized the importance of employing purpose-oriented architectures and conducting multi-centered studies during the AI training stage to enhance the success of these systems (Khan et al. 2021).

In a study by Chen et al. (2021), they examined the success of an AI system in diagnosing not only periodontal findings but also different dental issues such as caries and periapical lesions. The study involved 2900 digital periapical radiographs, and the AI system aimed to analyze the severity of each dental problem as mild, moderate, or severe. The researchers reported that the diagnostic success of the system increased as the severity level of each dental problem increased (Chen et al. 2021).

Chen et al. (2023) developed an AI algorithm based on the YOLOv5 model using 8000 periapical radiographs and detection/segmentation methods. In total, 27,964 teeth were evaluated. The study demonstrated that periodontal bone losses could be determined at a rate of 97%, and the bone level could be determined at a rate of 92.61% using this algorithm (Chen et al. 2023).

Bitewing Radiograph-Based Studies

Hildebolt and Vannier (1988) conducted a pioneering AI-based diagnostic study using a computer-controlled TV camera on bitewing radiographs. They reported that this computer-based system could determine the degree of periodontal disease with a success rate ranging from 78.8% to 91%. This study is a significant contribution, showcasing the early search for automated systems in the field, even in the 1990s (Hildebolt and Vannier 1988).

Kearney et al. (2022) utilized a large image archive consisting of 80,326 bitewing radiographs in their research. In this study, they demonstrated that periodontal bone destruction can be successfully detected from bitewing radiographs using artificial neural networks (ANN) (Kearney et al. 2022).

CBCT-Based Studies

CBCT is an imaging method used in dentistry for implant planning, orthodontic treatment planning, jaw pathologies, facial trauma, sinuses, and bone examination, allowing 3D imaging to be obtained (Macleod and Heath 2008). This imaging technique provides detailed information and high-quality images of the jawbones with a limited radiation dose (Correa et al. 2014; Bornstein et al. 2015; Fokas et al. 2018). Numerous studies in the literature have reported that CBCT images can be used to determine periodontal bone defects and other periodontal problems (Feijo et al. 2012; de Faria Vasconcelos et al. 2012; Braun et al. 2014; Li et al. 2015; Anter et al. 2016; Haas et al. 2018; Ozcan and Sekerci 2017; Suphanantachat et al. 2017; Choi et al. 2018; Jie and Ouyang 2016).

While there have been some studies aiming to automatically detect different anatomical variations, such as alveolar bones and apical lesions, on CBCT images using AI methods (Hung et al. 2022b; Ezhov et al. 2021; Orhan et al. 2022), as far as we know, there is no AI-based study on CBCT images for periodontal diagnosis yet. Filling this gap in the future could be revolutionary for periodontal diagnosis.

Photo-Based Studies

Photography was first used in dentistry in 1848 (Kalpana et al. 2018). Today, extraoral and intraoral photographs are widely used for dental diagnosis, treatment planning, and patient follow-up (Kalpana et al. 2018; Galante 2009; Vyas 2018). It has become an indispensable part of the routine workflow, especially in fields such as aesthetic dentistry, surgery, orthodontics, implantology, and periodontics (Ahmad 2009). There are academic studies exploring the use of AI systems to automatically detect certain periodontal conditions, pathologies, and anatomical formations from these images (Fig. 7.12). In the future, with the aid of these technologies,

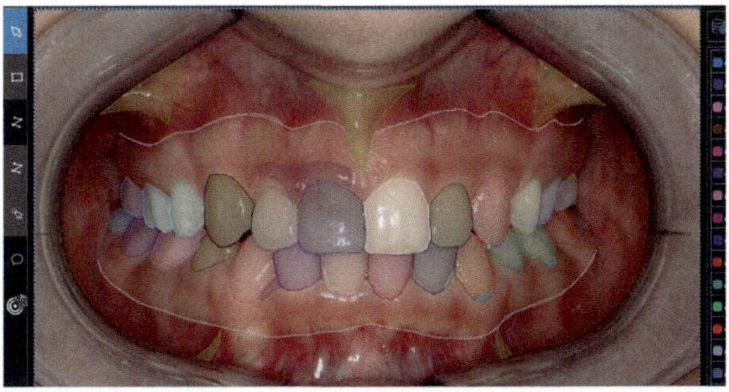

Fig. 7.12 Digital artificial intelligence model for detection of periodontal and mucosal conditions. (Courtesy of CranioCatch AI software)

high-performance computer software can be developed to automatically perform operations such as diagnosis, treatment planning, and monitoring of periodontics patients.

Rana et al. (2017) conducted a study using 405 intraoral photographs and developed a CNN-based AI algorithm. This pixel-based system successfully identified gingival inflammations through a segmentation method. They reported an area under the receiver operating characteristic curve (AUC) value of 0.746 for the AI algorithm in identifying healthy and inflamed gingiva (Rana et al. 2017).

Askarian et al. (2019) proposed a method of detecting periodontal disease with AI using smartphones and image processing techniques. Their model, based on images of 30 individuals, achieved a detection accuracy of 94.3%, sensitivity of 92.6%, and specificity of 93% for periodontal infection (Askarian et al. 2019).

Moriyama et al. (2019) utilized intraoral images and developed an AI model to estimate pocket depth from these images. This deep learning model also had the capability to assess the severity of pocket depths. Following the performance evaluation, they concluded that the algorithm's prediction accuracy ranged from 78.3% to 84.5% (Moriyama et al. 2019).

Alalharith et al. (2020) planned to develop a CNN system that automatically detects teeth and inflamed areas in intraoral photographs. This system was trained with 134 intraoral photographs and achieved a 77.12% accuracy in detecting inflamed gingival areas using the object detection method (Alalharith et al. 2020).

Chen and Chen (2020) developed an AI system using only 180 intraoral photographs in their study. The system was trained to automatically classify and diagnose gingivitis or healthy conditions. The gingivitis detection performance of the system (with the classification method) was evaluated, and the accuracy value was found to be 71%–75.44% (Chen and Chen 2020).

You et al. (2020) used the CNN method to detect dental plaque around primary teeth. They reported that this CNN algorithm, after being trained with 886 photographs, detected plaque at a higher accuracy rate than dentists. In this study, a plaque-disclosing agent was used for diagnosing plaque, and the plaque determination by the system was performed using the object detection method. This study is promising for the use of computer systems in oral hygiene monitoring (You et al. 2020).

Khaleel and Aziz (2021) developed an AI algorithm using 120 intraoral photos and reported an accuracy of 95% in gingival disease detection (Khaleel and Aziz 2021).

Shang et al. (2021) worked on an AI system that can detect dental calculus, dental caries, and gingivitis from photographs. The study, which used 7220 photographs, suggests that other conditions related to periodontics can also be detected by these systems (Shang et al. 2021). Similarly, in two different studies, it was proven that the diagnosis of gingivitis can be easily detected with AI systems through intraoral images (Li et al. 2021a,b).

Xu et al. (2022) designed an AI system that can be used for dental plaque detection. They reported that the system, trained using over 400 photographs by the

GoogLeNet model, could successfully detect dental plaque and debridements automatically (Xu et al. 2022).

Shen et al. (2022) evaluated a product in which periodontal disease findings can be detected with an AI system from intraoral images taken from smartphone cameras. The study aimed to evaluate the effectiveness of periodontal treatment results and follow up with patients. The 3-month periodontal parameters of the patients whose treatments were completed through this system were collected and followed up. They reported that this system will provide significant advantages in monitoring and early diagnosis of periodontal diseases and can be used safely in the future (Shen et al. 2022).

Ultrasound-Based Studies

In recent years, it has been accepted that ultrasound can be used as a complement to CBCT or alone in the detection of some periodontal conditions (Pan et al. 2022; Duong et al. 2019). Ultrasound provides a less traumatic and more comfortable examination. It facilitates the work of the patient and the physician in cases such as the presence of active wounds (Bains et al. 2008).

Duong et al. (2019) planned a study on an AI model that performs the automatic determination of alveolar bone from high-frequency ultrasound images by the segmentation method. As a result of the study, they reported that the algorithm developed with the U-net architecture had a high agreement (of 75% average decimetric) with the measurements of 15 observers (Duong et al. 2019).

Pan et al. (2022) performed an AI study that automatically segmented soft tissue, bone, and crown using the porcine model. They first evaluated 627 frames of ultrasound images of the maxilla and mandible premolar and molar tooth regions by readers. The model showed a Dice similarity coefficient of 83.7%–90.0% for the first test. They reported the high potential of using AI technologies for the evaluation of periodontal tissues from ultrasound images (Pan et al. 2022).

Chifor et al. (2021) conducted a study on performing periodontal tissue analysis by automatically processing ultrasound images with DL in a porcine model. They reported that automated systems could be used for this purpose (Chifor et al. 2021).

Chifor et al. (2022) segmented images from 11 patients using a 3D ultrasound scanner prototype and developed an algorithm using Mask R-CNN and U-Net architecture. The algorithm could be used to detect periodontal tissues automatically. The gingiva determination performance of the system was determined as the average intersection over union range value of 75.6% (Chifor et al. 2022).

Nguyen et al. (2021) showed that CNNs can detect cementum-enamel junctions with high performance on ultrasound images. The cementum-enamel junction points determined by the AI system were in high agreement with manually determined points ($R = 0.993$, $p < 0.001$). This study, which questioned the performance of AI systems in the automatic measurement of soft tissue height from ultrasound images, showed that DL could be effectively used in the recognition and measurement of periodontal structures (Nguyen et al. 2021).

Microbiological-Based Studies

Although clinical and radiographic findings are currently used in periodontal diagnosis, the detection of the periodontal pathogen (type/amount) from subgingival plaque is critical for disease detection. Therefore, in recent years, microbiology-based AI studies have focused on the automatic detection of plaque content. This field has the potential to accelerate the establishment of periodontal disease and health pathogen profiles.

Aberin and de Goma (2018) worked on a CNN-based algorithm that could automatically recognize dental plaque microscopy images. This system detected periodontal disease and health status with a 75% success rate (Aberin and de Goma 2018).

Feres et al. (2018) worked on computer-aided systems that examine 40 bacteria in dental plaque using checkerboard DNA–DNA hybridization and perform periodontal status determination (chronic/aggressive periodontitis, healthy) with machine learning. They stated that this system successfully detects periodontal disease in young individuals (AUC > 0.95) (Feres et al. 2018).

Na et al. (2020) found that AI was very successful in identifying potential oral microbial markers and microorganisms in the diagnosis of periodontitis. They even stated that possible disease-marking microorganisms, which are automatically detected at an early stage, are promising for early diagnosis of the disease (Na et al. 2020).

Similarly, there were some studies on the automatic microbiological evaluation of peri-implantitis patients. In these studies, it was stated that the amount of pathogens thought to play a role in the disease profile of peri-implantitis patients increased, and their automatic determination would provide a great advantage in disease diagnosis (Canullo et al. 2017).

Wang et al. (2021) reported that the microbial composition of the plaque could be successfully detected automatically with the help of these systems (Wang et al. 2021). In this study, it was reported that the AI system performed the prediction of the microbiological picture in peri-implantitis with a success rate of 82.7–97.5%. It has been noted that qualitative and quantitative microbiology profiles could be easily determined with AI and that such studies should be strengthened for clinical application (Wang et al. 2021).

Saliva/GCF/Plasma/Serum-Based Studies

Most of the biochemistry-based studies carried out in the field of periodontics are focused on determining host antibody and cytokine profiles (Brito et al. 2022; Tang et al. 2019). Consequently, one can infer the presence and severity of periodontal disease by detecting the inflammatory condition (Brito et al. 2022; Tang et al. 2019). This leads to practical and innovative diagnostic methods that automatically evaluate the analysis results of biological samples, such as GCF/saliva/plasma and serum, using AI.

Kim et al. (2020) examined the potential of an AI algorithm to automatically evaluate biomarkers in the saliva of healthy individuals and those with periodontitis, interpreting the presence and severity of the disease. They developed a machine learning system that identifies nine different bacteria (*Porphyromonas gingivalis, Tannerella forsythia, Treponema denticola, Prevotella intermedia, Fusobacterium nucleatum, Campylobacter rectus, Aggregatibacter actinomycetemcomitans, Peptostreptococcus anaerobic, and Eikenella corrodens*) from DNA samples isolated using mouthwashes of 692 participants and interprets disease severity. The system showed promising accuracy, ranging from 0.78 to 0.93, in diagnosing periodontal diseases. They emphasized that determining bacterial combinations from saliva can serve as a good marker for disease detection (Kim et al. 2020).

Kouznetsova et al. (2021) developed a system that automatically detects salivary metabolites and evaluated whether it could be used to diagnose periodontitis or oral cancer. They concluded that AI could detect oral cancer from saliva samples with 79.54% accuracy (Kouznetsova et al. 2021). Similarly, Romm et al. (2021) conducted a similar study and obtained successful results (Romm et al. 2021).

Huang et al. (2020b) designed an algorithm that automatically evaluates antibody arrays and determines periodontal disease using GCF. The success of the system in disease detection showed a high accuracy of 91–97.5% (Huang et al. 2020b).

It is known that reactive oxygen species, such as hydrogen peroxide and hypochlorous acid produced by bacteria, cause indirect tissue destruction (Chapple 1997; Valko et al. 2007). Based on this information, Bezruk et al. (2017) developed a CNN model that automatically interprets the high lipid peroxide levels of 141 subjects. Although the model was created successfully, no significant correlation could be established between peroxidase levels and inflammation (Bezruk et al. 2017).

Patient Data-Based Studies

Studies have shown that multiple patient information can be interpreted with the help of ANNs and used in stages such as disease diagnosis and classification.

Farhadian et al. (2020) recorded 11 different variables (age, sex, smoking, gingival index, plaque index, etc.) of 300 patients and attempted automatic periodontal disease classification using AI. When the performance of the system was evaluated, it was found to be successful in disease classification with an accuracy of 88.7%–91.2%. The study reported that these computer systems, which can process multiple and complex data, can significantly assist physicians in making diagnosis processes easier and faster (Farhadian et al. 2020).

It is evident that the new periodontal disease classification, especially, requires evaluating many parameters together. Therefore, automated systems capable of blending and interpreting multiple parameters, including clinical data, radiographic data, and patient anamnesis information, may enable physicians to perform these stages much more efficiently in the future.

Risk Estimation

AI can make predictions for future events and their consequences (Mesko 2017; Subramanian et al. 2020). AI can identify possible situations with new data using historical datasets to predict future events (Mesko 2017; Subramanian et al. 2020). For this purpose, some AI models such as regression, classification, time series, and DL models are used (Han et al. 2021). Although the estimation is not always completely accurate, physician judgment must be included in the evaluation. Nevertheless, AI can increase the quality of periodontal treatment at many stages, such as identifying risk groups, estimating prognosis, and determining patient appointment follow-up frequencies. For example, with accurate prognosis estimation, treatment costs can be reduced or the probability of less invasive treatment being preferred is increased (Troiano et al. 2023).

Sunmoo et al. (2018) evaluated 78 variables and tried to predict tooth mobility using a deep neural network in their study. In other words, they attempted to make a risk estimation about the probability of mobility using a DL algorithm. As a result of this study, they determined that the strongest markers affecting mobility are aging, general health status, flossing, soda consumption, and financial stress. They observed a significant correlation between aging and tooth mobility in this study, which was conducted with 4623 patient data (Sunmoo et al. 2018).

Troiano et al. (2023) conducted a study on the estimation of survival percentages and prognosis of teeth with periodontal damage. They used clinical and radiographic data from 515 patients and 3157 molars to train the machine learning model they developed. The best AUC value for estimation was found to be 0.724. They stated that the widespread use of such technologies will enable successful prediction of prognosis in multifactorial diseases (Troiano et al. 2023).

Lee et al. (2022) developed an AI algorithm to determine the prognosis of a tooth using five scales ranging from hopeless to good for the long-term. In this study, which used 94 cases and 2359 teeth, it was reported that determining the dental prognosis with AI made a significant contribution to the treatment decision (Lee et al. 2022).

Monsarrat et al. (2022) worked on an AI system that can predict periodontal situations using age, body mass index, smoking habits, systemic pathologies, diet, alcohol, education level, and hormonal status. They developed an AI system for this purpose and reported that its performance was evaluated with an F-1 score of 0.74 in predicting healthy periodontitis and 0.68 in predicting periodontitis (Monsarrat et al. 2022).

Treatment Planning

Studies are showing that AI systems can be used for treatment planning for various diseases in many fields of medicine (Bai and Xia 2021; Byrne et al. 2022). However, when the literature is examined, it becomes apparent that there has not been comprehensive research on this subject for periodontal treatment planning. There is limited information about the usability of these systems in dental implant planning (Kurt Bayrakdar et al. 2021; Mangano et al. 2023; Roongruangsilp and Khongkhunthian 2021). A computer system that provides a periodontal treatment plan by inquiring about the patient's diagnosis, age, systemic condition, oral hygiene habits, or interpreting radiology records will undoubtedly facilitate the physician's work.

For example, AI systems can interpret patient information or diagnostic records and generate reports on the need for specific surgeries such as regenerative surgery, mucogingival periodontal treatment, and gingivectomy. The developed AI-supported software may be integrated more effectively into treatment stages by utilizing it in application areas such as robotic or virtual technology.

In short, concepts such as deep learning, machine learning, and artificial neural networks (ANN) related to AI technologies are widely used in the field of periodontics today. Researchers have conducted periodontics-based studies aiming for automatic diagnosis and reporting from dental radiographs, ultrasound images, and intraoral photographs by harnessing the image processing and interpretation capacity of artificial neurons. Additionally, these AI systems have been employed to assist in the analysis and interpretation of saliva, gingival groove fluid, serum, and plasma samples, enabling a better understanding of the biological processes underlying periodontal disease (Romm et al. 2021; Bezruk et al. 2017).

Machine learning technology has demonstrated its analytical prediction ability and has found utility in stages such as periodontal disease estimation and determining patient risk groups (Liu et al. 2020). Already, AI systems are being used in numerous application areas of dentistry, including the creation of digital patient registration systems, automating secretariat operations, providing high-quality services through virtual technologies, and facilitating teledentistry and quality dentistry education processes (Schwendicke et al. 2020; Deshmukh 2018). The potential benefits, such as time-saving, enhanced patient and employee comfort, higher accuracy, reliability, and precise analysis of multiple and complex situations, predict that AI will find even more extensive use in routine dental work in the future (Bindushree et al. 2020). It is safe to say that these potential usage areas in the general workflow of dentistry are also valid and promising for the field of periodontics.

References

Abdolali F, Zoroofi RA, Otake Y, Sato Y. Automatic segmentation of maxillofacial cysts in cone beam CT images. Comput Biol Med. 2016;72:108–19.

Abdolali F, Zoroofi RA, Otake Y, Sato Y. Automated classification of maxillofacial cysts in cone beam CT images using contourlet transformation and spherical harmonics. Comput Methods Prog Biomed. 2017;139:197–207.

Aberin STA, de Goma JC, editors. Detecting periodontal disease using convolutional neural networks. 2018 IEEE 10th International Conference on Humanoid, Nanotechnology, Information Technology, Communication and Control, Environment and Management (HNICEM), IEEE; 2018.

Agbaje JO, de Casteele EV, Salem AS, Anumendem D, Lambrichts I, Politis C. Tracking of the inferior alveolar nerve: its implication in surgical planning. Clin Oral Investig. 2017;21:2213–20.
Agrawal P, Nikhade P. Artificial intelligence in dentistry: past, present, and future. Cureus. 2022;14(7):e27405.
Ahmad I. Digital dental photography. Part 1: an overview. Br Dent J. 2009;206(8):403–7.
Alalharith DM, Alharthi HM, Alghamdi WM, Alsenbel YM, Aslam N, Khan IU, et al. A deep learning-based approach for the detection of early signs of gingivitis in orthodontic patients using faster region-based convolutional neural networks. Int J Environ Res Public Health. 2020;17(22):8447.
Alami H, Lehoux P, Auclair Y, de Guise M, Gagnon MP, Shaw J, et al. Artificial intelligence and health technology assessment: anticipating a new level of complexity. J Med Internet Res. 2020;22(7):e17707.
Al-Helou N. The extra oral and intra oral examination. BDJ Team. 2021;8(5):20–2.
Almăşan O, Leucuţa DC, Hedeşiu M, Mureşanu S, Popa ŞL. Temporomandibular joint osteoarthritis diagnosis employing artificial intelligence: systematic review and meta-analysis. J Clin Med. 2023;12(3):942.
Amann J, Blasimme A, Vayena E, Frey D, Madai VI. Explainability for artificial intelligence in healthcare: a multidisciplinary perspective. BMC Med Inform Decis Mak. 2020;20(1):310.
Anter E, Zayet MK, El-Dessouky SH. Accuracy and precision of cone beam computed tomography in periodontal defects measurement (systematic review). J Indian Soc Periodontol. 2016;20(3):235–43.
Antonov AA. From artificial intelligence to human super-intelligence. Artif Intell. 2011;2(6):3560.
Ariji Y, Yanashita Y, Kutsuna S, Muramatsu C, Fukuda M, Kise Y, et al. Automatic detection and classification of radiolucent lesions in the mandible on panoramic radiographs using a deep learning object detection technique. Oral Surg Oral Med Oral Pathol Oral Radiol. 2019;128(4):424–30.
Ariji Y, Kise Y, Fukuda M, Kuwada C, Ariji E. Segmentation of metastatic cervical lymph nodes from CT images of oral cancers using deep-learning technology. Dentomaxillofac Radiol. 2022;51(4):20210515.
Armitage GC. The complete periodontal examination. Periodontol 2000. 2004;34:22–33.
Askarian B, Tabei F, Tipton GA, Chong JW, editors. Smartphone-Based Method for Detecting Periodontal Disease. 2019 IEEE Healthcare Innovations and Point of Care Technologies,(HI-POCT), IEEE; 2019.
Ayoub A, Pulijala Y. The application of virtual reality and augmented reality in oral & maxillofacial surgery. BMC Oral Health. 2019;19(1):238.
Baelum V, López R. Periodontal disease epidemiology - learned and unlearned? Periodontol 2000. 2013;62(1):37–58.
Bai E, Xia J. A knowledge based automatic radiation treatment plan alert system. Int J Artif Intellig Applic (IJAIA). 2021;12(6)
Bains VK, Mohan R, Bains R. Application of ultrasound in periodontics: part II. J Indian Soc Periodontol. 2008;12(3):55–61.
Başaran M, Çelik Ö, Bayrakdar IS, Bilgir E, Orhan K, Odabaş A, et al. Diagnostic charting of panoramic radiography using deep-learning artificial intelligence system. Oral Radiol. 2022;38(3):363–9.
Belibasakis GN, Belstrøm D, Eick S, Gursoy UK, Johansson A, Könönen E. Periodontal microbiology and microbial etiology of periodontal diseases: Historical concepts and contemporary perspectives. Periodontol 2000. 2023.
Beltrán-Aguilar ED, Eke PI, Thornton-Evans G, Petersen PE. Recording and surveillance systems for periodontal diseases. Periodontol 2000. 2012;60(1):40–53.
Bezruk V, Krivenko S, Kryvenko L, editors. Salivary lipid peroxidation and periodontal status detection in ukrainian atopic children with convolutional neural networks. 2017 4th International Scientific-Practical Conference Problems of Infocommunications Science and Technology (PIC S&T), IEEE; 2017.

Bianchi J, Ruellas A, Prieto JC, Li T, Soroushmehr R, Najarian K, et al. Decision support systems in temporomandibular joint osteoarthritis: a review of data science and artificial intelligence applications. Semin Orthod. 2021;27(2):78–86.
Bindushree V, Sameen R, Vasudevan V, Shrihari T, Devaraju D, Mathew NS. Artificial intelligence: In modern dentistry. J Dent Res Rev. 2020;7(1):27.
Bispo MS, Pierre Júnior M, Apolinário AL Jr, Dos Santos JN, Junior BC, Neves FS, et al. Computer tomographic differential diagnosis of ameloblastoma and odontogenic keratocyst: classification using a convolutional neural network. Dentomaxillofac Radiol. 2021;50(7):20210002.
Bornstein MM, Brügger OE, Janner SF, Kuchler U, Chappuis V, Jacobs R, et al. Indications and frequency for the use of cone beam computed tomography for implant treatment planning in a specialty clinic. Int J Oral Maxillofac Implants. 2015;30(5):1076–83.
Braun X, Ritter L, Jervøe-Storm PM, Frentzen M. Diagnostic accuracy of CBCT for periodontal lesions. Clin Oral Investig. 2014;18(4):1229–36.
Brito F, Curcio HFQ, da Silva Fidalgo TK. Periodontal disease metabolomics signatures from different biofluids: a systematic review. Metabolomics. 2022;18(11):83.
Bui FQ, Almeida-da-Silva CLC, Huynh B, Trinh A, Liu J, Woodward J, et al. Association between periodontal pathogens and systemic disease. Biom J. 2019;42(1):27–35.
Byrne M, Archibald-Heeren B, Hu Y, Teh A, Beserminji R, Cai E, et al. Varian ethos online adaptive radiotherapy for prostate cancer: early results of contouring accuracy, treatment plan quality, and treatment time. J Appl Clin Med Phys. 2022;23(1):e13479.
Canullo L, Radovanović S, Delibasic B, Blaya JA, Penarrocha D, Rakic M. The predictive value of microbiological findings on teeth, internal and external implant portions in clinical decision making. Clin Oral Implants Res. 2017;28(5):512–9.
Cao Z, Qin C, Fan S, Yu D, Wu Y, Qin J, et al. Pilot study of a surgical robot system for zygomatic implant placement. Med Eng Phys. 2020;75:72–8.
Cekici A, Kantarci A, Hasturk H, Van Dyke TE. Inflammatory and immune pathways in the pathogenesis of periodontal disease. Periodontol 2000. 2014;64(1):57–80.
Cha JY, Yoon HI, Yeo IS, Huh KH, Han JS. Panoptic segmentation on panoramic radiographs: deep learning-based segmentation of various structures including maxillary sinus and mandibular canal. J Clin Med. 2021a;10(12):2577.
Cha JY, Yoon HI, Yeo IS, Huh KH, Han JS. Peri-implant bone loss measurement using a region-based convolutional neural network on dental periapical radiographs. J Clin Med. 2021b;10(5):1009.
Chaiprasittikul N, Thanathornwong B, Pornprasertsuk-Damrongsri S, Raocharernporn S, Maponthong S, Manopatanakul S. Application of a multi-layer perceptron in preoperative screening for orthognathic surgery. Healthc Inform Res. 2023;29(1):16–22.
Chang HJ, Lee SJ, Yong TH, Shin NY, Jang BG, Kim JE, et al. Deep learning hybrid method to automatically diagnose periodontal bone loss and stage periodontitis. Sci Rep. 2020;10(1):7531.
Chapple IL. Reactive oxygen species and antioxidants in inflammatory diseases. J Clin Periodontol. 1997;24(5):287–96.
Chen Y, Chen X, editors. Gingivitis identification via GLCM and artificial neural network. Medical Imaging and Computer-Aided Diagnosis: Proceeding of 2020 International Conference on Medical Imaging and Computer-Aided Diagnosis (MICAD 2020), Springer; 2020.
Chen H, Li H, Zhao Y, Zhao J, Wang Y. Dental disease detection on periapical radiographs based on deep convolutional neural networks. Int J Comput Assist Radiol Surg. 2021;16:649–61.
Chen Z, Liu Y, Xie X, Deng F. Influence of bone density on the accuracy of artificial intelligence-guided implant surgery: an in vitro study. J Prosthet Dent. 2022.
Chen C-C, Wu Y-F, Aung LM, Lin JC-Y, Ngo ST, Su J-N, et al. Automatic recognition of teeth and periodontal bone loss measurement in digital radiographs using deep-learning artificial intelligence. J Dent Sci. 2023;18:1301–9.
Chifor R, Li M, Nguyen KT, Arsenescu T, Chifor I, Badea AF, et al. Three-dimensional periodontal investigations using a prototype handheld ultrasound scanner with spatial positioning reading sensor. Med Ultrason. 2021;23(3):297–304.

Chifor R, Hotoleanu M, Marita T, Arsenescu T, Socaciu MA, Badea IC, et al. Automatic segmentation of periodontal tissue ultrasound images with artificial intelligence: a novel method for improving dataset quality. Sensors (Basel). 2022;22(19):7101.

Choi IGG, Cortes ARG, Arita ES, Georgetti MAP. Comparison of conventional imaging techniques and CBCT for periodontal evaluation: a systematic review. Imaging Sci Dent. 2018;48(2):79–86.

Choi HI, Jung SK, Baek SH, Lim WH, Ahn SJ, Yang IH, et al. Artificial intelligent model with neural network machine learning for the diagnosis of orthognathic surgery. J Craniofac Surg. 2019;30(7):1986–9.

Choi E, Lee S, Jeong E, Shin S, Park H, Youm S, et al. Artificial intelligence in positioning between mandibular third molar and inferior alveolar nerve on panoramic radiography. Sci Rep. 2022;12(1):2456.

Chung M, Lee J, Song W, Song Y, Yang IH, Lee J, et al. Automatic registration between dental cone-beam CT and scanned surface via deep pose regression neural networks and clustered similarities. IEEE Trans Med Imaging. 2020;39(12):3900–9.

Corbet EF, Ho DK, Lai SM. Radiographs in periodontal disease diagnosis and management. Aust Dent J. 2009;54(Suppl 1):S27–43.

Correa LR, Spin-Neto R, Stavropoulos A, Schropp L, da Silveira HE, Wenzel A. Planning of dental implant size with digital panoramic radiographs, CBCT-generated panoramic images, and CBCT cross-sectional images. Clin Oral Implants Res. 2014;25(6):690–5.

Cui M, Zhang DY. Artificial intelligence and computational pathology. Lab Investig. 2021;101(4):412–22.

Danks RP, Bano S, Orishko A, Tan HJ, Moreno Sancho F, D'Aiuto F, et al. Automating periodontal bone loss measurement via dental landmark localisation. Int J Comput Assist Radiol Surg. 2021;16(7):1189–99.

De Ceulaer J, De Clercq C, Swennen GR. Robotic surgery in oral and maxillofacial, craniofacial and head and neck surgery: a systematic review of the literature. Int J Oral Maxillofac Surg. 2012;41(11):1311–24.

de Faria Vasconcelos K, Evangelista KM, Rodrigues CD, Estrela C, de Sousa TO, Silva MA. Detection of periodontal bone loss using cone beam CT and intraoral radiography. Dentomaxillofac Radiol. 2012;41(1):64–9.

Deshmukh S. Artificial intelligence in dentistry. J Int Clin Dent Res Organ. 2018;10(2):47.

Di Benedetto A, Gigante I, Colucci S, Grano M. Periodontal disease: linking the primary inflammation to bone loss. Clin Dev Immunol. 2013;2013:503754.

Duong DQ, Nguyen KT, Kaipatur NR, Lou EHM, Noga M, Major PW, et al. Fully automated segmentation of alveolar bone using deep convolutional neural networks from intraoral ultrasound images. Annu Int Conf IEEE Eng Med Biol Soc. 2019;2019:6632–5.

Etemad L, Wu TH, Heiner P, Liu J, Lee S, Chao WL, et al. Machine learning from clinical data sets of a contemporary decision for orthodontic tooth extraction. Orthod Craniofac Res. 2021;24(Suppl 2):193–200.

Ezhov M, Gusarev M, Golitsyna M, Yates JM, Kushnerev E, Tamimi D, et al. Clinically applicable artificial intelligence system for dental diagnosis with CBCT. Sci Rep. 2021;11(1):15006.

Farhadian M, Shokouhi P, Torkzaban P. A decision support system based on support vector machine for diagnosis of periodontal disease. BMC Res Notes. 2020;13(1):337.

Fatima A, Shafi I, Afzal H, Díez IT, Lourdes DRM, Breñosa J, et al. Advancements in dentistry with artificial intelligence: current clinical applications and future perspectives. Healthcare (Basel). 2022;10(11):2188.

Feijo CV, Lucena JG, Kurita LM, Pereira SL. Evaluation of cone beam computed tomography in the detection of horizontal periodontal bone defects: an in vivo study. Int J Periodontics Restorative Dent. 2012;32(5):e162–8.

Feres M, Louzoun Y, Haber S, Faveri M, Figueiredo LC, Levin L. Support vector machine-based differentiation between aggressive and chronic periodontitis using microbial profiles. Int Dent J. 2018;68(1):39–46.

Fokas G, Vaughn VM, Scarfe WC, Bornstein MM. Accuracy of linear measurements on CBCT images related to presurgical implant treatment planning: a systematic review. Clin Oral Implants Res. 2018;29(Suppl 16):393–415.

Friedland B, Donoff B, Dodson TB. The use of 3-dimensional reconstructions to evaluate the anatomic relationship of the mandibular canal and impacted mandibular third molars. J Oral Maxillofac Surg. 2008;66(8):1678–85.

Fu Q, Chen Y, Li Z, Jing Q, Hu C, Liu H, et al. A deep learning algorithm for detection of oral cavity squamous cell carcinoma from photographic images: a retrospective study. EClinicalMedicine. 2020;27:100558.

Fukuda M, Inamoto K, Shibata N, Ariji Y, Yanashita Y, Kutsuna S, et al. Evaluation of an artificial intelligence system for detecting vertical root fracture on panoramic radiography. Oral Radiol. 2020;36(4):337–43.

Galante DL. History and current use of clinical photography in orthodontics. J Calif Dent Assoc. 2009;37(3):173–4.

Garland J, Hu M, Kesha K, Glenn C, Duffy M, Morrow P, et al. An overview of artificial intelligence/deep learning. Pathology. 2021;53:S6.

Gasner NS, Schure RS. Periodontal disease. StatPearls. Treasure Island, FL: StatPearls Publishing. Copyright © 2023, StatPearls Publishing LLC.; 2023.

Haas LF, Zimmermann GS, De Luca Canto G, Flores-Mir C, Corrêa M. Precision of cone beam CT to assess periodontal bone defects: a systematic review and meta-analysis. Dentomaxillofac Radiol. 2018;47(2):20170084.

Hamet P, Tremblay J. Artificial intelligence in medicine. Metabolism. 2017;69s:S36–s40.

Han S, Mannan N, Stein DC, Pattipati KR, Bollas GM. Classification and regression models of audio and vibration signals for machine state monitoring in precision machining systems. J Manuf Syst. 2021;61:45–53.

Hashem M, Hassanein AS. Jaw fracture classification using meta heuristic firefly algorithm with multi-layered associative neural networks. Clust Comput. 2019;22:7079–86.

Hildebolt CF, Vannier MW. Automated classification of periodontal disease using bitewing radiographs. J Periodontol. 1988;59(2):87–94.

Huang J, Habib AR, Mendis D, Chong J, Smith M, Duvnjak M, et al. An artificial intelligence algorithm that differentiates anterior ethmoidal artery location on sinus computed tomography scans. J Laryngol Otol. 2020a;134(1):52–5.

Huang W, Wu J, Mao Y, Zhu S, Huang GF, Petritis B, et al. Developing a periodontal disease antibody array for the prediction of severe periodontal disease using machine learning classifiers. J Periodontol. 2020b;91(2):232–43.

Hung KF, Ai QYH, King AD, Bornstein MM, Wong LM, Leung YY. Automatic detection and segmentation of morphological changes of the maxillary sinus mucosa on cone-beam computed tomography images using a three-dimensional convolutional neural network. Clin Oral Investig. 2022a;26(5):3987–98.

Hung KF, Ai QYH, Wong LM, Yeung AWK, Li DTS, Leung YY. Current applications of deep learning and radiomics on CT and CBCT for maxillofacial diseases. Diagnostics (Basel). 2022b;13(1):110.

Ivanov SH, Webster C. Adoption of robots, artificial intelligence and service automation by travel, tourism and hospitality companies–a cost-benefit analysis. Artificial Intelligence and Service Automation by Travel, Tourism and Hospitality Companies–A Cost-Benefit Analysis. 2017.

Jalali A, Lonsdale H, Zamora LV, Ahumada L, Nguyen ATH, Rehman M, et al. Machine learning applied to registry data: development of a patient-specific prediction model for blood transfusion requirements during craniofacial surgery using the pediatric craniofacial perioperative registry dataset. Anesth Analg. 2021;132(1):160–71.

Jandali D, Barrera JE. Recent advances in orthognathic surgery. Curr Opin Otolaryngol Head Neck Surg. 2020;28(4):246–50.

Jaskari J, Sahlsten J, Järnstedt J, Mehtonen H, Karhu K, Sundqvist O, et al. Deep learning method for mandibular canal segmentation in dental cone beam computed tomography volumes. Sci Rep. 2020;10(1):5842.

Jeong SH, Yun JP, Yeom HG, Lim HJ, Lee J, Kim BC. Deep learning based discrimination of soft tissue profiles requiring orthognathic surgery by facial photographs. Sci Rep. 2020;10(1):16235.
Jiang J, Trundle P, Ren J. Medical image analysis with artificial neural networks. Comput Med Imaging Graph. 2010;34(8):617–31.
Jiang L, Chen D, Cao Z, Wu F, Zhu H, Zhu F. A two-stage deep learning architecture for radiographic staging of periodontal bone loss. BMC Oral Health. 2022;22(1):106.
Jie Z, Ouyang XY. Assessing maxillary molar furcation involvement by cone beam computed tomography. Chin J Dent Res. 2016;19(3):145–51.
Joda T, Zitzmann NU. Personalized workflows in reconstructive dentistry-current possibilities and future opportunities. Clin Oral Investig. 2022;26(6):4283–90.
Joda T, Waltimo T, Probst-Hensch N, Pauli-Magnus C, Zitzmann NU. Health data in dentistry: an attempt to master the digital challenge. Public Health Genomics. 2019;22(1–2):1–7.
Jubair F, Al-Karadsheh O, Malamos D, Al Mahdi S, Saad Y, Hassona Y. A novel lightweight deep convolutional neural network for early detection of oral cancer. Oral Dis. 2022;28(4):1123–30.
Kalpana D, Rao SJ, Joseph JK, Kurapati SKR. Digital dental photography. Indian J Dent Res. 2018;29(4):507–12.
Kearney VP, Yansane AM, Brandon RG, Vaderhobli R, Lin GH, Hekmatian H, et al. A generative adversarial inpainting network to enhance prediction of periodontal clinical attachment level. J Dent. 2022;123:104211.
Keser G, Bayrakdar İ, Pekiner FN, Çelik Ö, Orhan K. A deep learning algorithm for classification of oral lichen planus lesions from photographic images: a retrospective study. J Stomatol Oral Maxillofac Surg. 2023;124(1):101264.
Kesic L, Milasin J, Igic M, Obradovic R. Microbial etiology of periodontal disease-mini review. Med Biol. 2008;15(1):1–6.
Khaleel BI, Aziz MS, editors. Using artificial intelligence methods for diagnosis of gingivitis diseases. Journal of Physics: Conference Series, IOP Publishing; 2021.
Khan HA, Haider MA, Ansari HA, Ishaq H, Kiyani A, Sohail K, et al. Automated feature detection in dental periapical radiographs by using deep learning. Oral Surg Oral Med Oral Pathol Oral Radiol. 2021;131(6):711–20.
Khanagar SB, Al-Ehaideb A, Maganur PC, Vishwanathaiah S, Patil S, Baeshen HA, et al. Developments, application, and performance of artificial intelligence in dentistry—a systematic review. J Dent Sci. 2021;16(1):508–22.
Khanna SS, Dhaimade PA. Artificial intelligence: transforming dentistry today. Indian J Basic Appl Med Res. 2017;6(3):161–7.
Khechoyan DY. Orthognathic surgery: general considerations. Semin Plast Surg. 2013;27(3):133–6.
Kim DW, Kim H, Nam W, Kim HJ, Cha IH. Machine learning to predict the occurrence of bisphosphonate-related osteonecrosis of the jaw associated with dental extraction: a preliminary report. Bone. 2018;116:207–14.
Kim J, Lee HS, Song IS, Jung KH. DeNTNet: deep neural transfer network for the detection of periodontal bone loss using panoramic dental radiographs. Sci Rep. 2019a;9(1):17615.
Kim Y, Lee KJ, Sunwoo L, Choi D, Nam CM, Cho J, et al. Deep learning in diagnosis of maxillary sinusitis using conventional radiography. Investig Radiol. 2019b;54(1):7–15.
Kim EH, Kim S, Kim HJ, Jeong HO, Lee J, Jang J, et al. Prediction of chronic periodontitis severity using machine learning models based on salivary bacterial copy number. Front Cell Infect Microbiol. 2020;10:571515.
Kim YH, Park JB, Chang MS, Ryu JJ, Lim WH, Jung SK. Influence of the depth of the convolutional neural networks on an artificial intelligence model for diagnosis of orthognathic surgery. J Pers Med. 2021;11(5):356.
Kim KS, Kim BK, Chung MJ, Cho HB, Cho BH, Jung YG. Detection of maxillary sinus fungal ball via 3-D CNN-based artificial intelligence: fully automated system and clinical validation. PLoS One. 2022;17(2):e0263125.
Knoops PGM, Papaioannou A, Borghi A, Breakey RWF, Wilson AT, Jeelani O, et al. A machine learning framework for automated diagnosis and computer-assisted planning in plastic and reconstructive surgery. Sci Rep. 2019;9(1):13597.

Kong Z, Xiong F, Zhang C, Fu Z, Zhang M, Weng J, et al. Automated maxillofacial segmentation in panoramic dental x-ray images using an efficient encoder-decoder network. IEEE Access. 2020;8:207822–33.

Kouznetsova VL, Li J, Romm E, Tsigelny IF. Finding distinctions between oral cancer and periodontitis using saliva metabolites and machine learning. Oral Dis. 2021;27(3):484–93.

Krois J, Ekert T, Meinhold L, Golla T, Kharbot B, Wittemeier A, et al. Deep learning for the radiographic detection of periodontal bone loss. Sci Rep. 2019;9(1):8495.

Kurt Bayrakdar S, Çelik Ö, Bayrakdar IŞ, Orhan K, Bilgir E, Odabas A, et al. Success of artificial intelligence system in determining alveolar bone loss from dental panoramic radiography images. Cumhuriyet Dent J. 2020;23(4):318–24.

Kurt Bayrakdar S, Orhan K, Bayrakdar IS, Bilgir E, Ezhov M, Gusarev M, et al. A deep learning approach for dental implant planning in cone-beam computed tomography images. BMC Med Imaging. 2021;21(1):86.

Kuwada C, Ariji Y, Fukuda M, Kise Y, Fujita H, Katsumata A, et al. Deep learning systems for detecting and classifying the presence of impacted supernumerary teeth in the maxillary incisor region on panoramic radiographs. Oral Surg Oral Med Oral Pathol Oral Radiol. 2020;130(4):464–9.

Kuze LS, Fornari F, Collares K, Della Bona A. Association between masticatory dysfunction and gastroesophageal reflux disease: a population-based study in the elderly. J Oral Rehabil. 2023;50(2):150–6.

Kwon O, Yong TH, Kang SR, Kim JE, Huh KH, Heo MS, et al. Automatic diagnosis for cysts and tumors of both jaws on panoramic radiographs using a deep convolution neural network. Dentomaxillofac Radiol. 2020;49(8):20200185.

Lahoud P, Diels S, Niclaes L, Van Aelst S, Willems H, Van Gerven A, et al. Development and validation of a novel artificial intelligence driven tool for accurate mandibular canal segmentation on CBCT. J Dent. 2022;116:103891.

Lang NP, Bartold PM. Periodontal health. J Periodontol. 2018;89(Suppl 1):S9–s16.

Langdon JD, Patel MF, Ord R, Brennan PA. Operative oral and maxillofacial surgery. Boca Raton, FL: CRC Press; 2017.

Le Cun Y, Jackel LD, Boser B, Denker JS, Graf HP, Guyon I, et al., editors. Handwritten digit recognition: applications of neural net chips and automatic learning. Neurocomputing: Algorithms, Architectures and Applications, Springer; 1990.

Lee JH, Jeong SN. Efficacy of deep convolutional neural network algorithm for the identification and classification of dental implant systems, using panoramic and periapical radiographs: a pilot study. Medicine (Baltimore). 2020;99(26):e20787.

Lee JH, Kim DH, Jeong SN, Choi SH. Diagnosis and prediction of periodontally compromised teeth using a deep learning-based convolutional neural network algorithm. J Periodontal Implant Sci. 2018;48(2):114–23.

Lee JH, Kim DH, Jeong SN. Diagnosis of cystic lesions using panoramic and cone beam computed tomographic images based on deep learning neural network. Oral Dis. 2020;26(1):152–8.

Lee D-W, Kim S-Y, Jeong S-N, Lee J-H. Artificial intelligence in fractured dental implant detection and classification: evaluation using dataset from two dental hospitals. Diagnostics. 2021;11(2):233.

Lee SJ, Chung D, Asano A, Sasaki D, Maeno M, Ishida Y, et al. Diagnosis of tooth prognosis using artificial intelligence. Diagnostics (Basel). 2022;12(6):1422.

Leroy R, Eaton KA, Savage A. Methodological issues in epidemiological studies of periodontitis—How can it be improved? BMC Oral Health. 2010;10:8.

Li F, Jia PY, Ouyang XY. Comparison of measurements on cone beam computed tomography for periodontal intrabony defect with intra-surgical measurements. Chin J Dent Res. 2015;18(3):171–6.

Li G-H, Hsung T-C, Ling W-K, Lam WY-H, Pelekos G, McGrath C, editors. Automatic site-specific multiple level gum disease detection based on deep neural network. 2021 15th International Symposium on Medical Information and Communication Technology (ISMICT), IEEE; 2021a.

Li W, Liang Y, Zhang X, Liu C, He L, Miao L, et al. A deep learning approach to automatic gingivitis screening based on classification and localization in RGB photos. Sci Rep. 2021b;11(1):16831.

Liu C, Jiao D, Liu Z. Artificial intelligence (AI)-aided disease prediction. Bio Integration. 2020;1(3):130–6.

Liu M, Wang S, Chen H, Liu Y. A pilot study of a deep learning approach to detect marginal bone loss around implants. BMC Oral Health. 2022;22(1):11.

Luther F, Morris DO, Hart C. Orthodontic preparation for orthognathic surgery: how long does it take and why? A retrospective study. Br J Oral Maxillofac Surg. 2003;41(6):401–6.

Macleod I, Heath N. Cone-beam computed tomography (CBCT) in dental practice. Dent Update. 2008;35(9):590–2, 48

Mallikarjun SA, Tiwari S, Sathyanarayana S, Devi PR. Haptics in periodontics. J Indian Soc Periodontol. 2014;18(1):112–3.

Mangano FG, Admakin O, Lerner H, Mangano C. Artificial intelligence and augmented reality for guided implant surgery planning: a proof of concept. J Dent. 2023;133:104485.

Mesko B. The role of artificial intelligence in precision medicine. Taylor & Francis; 2017. p. 239–41.

Mikulka J, Gescheidtová E, Kabrda M, Peřina V. Classification of jaw bone cysts and necrosis via the processing of orthopantomograms. Radioengineering. 2013;22(1):114–22.

Miladinović M, Mihailović B, Mladenović D, Duka M, Živković D, Mladenović S, et al. Artificial intelligence in clinical medicine and dentistry. Vojnosanit Pregl. 2017;74(3):267–72.

Miller PD Jr, Allen EP. The development of periodontal plastic surgery. Periodontology 2000. 1996;11(1):7–17.

Mine Y, Iwamoto Y, Okazaki S, Nakamura K, Takeda S, Peng TY, et al. Detecting the presence of supernumerary teeth during the early mixed dentition stage using deep learning algorithms: a pilot study. Int J Paediatr Dent. 2022;32(5):678–85.

Minnema J, Ernst A, van Eijnatten M, Pauwels R, Forouzanfar T, Batenburg KJ, et al. A review on the application of deep learning for CT reconstruction, bone segmentation and surgical planning in oral and maxillofacial surgery. Dentomaxillofac Radiol. 2022;51(7):20210437.

Mladenovic R, Kalevski K, Davidovic B, Jankovic S, Todorovic VS, Vasovic M. The role of artificial intelligence in the accurate diagnosis and treatment planning of non-syndromic supernumerary teeth: a case report in a six-year-old boy. Children. 2023;10(5):839.

Mohaideen K, Negi A, Verma DK, Kumar N, Sennimalai K, Negi A. Applications of artificial intelligence and machine learning in orthognathic surgery: a scoping review. J Stomatol Oral Maxillofac Surg. 2022;123(6):e962–e72.

Mohammad-Rahimi H, Motamedian SR, Pirayesh Z, Haiat A, Zahedrozegar S, Mahmoudinia E, et al. Deep learning in periodontology and oral implantology: a scoping review. J Periodontal Res. 2022;57(5):942–51.

Mol A. Imaging methods in periodontology. Periodontol 2000. 2004;34:34–48.

Monsarrat P, Bernard D, Marty M, Cecchin-Albertoni C, Doumard E, Gez L, et al. Systemic periodontal risk score using an innovative machine learning strategy: an observational study. J Pers Med. 2022;12(2):217.

Monterubbianesi R, Tosco V, Vitiello F, Orilisi G, Fraccastoro F, Putignano A, et al. Augmented, virtual and mixed reality in dentistry: a narrative review on the existing platforms and future challenges. Appl Sci. 2022;12(2):877.

Moran MBH, Faria M, Giraldi G, Bastos L, da Silva Inacio B, Conci A, editors. On using convolutional neural networks to classify periodontal bone destruction in periapical radiographs. 2020 IEEE International Conference on Bioinformatics and Biomedicine (BIBM), IEEE; 2020.

Morgan N, Van Gerven A, Smolders A, de Faria Vasconcelos K, Willems H, Jacobs R. Convolutional neural network for automatic maxillary sinus segmentation on cone-beam computed tomographic images. Sci Rep. 2022;12(1):7523.

Moriyama Y, Lee C, Date S, Kashiwagi Y, Narukawa Y, Nozaki K, et al., editors. Evaluation of dental image augmentation for the severity assessment of periodontal disease. 2019 International Conference on Computational Science and Computational Intelligence (CSCI), IEEE; 2019.

Na HS, Kim SY, Han H, Kim HJ, Lee JY, Lee JH, et al. Identification of potential oral microbial biomarkers for the diagnosis of periodontitis. J Clin Med. 2020;9(5):1549.

Nazir MA. Prevalence of periodontal disease, its association with systemic diseases and prevention. Int J Health Sci (Qassim). 2017;11(2):72–80.

Nguyen KT, Le BM, Li M, Almeida FT, Major PW, Kaipatur NR, et al. Localization of cementoenamel junction in intraoral ultrasonographs with machine learning. J Dent. 2021;112:103752.

Nishiyama M, Ishibashi K, Ariji Y, Fukuda M, Nishiyama W, Umemura M, et al. Performance of deep learning models constructed using panoramic radiographs from two hospitals to diagnose fractures of the mandibular condyle. Dentomaxillofac Radiol. 2021;50(7):20200611.

Nurtanio I, Astuti ER, Purnama IKE, Hariadi M, Purnomo MH. Classifying cyst and tumor lesion using support vector machine based on dental panoramic images texture features. IAENG Int J Comput Sci. 2013;40(1):29–32.

Orhan K, Bilgir E, Bayrakdar IS, Ezhov M, Gusarev M, Shumilov E. Evaluation of artificial intelligence for detecting impacted third molars on cone-beam computed tomography scans. J Stomatol Oral Maxillofac Surg. 2021;122(4):333–7.

Orhan K, Shamshiev M, Ezhov M, Plaksin A, Kurbanova A, Ünsal G, et al. AI-based automatic segmentation of craniomaxillofacial anatomy from CBCT scans for automatic detection of pharyngeal airway evaluations in OSA patients. Sci Rep. 2022;12(1):11863.

Ossowska A, Kusiak A, Świetlik D. Artificial intelligence in dentistry—narrative review. Int J Environ Res Public Health. 2022;19(6):3449.

Ozcan G, Sekerci AE. Classification of alveolar bone destruction patterns on maxillary molars by using cone-beam computed tomography. Niger J Clin Pract. 2017;20(8):1010–9.

Pan YC, Chan HL, Kong X, Hadjiiski LM, Kripfgans OD. Multi-class deep learning segmentation and automated measurements in periodontal sonograms of a porcine model. Dentomaxillofac Radiol. 2022;51(3):20210363.

Papapanou PN, Sanz M, Buduneli N, Dietrich T, Feres M, Fine DH, et al. Periodontitis: consensus report of workgroup 2 of the 2017 world workshop on the classification of periodontal and peri-implant diseases and conditions. J Periodontol. 2018;89(Suppl 1):S173–s82.

Parahitiyawa NB, Scully C, Leung WK, Yam WC, Jin LJ, Samaranayake LP. Exploring the oral bacterial flora: current status and future directions. Oral Dis. 2010;16(2):136–45.

Park CW, Seo SW, Kang N, Ko B, Choi BW, Park CM, et al. Artificial intelligence in health care: current applications and issues. J Korean Med Sci. 2020;35(42):e379.

Parmar P, Habib AR, Mendis D, Daniel A, Duvnjak M, Ho J, et al. An artificial intelligence algorithm that identifies middle turbinate pneumatisation (concha bullosa) on sinus computed tomography scans. J Laryngol Otol. 2020;134(4):328–31.

Poedjiastoeti W, Suebnukarn S. Application of convolutional neural network in the diagnosis of jaw tumors. Healthc Inform Res. 2018;24(3):236–41.

Preshaw PM. Host response modulation in periodontics. Periodontol 2000. 2008;48:92–110.

Rana M, Modrow D, Keuchel J, Chui C, Rana M, Wagner M, et al. Development and evaluation of an automatic tumor segmentation tool: a comparison between automatic, semi-automatic and manual segmentation of mandibular odontogenic cysts and tumors. J Craniomaxillofac Surg. 2015;43(3):355–9.

Rana A, Yauney G, Wong LC, Gupta O, Muftu A, Shah P, editors. Automated segmentation of gingival diseases from oral images. 2017 IEEE Healthcare Innovations and Point of Care Technologies (HI-POCT), IEEE; 2017.

Rasteau S, Ernenwein D, Savoldelli C, Bouletreau P. Artificial intelligence for oral and maxillofacial surgery: a narrative review. J Stomatol Oral Maxillofac Surg. 2022;123(3):276–82.

Real AD, Real OD, Sardina S, Oyonarte R. Use of automated artificial intelligence to predict the need for orthodontic extractions. Korean J Orthod. 2022;52(2):102–11.

Romm E, Li J, Kouznetsova VL, Tsigelny IF, editors. Machine learning strategies to distinguish oral cancer from periodontitis using salivary metabolites. Intelligent Systems and Applications: Proceedings of the 2020 Intelligent Systems Conference (IntelliSys) Volume 3, Springer; 2021.

Roongruangsilp P, Khongkhunthian P. The learning curve of artificial intelligence for dental implant treatment planning: a descriptive study. Appl Sci. 2021;11(21):10159.

Saini R, Marawar PP, Shete S, Saini S. Periodontitis, a true infection. J Glob Infect Dis. 2009;1(2):149–50.
Sakai T, Li H, Shimada T, Kita S, Iida M, Lee C, et al. Development of artificial intelligence model for supporting implant drilling protocol decision making. J Prosthodont Res. 2022;67:360–5.
Sayin I, Fakhoury R, Prasad VM, Remacle M, Lawson G. Transoral robotic surgery for base of tongue neoplasms. B-ENT. 2015;Suppl 24:45–50.
Scannapieco FA, Gershovich E. The prevention of periodontal disease-an overview. Periodontol 2000. 2020;84(1):9–13.
Schramm A, Suarez-Cunqueiro MM, Rücker M, Kokemueller H, Bormann KH, Metzger MC, et al. Computer-assisted therapy in orbital and mid-facial reconstructions. Int J Med Robot. 2009;5(2):111–24.
Schwalbe N, Wahl B. Artificial intelligence and the future of global health. Lancet. 2020;395(10236):1579–86.
Schwendicke F, Samek W, Krois J. Artificial intelligence in dentistry: chances and challenges. J Dent Res. 2020;99(7):769–74.
Scott J, Biancardi AM, Jones O, Andrew D. Artificial intelligence in periodontology: a scoping review. Dent J (Basel). 2023;11(2):43.
Seo J, Yang IH, Choi JY, Lee JH, Baek SH. Three-dimensional facial soft tissue changes after orthognathic surgery in cleft patients using artificial intelligence-assisted landmark autodigitization. J Craniofac Surg. 2021;32(8):2695–700.
Shamim MZM, Syed S, Shiblee M, Usman M, Ali SJ, Hussein HS, et al. Automated detection of oral pre-cancerous tongue lesions using deep learning for early diagnosis of oral cavity cancer. Comput J. 2022;65(1):91–104.
Shang W, Li Z, Li Y, editors. Identification of common oral disease lesions based on U-Net. 2021 IEEE 3rd International Conference on Frontiers Technology of Information and Computer (ICFTIC), IEEE; 2021.
Shen KL, Huang CL, Lin YC, Du JK, Chen FL, Kabasawa Y, et al. Effects of artificial intelligence-assisted dental monitoring intervention in patients with periodontitis: a randomized controlled trial. J Clin Periodontol. 2022;49(10):988–98.
Shin W, Yeom HG, Lee GH, Yun JP, Jeong SH, Lee JH, et al. Deep learning based prediction of necessity for orthognathic surgery of skeletal malocclusion using cephalogram in Korean individuals. BMC Oral Health. 2021;21(1):130.
Shujaat S, Jazil O, Willems H, Van Gerven A, Shaheen E, Politis C, et al. Automatic segmentation of the pharyngeal airway space with convolutional neural network. J Dent. 2021;111:103705.
Shujaat S, Riaz M, Jacobs R. Synergy between artificial intelligence and precision medicine for computer-assisted oral and maxillofacial surgical planning. Clin Oral Investig. 2023;27(3):897–906.
Silva N, Abusleme L, Bravo D, Dutzan N, Garcia-Sesnich J, Vernal R, et al. Host response mechanisms in periodontal diseases. J Appl Oral Sci. 2015;23(3):329–55.
Songa VM, Jampani ND, Babu V, Buggapati L, Mittapally S. Accuracy of cone beam computed tomography in diagnosis and treatment planning of periodontal bone defects: a case report. J Clin Diagn Res. 2014;8(12):Zd23–5.
Sroussi HY, Epstein JB, Bensadoun RJ, Saunders DP, Lalla RV, Migliorati CA, et al. Common oral complications of head and neck cancer radiation therapy: mucositis, infections, saliva change, fibrosis, sensory dysfunctions, dental caries, periodontal disease, and osteoradionecrosis. Cancer Med. 2017;6(12):2918–31.
Stehrer R, Hingsammer L, Staudigl C, Hunger S, Malek M, Jacob M, et al. Machine learning based prediction of perioperative blood loss in orthognathic surgery. J Craniomaxillofac Surg. 2019;47(11):1676–81.
Subramanian M, Wojtusciszyn A, Favre L, Boughorbel S, Shan J, Letaief KB, et al. Precision medicine in the era of artificial intelligence: implications in chronic disease management. J Transl Med. 2020;18(1):472.

Sukegawa S, Yoshii K, Hara T, Matsuyama T, Yamashita K, Nakano K, et al. Multi-task deep learning model for classification of dental implant brand and treatment stage using dental panoramic radiograph images. Biomol Ther. 2021;11(6):815.

Sukegawa S, Yoshii K, Hara T, Tanaka F, Yamashita K, Kagaya T, et al. Is attention branch network effective in classifying dental implants from panoramic radiograph images by deep learning? PLoS One. 2022;17(7):e0269016.

Sunmoo Y, Odlum M, Lee Y, Thomas C, Kronish IM, Davidson KW, et al. Applying deep learning to understand predictors of tooth mobility among Urban Latinos. Stud Health Technol Inform. 2018;251:241.

Suphanantachat S, Tantikul K, Tamsailom S, Kosalagood P, Nisapakultorn K, Tavedhikul K. Comparison of clinical values between cone beam computed tomography and conventional intraoral radiography in periodontal and infrabony defect assessment. Dentomaxillofac Radiol. 2017;46(6):20160461.

Tang H, Yuan C, Ma Z, Zhu C, Tong P, Gallagher JE, et al. The potentiality of salivary peptide biomarkers for screening patients with periodontal diseases by mass spectrometry. Clin Chim Acta. 2019;495:278–86.

Tanriver G, Soluk Tekkesin M, Ergen O. Automated detection and classification of oral lesions using deep learning to detect oral potentially malignant disorders. Cancers (Basel). 2021;13(11):2766.

Thanathornwong B, Suebnukarn S. Automatic detection of periodontal compromised teeth in digital panoramic radiographs using faster regional convolutional neural networks. Imaging Sci Dent. 2020;50(2):169–74.

Theilade J. An evaluation of the reliability of radiographs in the measurement of bone loss in periodontal disease. Univ Toronto Undergrad Dent J. 1965;2:19–27.

Troiano G, Nibali L, Petsos H, Eickholz P, Saleh MHA, Santamaria P, et al. Development and international validation of logistic regression and machine-learning models for the prediction of 10-year molar loss. J Clin Periodontol. 2023;50(3):348–57.

Tugnait A, Clerehugh V, Hirschmann PN. Use of the basic periodontal examination and radiographs in the assessment of periodontal diseases in general dental practice. J Dent. 2004;32(1):17–25.

Valko M, Leibfritz D, Moncol J, Cronin MT, Mazur M, Telser J. Free radicals and antioxidants in normal physiological functions and human disease. Int J Biochem Cell Biol. 2007;39(1):44–84.

van Staveren HJ, van Veen RL, Speelman OC, Witjes MJ, Star WM, Roodenburg JL. Classification of clinical autofluorescence spectra of oral leukoplakia using an artificial neural network: a pilot study. Oral Oncol. 2000;36(3):286–93.

Vandenberghe B, Jacobs R, Yang J. Diagnostic validity (or acuity) of 2D CCD versus 3D CBCT-images for assessing periodontal breakdown. Oral Surg Oral Med Oral Pathol Oral Radiol Endod. 2007;104(3):395–401.

Vicini C, Dallan I, Canzi P, Frassineti S, Nacci A, Seccia V, et al. Transoral robotic surgery of the tongue base in obstructive sleep apnea-hypopnea syndrome: anatomic considerations and clinical experience. Head Neck. 2012;34(1):15–22.

Vikram K, Karjodkar FR. Decision support systems in dental decision making: an introduction. J Evid Based Dent Pract. 2009;9(2):73–6.

Vollmer A, Saravi B, Vollmer M, Lang GM, Straub A, Brands RC, et al. Artificial intelligence-based prediction of oroantral communication after tooth extraction utilizing preoperative panoramic radiography. Diagnostics (Basel). 2022;12(6):1406.

Vuorjoki-Ranta TR, Lobbezoo F, Vehkalahti M, Tuomilehto H, Ahlberg J. Treatment of obstructive sleep apnoea patients in community dental care: knowledge and attitudes among general dental practitioners and specialist dentists. J Oral Rehabil. 2016;43(12):937–42.

Vyas M. Photography: a diagnostic tool. J Int Clin Dent Res Organization. 2018;10(2):59.

Walvekar RR, Peters G, Hardy E, Alsfeld L, Stromeyer FW, Anderson D, et al. Robotic-assisted transoral removal of a bilateral floor of mouth ranulas. World J Surg Oncol. 2011;9:78.

Wang SY, Pershing S, Lee AY. Big data requirements for artificial intelligence. Curr Opin Ophthalmol. 2020;31(5):318–23.

Wang C-W, Hao Y, Di Gianfilippo R, Sugai J, Li J, Gong W, et al. Machine learning-assisted immune profiling stratifies peri-implantitis patients with unique microbial colonization and clinical outcomes. Theranostics. 2021;11(14):6703.

Warin K, Limprasert W, Suebnukarn S, Jinaporntham S, Jantana P. Automatic classification and detection of oral cancer in photographic images using deep learning algorithms. J Oral Pathol Med. 2021;50(9):911–8.

Warin K, Limprasert W, Suebnukarn S, Paipongna T, Jantana P, Vicharueang S. Maxillofacial fracture detection and classification in computed tomography images using convolutional neural network-based models. Sci Rep. 2023;13(1):3434.

Weiss R 2nd, Read-Fuller A. Cone beam computed tomography in oral and maxillofacial surgery: an evidence-based review. Dent J (Basel). 2019;7(2):52.

Wu Y, Wang F, Fan S, Chow JK. Robotics in dental implantology. Oral Maxillofac Surg Clin North Am. 2019;31(3):513–8.

Xiang X, Sowa MG, Iacopino AM, Maev RG, Hewko MD, Man A, et al. An update on novel non-invasive approaches for periodontal diagnosis. J Periodontol. 2010;81(2):186–98.

Xiao Y, Liang Q, Zhou L, He X, Lv L, Chen J, et al. Construction of a new automatic grading system for jaw bone mineral density level based on deep learning using cone beam computed tomography. Sci Rep. 2022;12(1):12841.

Xu J, Wang L, Sun H, Liu S. Evaluation of the effect of comprehensive nursing interventions on plaque control in patients with periodontal disease in the context of artificial intelligence. J Healthc Eng. 2022;2022:6505672.

Yan K-X, Liu L, Li H. Application of machine learning in oral and maxillofacial surgery. Artific Intellig Med Imaging. 2021;2(6):104–14.

Yang H, Jo E, Kim HJ, Cha I-h, Jung Y-S, Nam W, et al. Deep learning for automated detection of cyst and tumors of the jaw in panoramic radiographs. J Clin Med. 2020;9(6):1839.

Yilmaz E, Kayikcioglu T, Kayipmaz S. Computer-aided diagnosis of periapical cyst and keratocystic odontogenic tumor on cone beam computed tomography. Comput Methods Prog Biomed. 2017;146:91–100.

Yoo JH, Yeom HG, Shin W, Yun JP, Lee JH, Jeong SH, et al. Deep learning based prediction of extraction difficulty for mandibular third molars. Sci Rep. 2021;11(1):1954.

Yoon S, Odlum M, Lee Y, Choi T, Kronish IM, Davidson KW, et al. Applying deep learning to understand predictors of tooth mobility among Urban Latinos. Stud Health Technol Inform. 2018;251:241–4.

You W, Hao A, Li S, Wang Y, Xia B. Deep learning-based dental plaque detection on primary teeth: a comparison with clinical assessments. BMC Oral Health. 2020;20(1):141.

Zhang W, Li J, Li ZB, Li Z. Predicting postoperative facial swelling following impacted mandibular third molars extraction by using artificial neural networks evaluation. Sci Rep. 2018;8(1):12281.

Zhang YN, Xia KR, Li CY, Wei BL, Zhang B. Review of breast cancer pathologigcal image processing. Biomed Res Int. 2021;2021:1994764.

Zhu T, Chen D, Wu F, Zhu F, Zhu H. Artificial intelligence model to detect real contact relationship between mandibular third molars and inferior alveolar nerve based on panoramic radiographs. Diagnostics (Basel). 2021;11(9):1664.

AI in Orthodontics

8

Kaan Orhan and Hakan Amasya

Introduction

The remnants of the Neanderthal man who lived in about 50,000 BC represent the primal evidence for crooked teeth. The first written document regarding attempts to correct the crooked teeth belongs to 3000 years ago. Archeological findings revealed that in some of the Egyptian mummies, there were metal bands wrapped around individual teeth. Considering the material options of that period, catgut was speculated to be used for closing the gaps between teeth. Greek and Etruscan artifacts are the examples of primitive orthodontic appliances, which were well designed considering their period. Celcus (25 BC–AD 50) proposed the removal of the retaining deciduous teeth and using finger pressure to correct the position of the permanent tooth. Over time, new techniques and tools such as brackets and appliances were discovered that can be used to correct the teeth. While the early motivation for regulating the teeth was a good smile, orthodontics became a scientific foundation with the inclusion of occlusion in treatment planning. Nowadays, the expectation of the patients stands out as a better facial aesthetics (Wahl 2005). As the expectations of the patients have changed over time, there have also been major changes in the tools that can be used to achieve such goals. With spread of the digital technologies in practice of orthodontics, the volume of the digital data produced per patient is increasing. Machine learning tools can provide clinicians' patient-specific solutions. In this chapter, common study topics regarding the use of AI or ML in orthodontics is defined under four categories to provide information about the general

K. Orhan
Faculty of Dentistry, Department of Dentomaxillofacial Radiology, Ankara University, Ankara, Turkey

H. Amasya (✉)
Faculty of Dentistry, Department of Dentomaxillofacial Radiology, Istanbul University-Cerrahpaşa, Istanbul, Turkey

K. Orhan, R. Jagtap (eds.), *Artificial Intelligence in Dentistry*,
https://doi.org/10.1007/978-3-031-43827-1_8

concepts and how to implement such AI tools into the clinical practice of orthodontics.

1. Diagnosis and Treatment Planning
   (a) Image Analysis and Interpretation
   (b) Computer-Aided Diagnosis
   (c) Treatment Simulation and Outcome Prediction
2. Treatment Monitoring and Adjustment
   (a) Remote Monitoring
   (b) Intelligent Appliances and Devices
   (c) Adaptive Treatment Planning
3. Predictive Analytics and Outcome Assessment
   (a) Treatment Duration Prediction
   (b) Treatment Success Assessment
   (c) Long-term Stability Analysis
4. Patient Experience and Engagement
   (a) Virtual Consultations and Follow-Ups
   (b) Personalized Treatment Progress Tracking
   (c) Gamification and AR/VR in Orthodontics

Diagnosis and Treatment Planning

Image Analysis and Interpretation

Developing machine learning tools and using them for patient-specific solutions are possible only with the digital patient data. The system may analyze digital data from a single source or may combine multiple sources to produce an output. Information such as gender or chronological age can be available in text format. In orthodontics, digital radiographic data may be obtained as lateral or frontal cephalograms or orthopantomogram for plain imaging or cone-beam computed tomography (CBCT) for volumetric imaging, commonly. In addition, volumetric optical scanning technology provides a more precise information for both intraoral and extraoral surfaces, with intraoral or extraoral scanning devices. Medical imaging devices, such as CBCT and cephalometric, ultrasonic, and magnetic resonance imaging, are compatible with digital imaging and communication in medicine (DICOM) format defined in ISO 12052:2017, currently. Radiography provides information regarding the internal structure of objects. Optical scanning is another solution to obtain the surface data; however, the information is limited to the surface of the total object volume and limited as the human visual system. Optical scanners can be classified as intraoral and extraoral devices. Intraoral devices can be used to record the status of the present teeth directly, which eliminates the need for conventional dental impression or cast models. Extraoral devices may be used to scan the cast models optically or scan the face profile of the patient. Some CBCT devices may have integrated optical cameras to record the facial profile of the patient during radiographic image acquisition. Most CBCT devices can digitize the physical cast models radiographically. Volumetric surface information can be in several file formats such as .STL, .PLY, and .OBJ, awaiting to be combined with such radiographic data.

As digital technologies became widespread, various machine learning tools began to be used to process the patient data more efficiently. Such tools can be integrated into the clinical workflow as fully automatic, or it can give partial or complete control to its user. Thus, it is possible for the clinician to choose the system most suitable for the clinical workflow and implement the system effectively. For example, cephalometric analysis is based on identifying the anatomical landmarks on radiographs and then measuring the distances, angles, and ratios to evaluate the sagittal and vertical relationships of the anatomical structures. A system developed for cephalometric analysis may require manual marking of the landmarks, or may provide fully automatic landmark detection, or the user may validate or revise the position of landmarks suggested by the system. An important issue here is that these systems do not represent a superior decision that never makes mistakes, and they do make mistakes just like the humans. It is clear that a fully automated workflow will save time, but it is up to the user to decide how tolerable the mistakes made by the system will be in the clinic. There are also variances among clinicians in determining the location of cephalometric points, and it may be wise to be skeptical about this part of the system; however, it is possible to leave the work to the computer in the calculations after the location of the points is determined, more confidently. Computer-assisted cephalometric analysis of two-dimensional cephalometric images and volumetric CBCT images has always attracted the attention of researchers, and today, it is possible to find various commercial software that can be used for this task. Advances in cloud technology have made it possible to develop online-based systems. The advantages of these systems are that they do not require a powerful computer in the clinic as the analyses are calculated on a central computer and can be accessed from different platforms such as personal computers and mobile phones; however, it has some limitations such as internet access is required for its use (Leonardi et al. 2008; Alsubai 2022).

Evaluation of skeletal bone development has a critical role in orthodontic treatment planning. Skeletal maturity indicators can be found on various radiographic, such as lateral cephalograms or hand-wrist radiographs. Radiographic bone age assessment with machine learning is another popular subject for researchers. Similar to cephalometric analysis, the maturation indicators can be segmented automatically, or user-assisted, and the system generates an output according to the input data and the established mathematical model. Such systems can analyze with a single-image type as well as combine different images and data. The extent of trust in these systems depends on the ability of the clinician to explain the final decisions made, and combining more than one type of indicator for a final decision is always suggested (Dallora et al. 2019; Amasya et al. 2020; Amasya et al. 2023).

Digital radiography provides a wide range of applications of machine learning tools as the data is produced in numerical format, already. In theory, it is possible to transfer all radiographic examinations to machine learning. Deep learning and convolutional neural network models have gained popularity with their superior performances in image processing over time; however, lack of the explainability of the results should not be ignored. Systems for evaluating asymmetry or measuring the sinus and airway volume can be developed for both two- or three-dimensional imaging. Image processing applications are not limited to just radiographic data, digital facial photos and surface scan data of intraoral or extraoral regions can be processed for suggestions regarding the functional and aesthetic expectations. While some repetitive work may be acceptable to be done by these systems, the clinician plays an active role in the final decision phase, and it is the clinician's responsibility for how much of the analysis process is delegated to automation. Parameters such as the margins of error of the systems and their effects in the clinic should be well decided. It may be beneficial for the clinician to take control, especially in decisions that will have a major impact on the diagnosis, treatment, and patient benefit (Orhan et al. 2022).

Computer-Aided Diagnosis

Computer-aided diagnosis (CAD) systems analyze the digital input data, which may represent various features, and generate an output to aid the physician in clinical decision-making process. Most CAD systems exploit radiographic data, but not all CAD systems are dependent on it. For example, in orthodontic treatment planning, a suggestion can be produced by entering only manual measurements in text format, without involving any radiographic procedure, in making the decision of tooth extraction. CAD systems may accept data from a single source or can combine several sources such as the gender, chronological age, geographic location, laboratory results, medical history, and more.

How reliable such CAD systems in determining diagnosis, treatment planning, predicting the prognosis, monitoring the treatment, motivating the patient, and improving the execution of orthodontics? Parameters such as the clinician's training and experience play a critical role in conventional clinical decision process; however, what is the role of CAD systems in final decision at current digital era? The perception of an intelligent machine is limited to what was provided in the developing, and the resulting suggestions may represent what the clinicians' been missing or may be biased due to limited perception. Perhaps the ideal solution is neither to hand over all the work entirely to the machines nor to ignore such improvements, but ideally, it is to understand why the software came up with this suggestion and how to implement it into the clinical setting for the patient's benefit.

CAD systems can analyze large volumes of patient data at an incredible speed, which can be turned into an advantage especially when time is limited. Thus, useful suggestions for diagnosis and treatment can be generated, for example, from some archival records that would not even be considered without CAD. In cases where the training and experience of the clinician is insufficient, the recommendations of a CAD system prepared by experts can guide the clinician. In this scenario, the final decision about the accuracy and applicability of the suggestions of the CAD is again with the practitioner. It may be rational for the clinician to consider the suggestions that he can explain as primary, and what he cannot explain as secondary, in establishing a diagnosis and treatment plan. However, adding annotation modules to

CAD systems is beneficial both for clinician understanding of recommendations and for the postgraduate education concept (Alam et al. 2023; Baxi et al. 2022; Gupta 2020).

Treatment Simulation and Outcome Prediction

Various tools can be used to digitize information such as teeth, jaws, or soft tissue profile of a patient in the clinic, and AI tools can be involved to enhance the process. The data sources can be text based, as well as planar and volumetric radiographic and optical information, and more. Clinical recordings can be an example to text-based data, may be automatically retrieved from a source as allowed, or may require manual input. Virtual models and digital impressions, created through intraoral scanners and 3D imaging, provide volumetric representations of the patient's teeth and oral structures in digital environment. AI algorithms combine different patient data, such as digital models, facial scans, radiographs, and clinical records, to create a comprehensive picture of the patient's orthodontic state in a holistic view and support treatment planning decisions.

Electronic storage of virtual models and digital impressions allows for quick access, retrieval, as well as improved communication and teamwork among orthodontic specialists. Moreover, alternative treatment scenarios can be simulated using AI-based treatment planning tools, to decide the best treatment strategy depending on the unique requirements and objectives of the patient by taking into account variables like treatment time, complexity, and anticipated effects. Algorithms may be used to analyze patient data to predict treatment duration, assess treatment success, and evaluate long-term stability and pave the way for an individualized treatment planning. With the use of these tools in the clinic, the patient better understands the process that will take place in the orthodontic treatment journey and, in a sense, offers the opportunity to make shared decisions for more predictable results.

Each individual's growth and development are unique and may not be predicted definitely. Similarly, each patient's reaction to treatment is different, influenced by many factors. The use of such systems in determining the right treatment plan can contribute to improving predictions, and it can make the results closer to patient expectation. Indeed, it should be clarified that simulations in these systems are only an estimate and may not reflect the final treatment outcomes definitely (Elnagar et al. 2020).

Treatment Monitoring and Adjustment

Remote Monitoring

In a routine orthodontic treatment process, the changes caused by the treatments applied to the individual are followed by consecutive examinations. Today, with the spread of digital technologies in daily lives, cameras such as personal cell phones are widely available to patients. Real-time data on treatment outcomes, such as tooth movement, occlusal alterations, and patient compliance, can be collected using such devices remotely. Apparatuses such as a mouth opener or camera stabilizer can be used to improve standardization in the images that the patient will produce at home. With various ML tools, the user can be guided in image acquisition, and the changes in the produced images can be recorded.

Such systems are not a substitute for a detailed physical examination but can contribute to the physician's remote monitoring of changes in the patient. With applications such as self-ligating brackets, its use may be beneficial in cases where follow-up sessions need to be long. Also, remote monitoring makes it possible to identify issues or anomalies early on, allowing orthodontists to take immediate action and modify the treatment plan as needed. The variety of remote monitoring instruments is increasing along with the developments in wearable orofacial and tele-orthodontic technologies (Caruso et al. 2021).

Intelligent Appliances and Devices

The idea of monitoring the patient's treatment compliance with wearable electronic circuits and sensors started in 1970s. The primal studies focused on recording the duration of the patients' extraoral headgear usage with electronic timer and memory circuits. It was reported that the patients who were reported to be followed up used their appliances for a longer period of time. In a study using Aledyne timer, it was learned that young patients used their appliances for a longer time. Due to the technology of that period, intraoral applications remained after the 1990s, and the use of these circuits was uncomfortable due to their size and weight. Over time, microelectronic sensors with the sizes enabling the embedded use in functional appliances, retainers, and other intraoral applications have evolved. Most of the intraoral microelectronic sensors are temperature sensitive to monitor wear time. Also, the spatial orientation/position can be recorded, and sensor readings can be received using static stations or may be transferred via Bluetooth. As microelectronic sensors that are even smaller, have longer battery lives, and are more reliable will be produced, the use of these technologies in orthodontics will increase.

The diagnosis, treatment planning, and monitoring can be improved in obstructive sleep apnea (OSA), by combining all the available data from several sensors such as the internal measuring unit in a mobile phone. Overnight polysomnography is considered as the gold standard in diagnosis of OSA; however, such concepts enable the tracking of more than just a night to improve the patient benefit. Real-time monitoring systems can assess bite forces and occlusion, identifying imbalances or abnormal patterns. Masticatory muscle forces can be monitored using portable surface electromyography equipment, which can provide improvements in the sleep bruxism diagnosis and treatment outcomes. Several sensor technologies are studied to track the mandibular motion, such as mechanical, inertial, acoustic, magnetic, optical, or radio frequency sensors. Among them, optical, inertial, and magnetic sensors have been successfully used lab-based, hospital-based, home-based, or ambulatory subjects (Prasad et al. 2023).

Digital data from the developed intraoral and extraoral sensors can be used to develop ML tools. For example, a potential 3D sensor inside a bracket to monitor orthodontic forces may provide data to optimize the forces. A sensor to detect pH changes in the mouth can give feedback to both the physician and the patient about the risk of caries. Patients can track their treatment progress, and as a result, patient engagement and motivation can be increased throughout the course of treatment. Sensor fusion is the process of combining data from multiple sensors; thus, uncertainty relative to data from an individual sensor can be reduced with ML tools. As sensor technologies progress, different applications will develop in this area, so for now, limitations such as sensor size and battery need to be overcome to be used widely.

Adaptive Treatment Planning

Pretreatment simulations with digital systems may not be realized exactly. Treatment progress can be evaluated considering changes in tooth positions, facial profile, occlusal relationships, patient compliance, or tooth mobility, using ML tools to help in identifying the need for treatment adjustments or modifications. Based on the analysis of patient data and treatment progress, AI systems may provide personalized treatment recommendations and modifications, which include adjustments in appliance mechanics, treatment mechanics, or changes in treatment protocols. Transferring the differences between the planned and the actual allows the early predicted treatment output to be updated, and the treatment plan can be optimized by the orthodontists' decisions with data-driven suggestions to direct the treatment outcomes towards the desired results.

Technologies such as adaptive treatment planning help achieve more predictable treatment outcomes and improve physician-patient communication. However, these tools are not available in all of the systems which contain AI elements. For example, a system developed for simulating treatment and estimating treatment outcomes can be used in adaptive treatment planning only if its developer includes it in the system; otherwise, it will not be possible to transfer the data generated during the treatment and analyze it. In adaptive treatment planning, the effect of new information given to the system on the treatment plan and results should be well analyzed, the differences should be explained to the patient using an appropriate language, and it should be reminded that the actual treatment results may differ from the simulated outcomes.

Predictive Analytics and Outcome Assessment

Treatment Duration Prediction

AI tools can improve the process of treatment duration estimation. In addition to the past treatment data, patient characteristics, and treatment plans, input data may contain various elements, including patient compliance, intricacy of the treatment, and tooth movement patterns, to make more precise predictions. AI tools can be used to compare the patient's predicted simulation and current status for the relevant examination date, to reveal the change in estimated treatment time earlier. This enables orthodontists to identify any deviations earlier and make necessary adjustments to keep treatment on track. In this way, the practitioner can take precautions earlier if there is a lack of information or motivation about the patient and may have the opportunity to make a decision of changing treatment parameters earlier when required.

Each individual's response to treatment is different, and simulations can be revised and improved with the new data obtained at consecutive examinations. In cases where planned and actual are different, algorithms can analyze to the current status and make recommendations that can shorten the treatment time while maintaining the optimal outcomes. Thus, patient satisfaction can be increased as the treatment time is shortened. Moreover, these simulations can be visualized, making it easier for the patient to understand the variances.

Treatment Success Assessment

The success of an orthodontic treatment experience can be determined not by a single criterion but by evaluating many factors together. When a treatment planned with AI support in the digital workflow and carried out with the decisions taken by the orthodontist within the doctor-patient relationship, the comparison of these with the previously planned factors such as the resulting tooth position, occlusion, or treatment duration can give an idea in determining the success of the applied treatment. In AI-assisted orthodontic treatment process, the simulation is not expected to realize exactly, and minor differences between the simulated and the actual outcomes are acceptable. However, especially in cases where there are major deviations, it is useful to analyze the reason for this by the clinician and to take the necessary precautions for the future treatments. Predictive analytics can also incorporate patient feedback through surveys or questionnaires to evaluate subjective criteria like patient contentment, changes in quality of life, and functional results.

Long-Term Stability Analysis

Some relapse or instability may occur after terminating the application of the orthodontic forces in variable magnitude. The amount and pattern of this occurrence may be predicted using ML tools, by analyzing the patients' treatment recordings and finding the elements causing treatment instability or relapse. This aids in creating individualized retention programs to improve in maintaining treatment results over the long term. Risk of relapse can be predicted based on elements including bone discrepancies, dental anomalies, and treatment features and enables orthodontists to take preventative steps to lessen the chance of relapse. AI-powered remote monitoring systems can track treated patients over an extended period of time to gauge how consistently positive treatment outcomes are. This makes it easier to spot any changes or prospective problems that might call for more assistance. These technologies aid the orthodontists to optimize treatment process, develop personalized retention strategies, and apply improved treatment strategies for the patient's benefit. Creating 3D virtual simulations of how the patient's dentition and facial appearance will change in case of relapse may enhance the awareness of the patient to the possible scenarios and may enable early detection (Li et al. 2021).

Patient Experience and Engagement

Virtual Consultations and Follow-Ups

Some of the communication systems that are especially designed for virtual follow-ups and consultations can have integrated AI tools and provide user-friendly and secure remote communication between the patient and the orthodontist. These technologies allow orthodontists and patients to collaborate effectively by enabling real-time videoconferencing, messaging, and file sharing. Such tools can be used for remote monitoring of patients, can be used to make personalized recommendations according to the protocol chosen by the physician, and can be used to reduce the number of clinical visits required. During virtual consultations, patient information can be kept private and secure with various AI technologies. Sensitive data can be protected by encryption and authentication systems, while AI algorithms may help to discover and stop unwanted access or data breaches.

Personalized Treatment Progress Tracking

Patient portals or mobile applications where the patient can access the pre-planned progress throughout the treatment are developed for some orthodontic applications. With these mobile applications, the entire planned treatment process can be shown to the patient with 3D virtual models, and the changes that will occur over time in tooth alignment or occlusion can be visually presented to the patient to be compared with the current situation. The patient can be reminded of their future visits or can be informed when the milestones in the treatment are reached. Patients can visually see their improvements, fostering motivation and engagement throughout the treatment journey.

Gamification and AR/VR in Orthodontics

Gamification techniques, such as rewards or challenges, can be included in the mobile orthodontics applications to increase the motivation and compliance of the patients. Users can earn points or badges for following treatment guidelines, practicing good oral hygiene, or attending appointments, which makes their orthodontic experience more enjoyable and motivating. It can be used to remind patients in a game concept what they need to do routinely. These systems can be customized by the user with cosmetic features and made more fun, but the system must stick to the protocols determined by the practitioner.

Virtual reality (VR) and augmented reality (AR) technologies can be used for both educational purposes or providing care to patients. In educational applications, possible treatment scenarios can be experienced in a virtual space, this experience can be advanced one step further implementing haptic devices, and education can be reinforced with simulations based on real patient data. Patients can experience virtual simulations in 3D and see the prediction for how their teeth alignment will change over time and better comprehend their course of treatment. Orthodontic practices improve patient experience and engagement by using virtual consultations, tailored treatment progress tracking, gamification, and virtual reality. Moreover, such systems can be beneficial in pain and anxiety management

(Gandedkar et al. 2021). Various medical products can be designed using the digital volumetric data in this process and can be converted into physical products with additive manufacturing technologies.

Of course, all these dazzling processes can be misleading, especially for patients. The various possibilities and tools offered by the systems may lead to overconfidence in the system, increased expectations for the predictability of treatment results, and disappointment at the end of the process. It should be ensured that patients understand well that the simulations offered by these systems are only an estimate and the actual treatment experience may differ. Similarly, orthodontists who make clinical decisions should not surrender themselves to the suggestions and plans made by the systems and should not hesitate to intervene for the benefit of the patient, when necessary, by analyzing the whole process well and being aware of treatment-induced changes.

References

Alam MK, Abutayyem H, Kanwal B, Shayeb MAL. Future of orthodontics—a systematic review and meta-analysis on the emerging trends in this field. J Clin Med. 2023;12(2):532.

Alsubai S. A critical review on the 3D cephalometric analysis using machine learning. Computers. 2022;11(11):154.

Amasya H, Cesur E, Yıldırım D, Orhan K. Validation of cervical vertebral maturation stages: artificial intelligence vs human observer visual analysis. Am J Orthod Dentofac Orthop. 2020;158(6):e173–e9.

Amasya H, Aydoğan T, Cesur E, Kemaloğlu Alagöz N, Uğurlu M, Bayrakdar İŞ, et al. Using artificial intelligence models to evaluate envisaged points initially: a pilot study. Proc Inst Mech Eng H J Eng Med. 2023;237:09544119231173165.

Baxi S, Shadani K, Kesri R, Ukey A, Joshi C, Hardiya H. Recent advanced diagnostic aids in orthodontics. Cureus. 2022;14(11):e31921.

Caruso S, Caruso S, Pellegrino M, Skafi R, Nota A, Tecco S. A knowledge-based algorithm for automatic monitoring of orthodontic treatment: the dental monitoring system. Two cases. Sensors. 2021;21(5):1856.

Dallora AL, Anderberg P, Kvist O, Mendes E, Diaz Ruiz S, Sanmartin Berglund J. Bone age assessment with various machine learning techniques: a systematic literature review and meta-analysis. PLoS One. 2019;14(7):e0220242.

Elnagar MH, Aronovich S, Kusnoto B. Digital workflow for combined orthodontics and orthognathic surgery. Oral Maxillofac Surg Clin. 2020;32(1):1–14.

Gandedkar NH, Wong MT, Darendeliler MA, editors. Role of virtual reality (VR), augmented reality (AR) and artificial intelligence (AI) in tertiary education and research of orthodontics: An insight. Seminars in Orthodontics, Elsevier; 2021.

Gupta A. Challenges for computer aided diagnostics using X-ray and tomographic reconstruction images in craniofacial applications. Int J Comput Vision Robot. 2020;10(4):360–71.

Leonardi R, Giordano D, Maiorana F, Spampinato C. Automatic cephalometric analysis: a systematic review. Angle Orthod. 2008;78(1):145–51.

Li Y, Shao Y, Yu Y, Ye Y, Lu Y, Chang S. Finite element analysis of orthodontic relapse in different maxillary arch form. BIO Integrat. 2021;2(4):152–60.

Orhan K, Shamshiev M, Ezhov M, Plaksin A, Kurbanova A, Ünsal G, et al. AI-based automatic segmentation of craniomaxillofacial anatomy from CBCT scans for automatic detection of pharyngeal airway evaluations in OSA patients. Sci Rep. 2022;12(1):1–9.

Prasad S, Arunachalam S, Boillat T, Ghoneima A, Gandedkar N, Diar-Bakirly S. Wearable orofacial technology and orthodontics. Dent J. 2023;11(1):24.

Wahl N. Orthodontics in 3 millennia. Chapter 1: antiquity to the mid-19th century. Am J Orthod Dentofac Orthop. 2005;127(2):255–9.

AI on Oral Mucosal Lesion Detection

9

Gaye Keser, Filiz Namdar Pekiner, and Kaan Orhan

Artificial Intelligence: Concepts and Terminology

In recent years, the application of deep machine learning, an artificial intelligence discipline, has been a rising focus of interest in prognostic medicine (Alabi et al. 2021; Pai and Pai 2021; Hogarty et al. 2019). Artificial intelligence is an area of computer science that deals with decision-making or classification in broad terms. AI aspires to outperform human cognitive abilities so that automated decisions may be made. Image identification frequently employs machine learning, an artificial intelligence application. In general, a huge dataset exposes the machine, or algorithm, to new information. The method may then be applied to previously unknown data once it has been learned. The potential benefits of this technique in healthcare are obvious: robots can learn from enormous datasets in a short amount of time and apply what they've learned to fresh data without becoming fatigued or experiencing intra-observer replication error (Wada et al. 2020; Saba et al. 2019).

Artificial Intelligence Terminologies

AI is described as "the scientific study of the concepts underlying cognition and intelligent behavior and their application in computers." In its most basic form, AI is a discipline of computer science that involves developing systems with the

G. Keser (✉) · F. Namdar Pekiner
Faculty of Dentistry, Department of Dentomaxillofacial Radiology, Marmara University, İstanbul, Turkey
e-mail: gaye.sezgin@marmara.edu.tr

K. Orhan
Faculty of Dentistry, Department of Dentomaxillofacial Radiology, Ankara University, Ankara, Turkey

Ankara University Medical Design Application and Research Center (MEDITAM), Ankara, Turkey

K. Orhan, R. Jagtap (eds.), *Artificial Intelligence in Dentistry*,
https://doi.org/10.1007/978-3-031-43827-1_9

objective of emulating human cognition and data processing operations (Quer et al. 2017; Hogarty et al. 2019; De et al. 2020; Schwendicke et al. 2020; Huang et al. 2017; Silver et al. 2016).

Machine Learning

It is challenging to exactly characterize AI. In Alan Turing's landmark article "Computing Machinery and Intelligence," he developed the well-known Turing test, according to which a computer is regarded intelligent if it is indistinguishable from a person in conversation to an unbiased observer. In contemporary vernacular, artificial general intelligence refers to a machine's capacity to communicate, think, and act autonomously in both known and unfamiliar situations in a way comparable to that of a person. This remains much beyond the capabilities of existing approaches

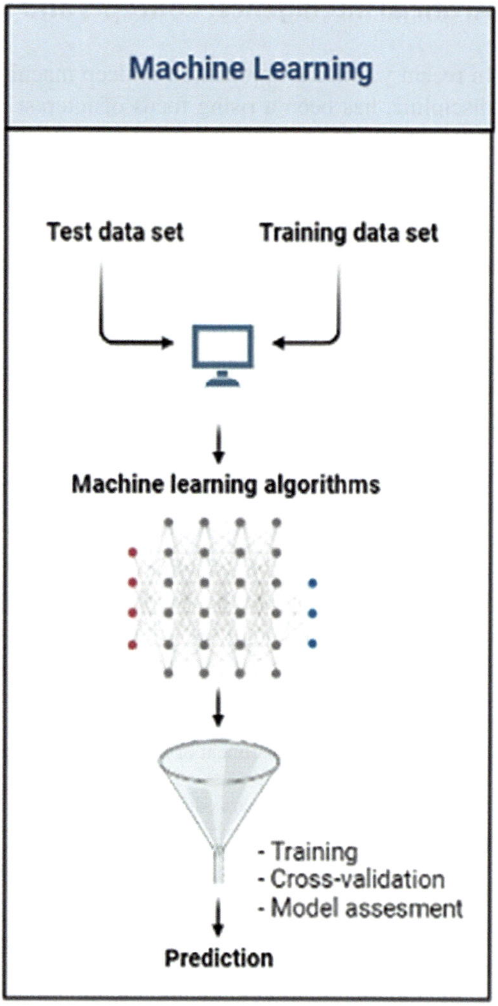

Fig. 9.1 ML workflows define which steps of a machine learning project are carried out. Normal procedures include data collection, data preparation, dataset construction, model training and refining, assessment, and production deployment. (Created with BioRender.com)

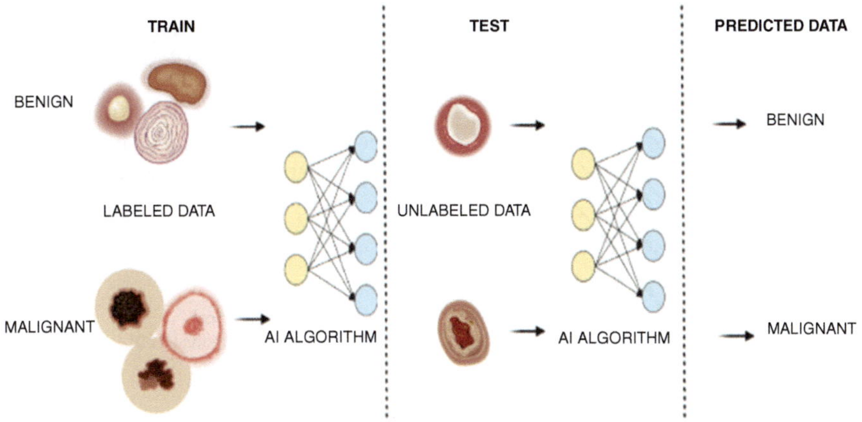

Fig. 9.2 Graphic showing how a ML algorithm is trained on a big dataset in order to be able to correlate data to label (supervised learning), after which its performance may be evaluated. (Created with BioRender.com)

and is not what is typically referred to when the phrase "artificial intelligence" is employed (Chartrand et al. 2017; Hogarty et al. 2020). Machine learning (ML) refers to algorithms and statistical models that detect and infer patterns from training data that has been labeled (Fig. 9.1).

During the training of a ML model, a subset of the data is typically "kept back" and later utilized to evaluate the model's accuracy. On this test dataset, the accuracy of the model is evaluated based on its ability to accurately match a picture with its label, such as malign or benign (Fig. 9.2). In any classification system, there will be a trade-off between sensitivity and specificity. For instance, an AI system may output a probability score between 0 and 1 for a skin lesion requiring the operator to specify a threshold for the decision border. At a low threshold, a greater proportion of melanomas will be detected (high sensitivity), but there is a danger of misclassifying benign lesion as cancerous (low specificity). As the threshold is raised, the sensitivity will fall, while the specificity will increase (Du-Harpur et al. 2020). The reaction of a ML classifier to a change in the threshold can be represented by a receiver operating characteristic (ROC) curve (Fig. 9.3).

ML is a category of artificial intelligence in which computer systems learn organically from their experiences rather than being programmed (Chartrand et al. 2017). ML can occur in supervised, semi-supervised, or unsupervised environments. In a supervised setting, the computer is fed datasets containing questions and responses. Machines learn to detect right responses through trial and error. In unsupervised learning, machines analyze incoming data with no predefined answer. Semi-supervised data analysis uses both labeled and unlabeled data (Hogarty et al. 2020).

Artificial Neural Network and Deep Learning

Artificial neural networks are multi-algorithm mathematical models that uncover complicated nonlinear correlations in massive datasets (analytics) (Miller and Brown 2018). The input layer feeds information into the artificial neural network,

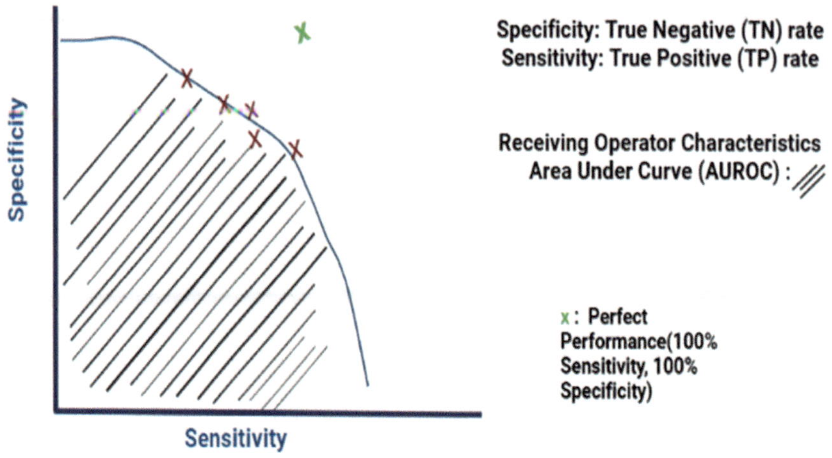

Fig. 9.3 ROC curve is a graphical representation of the sensitivity and specificity of a trained model. ROC curves and measurements of the area under the curve (AUC or AUROC) are typically employed to measure accuracy in machine learning research. The dashed line shows the optimal performance where both sensitivity and specificity are 100%; in this case, the AUROC would equal 1.0. In practice, there is an exchange between sensitivity and specificity, resulting in a curve. (Created with BioRender.com)

which is subsequently passed via numerous levels of hidden algorithmic operations. The weights learned in the machine learning procedures are used to apply these operations. Finally, the output layer produces the processed data. Artificial neural networks assist the machine in deep learning. Deep learning is a sort of machine learning in which artificial neural networks are used (Hogarty et al. 2020). It is a subfield of artificial intelligence that extracts patterns from raw data by using computer systems inspired by the human brain.

Neural networks route incoming information through a number of linked nodes (analogous to biological neurons). Each node works as a mathematical operation (addition, multiplication, etc.), and a set of interconnected nodes inside a network is known as a "layer," with the overall structure of the layers known as the "architecture." During training, every node is changed and refined by an iterative process known as "backpropagation," allowing the neural network's classification accuracy to improve (LeCun et al. 1990; LeCun et al. 2015).

Neural networks with several "hidden layers" of nodes are referred to as "deep" neural networks and are capable of "deep learning." Although the notion of deep neural networks was introduced decades ago, the inability to train them properly was hampered by the absence of inexpensive and efficient processing power. However, in 2013 it became apparent that graphical processing units (GPUs), which were initially built for three-dimensional visuals in computer games, might be repurposed to power the repeated training necessary for neural networks. Notably, convolutional neural networks (CNNs) are a special type of deep learning architecture that has shown useful for picture data categorization (Cireşan et al. 2010; Krizhevsky et al. 2012). After the success of the GPU-powered CNN AlexNet in 2012, which won the ImageNet competition with a top 5 error rate of 15.3%, a stunning 10% improvement over the next best competitor, CNNs have gained immense appeal as a technique for computer-based image categorization (Krizhevsky et al. 2012).

Artificial intelligence-powered medical technology is fast becoming practical clinical practice solutions. The increasing amounts of data generated by mobile monitoring sensors found in wearables, smartphones, and other medical equipment may be handled by deep learning algorithms. Machine learning models are used in medicine to scan medical data and reveal insights to help enhance patient experiences and health outcomes. Artificial intelligence (AI) has recently made significant strides in computer science and informatics, and it is now becoming a crucial component of contemporary healthcare. Medical practitioners are supported by AI algorithms and other applications driven by AI in clinical settings and current research.

The Current State of Artificial Intelligence in Dermatology

The epidermis, dermis, and hypodermis make up the structure of the human skin. Melanocytes in the epidermis can create melanin at an abnormally high rate when exposed to, for example, intense UV light. Melanoma is the malignant tumor caused by the aberrant development of melanocytes. As soon as pigmented lesions emerge on the skin's surface, melanoma can be identified by a clinical specialist through adequate visual assessment (Li et al. 2019; Cullell-Dalmalu et al. 2020; Pai and Pai 2021).

Dermatology is a science that relies on morphological characteristics, and the bulk of diagnoses are based on the detection of visual patterns. This branch of medicine is ideally suited for aided diagnosis using AI image recognition skills. Presently, dermoscopy, very high-frequency (VHF) ultrasound, and reflectance confocal microscopy (RCM) constitute skin imaging technologies. Each skin imaging technique has its own advantages and disadvantages. Dermatologists must select several imaging techniques based on the status of skin lesions. The worldwide acceptance and application of skin imaging technology has elevated its significance for the clinical diagnosis of skin disorders (Li et al. 2019; Masood and Al- Jumaily 2013).

AI in radiology has served as a model for dermatological AI. Early on, AI in medicine did not gain a great deal of attention or application for a variety of reasons (Mahmood et al. 2021). Due to a difficulty with data capture, there are insufficient quantities of labeled data, and there are insufficient samples to match the parameters of the complicated network model. Local extremum concerns, gradient dispersion issues, and inadequate hardware requirements have hindered the development of artificial intelligence in medicine (Polesie et al. 2020). In the last several decades, artificial neural networks (ANNs) have been developed for a variety of medical applications. However, its application in dermatology remains somewhat restricted. Although many dermatologists and patients are optimistic about AI/ML algorithms, these algorithms must be carefully evaluated to ensure that they are accurate, effective, cost-effective, and safe enough for clinical use and that increased access to skin lesion assessment does not increase the biopsy burden on specialist care providers or contribute to melanoma overdiagnosis (Jutzi et al. 2020; Welch et al. 2021).

Modern classifiers based on machine learning are superior to human specialists in the identification of pigmented skin lesions and should play a larger role in clinical practice. Clinicians with years of experience require routine training. It is challenging to deliver high-quality medical services to a big population using the traditional paradigm of medical care. There is a large gap between the supply and demand of doctor resources and the high cost of medical expenses. Medical AI technology relies on highly efficient computing ability and imitates through deep learning to provide high-quality medical services and address the issue of the uneven distribution of medical resources. In light of the aforementioned issues, it is certain that dermatological AI will be developed extensively.

AI in Skin Malignancies

Melanoma is a dangerous skin cancer that is becoming more common in various cultures. Since the mid-twentieth century, the incidence among white populations has climbed by 3–5% each year, with rates today at 20–60 instances per 100,000 people per year. Nonmelanoma skin malignancies that are more frequent include squamous cell carcinoma and basal cell carcinoma, which are increasingly considered as keratinocyte carcinomas. Nonetheless, earlier detection of skin cancer results in better outcomes (Jones et al. 2022; Garbe et al. 2021; Karimkhani et al. 2015; Marka et al. 2019).

Researchers have been investigating the use of AI to improve or complement current melanoma and nonmelanoma skin cancer (NMSC) screening techniques. Nasr-Esfahani et al. (2016) were the first to train a neural network for melanoma detection, with sensitivity and specificity of 0.81 and 0.80, respectively. A research on deep learning of skin cancers was released in 2017 at Stanford University. They used a single convolutional neural network that was trained end-to-end from photos, with just pixels and disease labels as inputs, to classify skin lesions. The researchers introduced a dataset of 129,450 clinical photos from 2032 various diseases to train a convolutional neural network. They put it to the test on biopsy-proven clinical pictures with two important binary classifications of cases: keratinocyte carcinomas vs. benign seborrheic keratoses and malignant melanomas versus benign nevi. The first example included identifying the most prevalent malignancies, while the second involved identifying the worst skin cancer. In terms of recognizing and categorizing skin cancer, the machine was found to be on par with board-certified dermatologists. This was a pioneering study in the field of dermatological AI. However, because they did not incorporate demographic data, the external validity of their study is questionable. Another study limitation was that, while it was widely acknowledged that applying deep learning technology to skin cancer classification could potentially improve the sensitivity and specificity of skin cancer screening, it was widely portrayed that the number of training images required for such a system would be enormous.

Fujisawa et al. (2019) released a research in which they investigated whether deep learning technology might be utilized to construct a reliable skin cancer classification system using a limited dataset of clinical photos. They used a dataset of 4867 clinical photos from 1842 patients diagnosed with skin cancers at the University of Tsukuba Hospital from 2003 to 2016 to train a deep convolutional neural network (DCNN). There were 14 diagnoses in all, including both malignant and benign conditions. The trained DCNN's total classification accuracy was 76.5%. The DCNN has a sensitivity of 96.3% and a specificity of 89.5%. Although the accuracy of malignant or benign categorization by board-certified dermatologists was statistically higher than that of dermatology trainees (85.3% ± 3.7% and 74.4% ± 6.8%, $p < 0.01$, respectively), the DCNN obtained even greater accuracy, reaching 92.4% ± 2.1% ($p < 0.001$).

Another area where AI can help with skin cancer diagnosis is at the histological level. Hekler et al. (2019) examined a total of 695 lesions that were categorized according to current recommendations by an expert histopathologist (350 nevi/345 melanoma). A CNN was trained using 595 of the generated pictures, and a total of 100 H&E (hematoxylin and eosin) segment images were utilized to compare the CNN's results to those of 11 histopathologists. To test for significance ($p < 0.05$), three combined McNemar tests comparing the outcomes of the CNN test runs in terms of sensitivity, specificity, and accuracy were established. Over 11 test cycles, the CNN obtained a mean sensitivity/specificity/accuracy of 76%/60%/68%. The 11 pathologists, on the other hand, had a mean sensitivity, specificity, and accuracy of 51.8%, 66.5%, and 59.2%, respectively. As a result, they determined that CNN outperformed 11 histopathologists in classifying histological melanoma images, indicating that it has the potential to aid human melanoma diagnosis. Though the application of artificial intelligence in the detection of skin cancer using clinical images, dermatoscopic images, and histopatholgic images is still in its early stages of development, it shows great potential.

Beginning in 1990, CAD systems and its components devoted to skin lesion detection were released. Since then, a variety of techniques have been presented to approach this difficult problem. Several algorithms employ a manual assessment technique based on the ABCD principles provided by Nachbar et al. (1994). The requirements for this technique include asymmetry (A), border (B), color (C), and differential structure (D). For the correct integration of this rule-based technology into a CAD system, a number of issues must be resolved.

The first and maybe most crucial stage is the exact segmentation of the skin lesion, which serves as the foundation for the examination of asymmetry and the lesion's boundary. Regarding this job, several proposals are available, including thresholding, region- and edge-based methods, soft computing techniques, and deformable models (Nachbar et al. 1994; Kasmi and Mokrani 2016; Abbas et al. 2013).

The approaches suggested in papers by Celebi et al. (2007), Faziloglu et al. (2003); and Hajdu et al. (2016) for classifying photos of skin lesions employ typical handcrafted feature sets; nevertheless, the supremacy of self-extracted, strong, deep convolutional neural network-based features is barely debatable at this time. Twenty-two out of 23 participants in the 2017 ISBI Challenge on Skin Lesion Analysis Towards Melanoma Detection considered deep neural network-based methods for an image classification problem, which is a strong indicator of the current superiority of CNN-based approaches in the field of dermoscopy image analysis (Codella et al. 2017).

Considering common measures, the classification accuracies of the different solutions are nearly identical. The modest variation in performance is likely due to the various sizes of picture sets used to train CNNs.

In a work reported by Esteva et al. (2017), a GoogLeNet Inception V3 CNN architecture was trained using 129,450 dermatologist-labeled clinical pictures. The scientists demonstrated that if the training dataset was sufficiently big, a deep neural network-based technique may surpass clinical specialists in terms of dermoscopy picture categorization accuracy. In the majority of medical domains, a sufficient quantity of humanly annotated training pictures is not currently available for a single CNN to extract and learn all the discriminative texture-based descriptors necessary for good classification accuracy.

In the previous decade, the development and implementation of deep learning algorithms for image analysis, such as classification, segmentation, and restoration, has increased. These methods have gradually been integrated into a variety of study domains, offering up new possibilities for biomedical imaging analysis. Deep learning has recently showed considerable promise when used to dermatological photos. In categorizing skin lesion photos into distinct skin cancer categories, deep learning systems have exhibited performance equivalent to humans (Fig. 9.4). Deep learning's potential therapeutic use necessitated the understanding of its basics by academics from fields other than computer science (Du-Harpur et al. 2020).

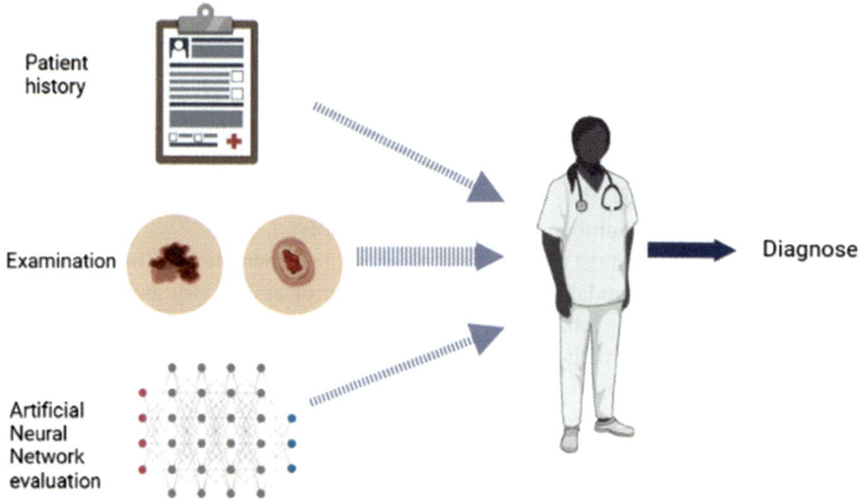

Fig. 9.4 Schematic demonstrating the prospective application of a machine learning system to assist nonexpert doctors in risk stratifying lesions and making clinical decisions. CNNs might represent a new form of decision aid that could assist nonexpert doctors triage correctly and narrow differential diagnoses. (Created with BioRender.com)

Computer-based image analysis aids in the elimination of subjective inter- and intra-observer variability, allowing for objective parameter assessment. In dermatology, artificial intelligence is rapidly being employed as a diagnostic tool. Computer technologies are being employed in dermatology to speed up data processing and give better outcomes. Over the last three decades, much research has been conducted on the use of machine learning models to assess and categorize data from skin lesions (Tchandl et al. 2018; Goyal et al. 2020; Young et al. 2020).

Artificial Intelligence in Dermoscopic Images

Dermoscopy is the screening and evaluation of skin lesions using a dermatoscope instrument comprised of a high-quality magnification lens and a (polarizable) lighting system (Tchandl et al. 2018; Goyal et al. 2020; Sadeghi et al. 2011; Stoecker et al. 2005; Yu et al. 2017). Dermoscopic pictures are obtained using digital single-lens reflex (DSLR) or smartphone camera attachments with high resolution (Fig. 9.5). The use of dermoscopic pictures for AI algorithms is becoming an increasingly popular area of research with the advent of several huge publically accessible dermoscopic datasets containing various types of benign and malignant skin diseases. There have been several AI experiments on lesion diagnosis with dermoscopic skin lesion datasets (Table 9.1).

Dermoscopic images were included in a study by Codella et al. (2017) who created an ensemble of deep learning algorithms using the ISIC-2016 dataset and compared the results of this network to that of 8 dermatologists in classifying 100 skin lesions as benign or malignant. The ensemble technique beats the average performance of dermatologists with an accuracy of 76% and a specificity of 62%, compared to 70.5% and 59%, respectively, for dermatologists.

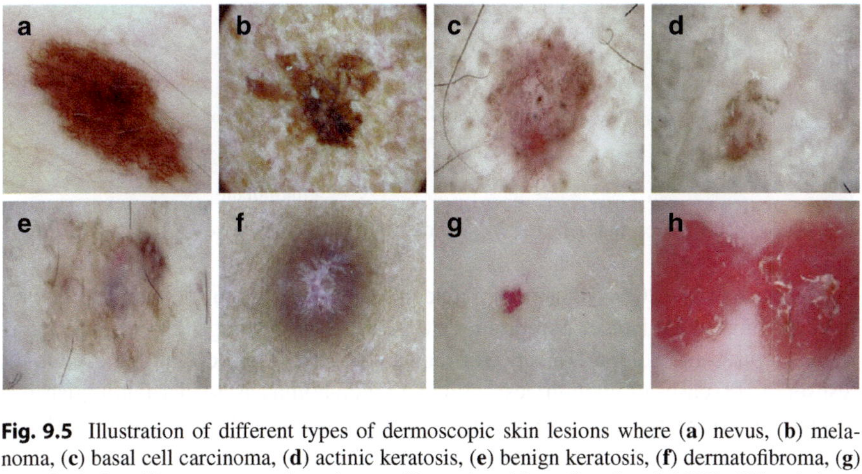

Fig. 9.5 Illustration of different types of dermoscopic skin lesions where (**a**) nevus, (**b**) melanoma, (**c**) basal cell carcinoma, (**d**) actinic keratosis, (**e**) benign keratosis, (**f**) dermatofibroma, (**g**) vascular lesion, (**h**) squamous cell carcinoma. (Reproduced from Goyal et al. 2020). Abbreviations: *AK* actinic keratosis, *AUC* area under the receiver operating characteristic curve, *BCC* basal cell cancer, *LPLK* lichen planus-like keratosis, *SCC* squamous cell cancer, *SK* seborrheic keratosis

Table 9.1 A summary of studies looking into the use of artificial intelligence on lesion diagnosis with dermoscopic skin lesion datasets

Study	Location	Dataset	Classification task	Algorithm performance	Clinician performance
Codella et al. (2017)	USA	1279 images (900 train and 379 test)	Melanoma versus melanocytic nevi	82% sensitivity and 62% specificity AUC 0.84	82% sensitivity and 59% specificity, 8 expert dermatologists
Haenssle et al. (2018)	Germany	>100,000 dermoscopic images	Melanoma versus benign melanocytic nevi	AUC 0.86 (more difficult test-set-100); AUC 0.95 (test-set-300)	AUC 0.79, international group of 58 dermatologists
Brinker et al. (2019)	Germany	12,378 open-source dermoscopic images	Melanoma versus atypical nevi	74.1% sensitivity and 86.5% specificity	74.1% sensitivity and 60% specificity, 157 dermatologists
Tschandl et al. (2019a)	Austria, Australia	Training set: 7895 dermoscopic and 5829 close-up images Test set: 2072 dermoscopic and clinical close-up images	Malignant versus benign nonpigmented skin lesions	80.5% sensitivity and 51.3% specificity AUC 0.74	77.6% sensitivity and 51.3% specificity AUC 0.70, 95 dermatologists
Maron et al. (2019)	Germany	11,444 dermoscopic images from the International Skin Imaging Collaboration (ISIC) archive	Malignant versus benign skin lesions	AUC 0.96 AUC 0.93 for benign versus malignant	112 dermatologists; performance was below the model's average performance
Haenssle et al. (2020)	Multiple countries	Dermoscopic images from multiple sources	Benign lesions In situ melanomas Invasive melanomas	95.0% sensitivity, 80.4% specificity for benign versus malignant	94.1% sensitivity, 80.4% specificity by 96 dermatologists

Abbreviations: *AUC* area under the receiver operating characteristic curve

Haenssle et al. (2018) constructed a deep learning technique (InceptionV4) on a huge dermoscopic dataset comprising of over 100,000 benign lesions and melanoma pictures and compared its performance with that of 58 dermatologists. On the test set of 100 cases (75 benign lesions and 25 melanoma cases), dermatologists had a sensitivity of 86.6% and a specificity of 71.3%, whereas deep learning reached a sensitivity of 95% and a specificity of 63.8%. In another study, Haenssle et al. (2020) contrasted the deep learning architecture based on InceptionV4 (licensed as a medical device by the European Union) with dermatologists on a 100-case dermoscopic test set (60 benign and 40 malignant lesions). This investigation was conducted on two levels, namely, level I: dermoscopic image and level II: additional clinical close-up photographs, dermoscopic image, and clinical data. The deep learning method attained sensitivity and specificity scores of 95% and 76.7%, respectively, whereas the average sensitivity and specificity scores for level I dermatologists were 89% and 80%, respectively. With additional level II information, the average sensitivity of dermatologists climbed to 94.1%, but the average specificity remained unchanged. As it is seen, dermatologists currently assess patients combining AI and the visual tool, dermoscopy.

Brinker et al. (2019) examined the performance of 157 board-certified dermatologists at 12 German university hospitals using a deep learning algorithm (ResNet50) using 100 dermoscopic pictures with 80 nevi and 20 melanoma cases. On the dermoscopic dataset, dermatologists obtained a sensitivity of 74.1% and a specificity of 60%, whereas a deep learning approach produced a specificity of 69.2% and a sensitivity of 84.2%. In another study, Maron et al. (2019) compared the sensitivity and specificity of a deep learning system (ResNet50) with those of 112 German doctors for multiclass categorization of skin diseases, including nevi, melanoma, benign keratosis, basal cell carcinoma (BCC), and SCC (including solar keratosis and intraepithelial carcinoma). Significantly ($p < 0.001$), the deep learning technique beat dermatologists (Fig. 9.6). In addition, Tschandl et al. (2019a) demonstrated the diagnosis accuracy of the most advanced machine learning algorithms and human readers for all clinically significant benign and malignant pigmented skin lesions.

Current findings have effectively proved the application of deep learning algorithms for dermatologist-level categorization of questionable lesions using large proprietary image datasets and a restricted number of dermatologists. The performance of a deep learning algorithm trained only on open-source photos is compared to that of a large number of dermatologists encompassing all levels of the clinical hierarchy. Modern machine learning classifiers that outperformed human specialists in the identification of pigmented skin lesions should play a larger role in clinical practice.

Artificial Intelligence in Clinical Imaging

A plentiful amount of datasets is required for deploying machine learning. Data can relate to a range of inputs, including visuals such as clinical photos and radiographs, as well as words such as patient data and symptoms information (Yang et al. 2018; Adoeye et al. 2021; Tschandl et al. 2019b; Chan et al. 2020; Esteva et al. 2017; Ferrer-Sánchez et al. 2022). Yang et al. (2018) diagnosed clinical skin lesions using an ABCD-inspired representation on the dataset. They compared the performance of the suggested techniques to those of deep learning techniques and dermatologists. It earned a score of 57.62% (accuracy) compared to ResNet's 53.35%. In comparison with other physicians, only senior clinicians with extensive expertise in skin disease had an average accuracy of 83.29%.

Han et al. (2018) constructed a deep learning architecture (ResNet-152) to identify clinical photos of 12 skin disorders using an Asan training dataset, a MED-NODE dataset, and atlas site images and then evaluated it using an Asan testing set

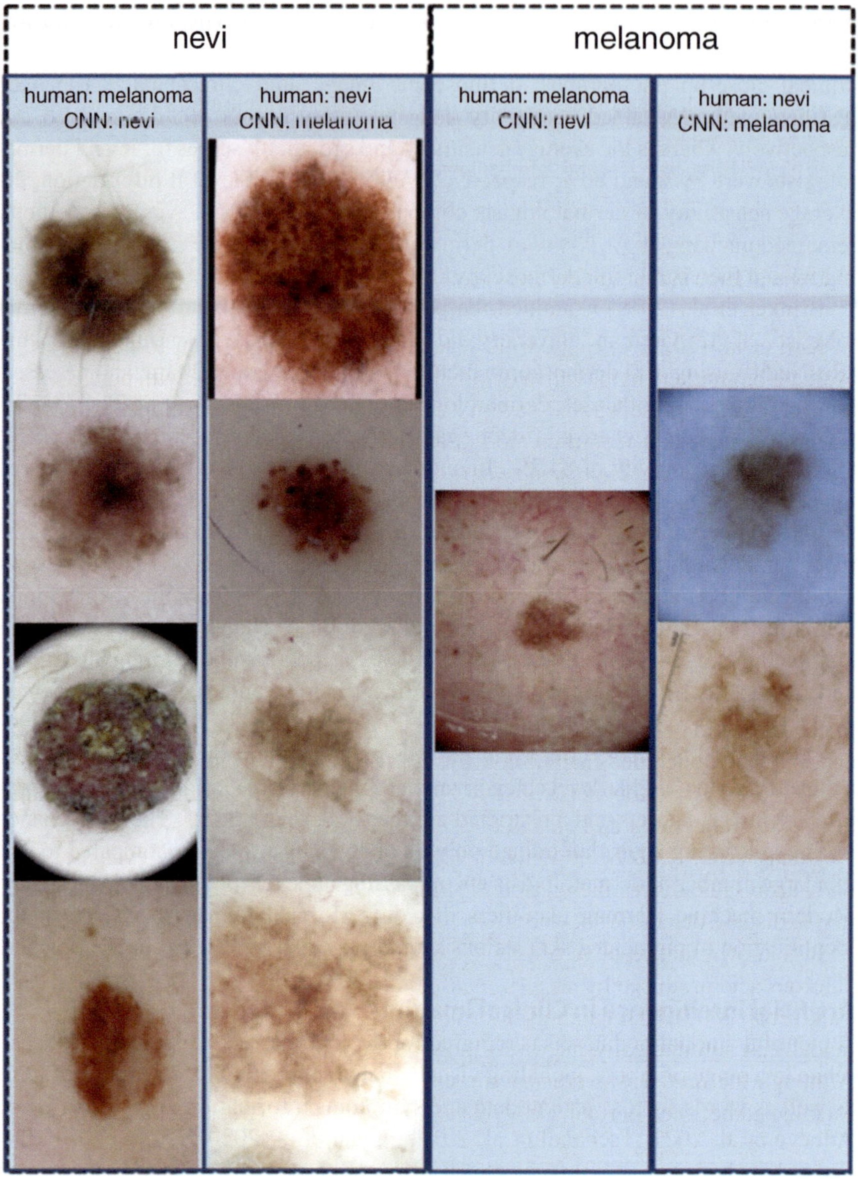

Fig. 9.6 The majority of human raters and the majority of CNN tests performed disagreed on some lesions. (Reproduced from Brinker et al. 2019a)

and an Edinburgh dataset (Dermofit). On 480 randomly selected photographs from the Asan test dataset (260 images) and the Edinburgh dataset (220 images), the algorithm performed similarly to the team of 16 dermatologists; however, the AI system excelled dermatologists in the diagnosis of BCC. Brinker et al. (2019b) assessed the performance of 145 dermatologists and a deep learning approach (ResNet50) on 100 clinical skin lesion photos (MClass-ND) comprised of 80 nevi cases and 20 biopsy-verified melanoma cases. The dermatologists obtained a sensitivity of 89.4%, a specificity of 64.4%, and an AUROC of 0.769, whereas a deep learning technique acquired the same sensitivity but a specificity score of 69.2%.

When comparing the outcomes of several training runs, it is clear that the categorization quality varies only little. Dermatologists' performance, on the other hand, varied greatly. Clinical contacts with live patients give more information than photographs alone can. It has previously been demonstrated that more clinical data improves dermatologists' sensitivity and specificity considerably. This information may also be used by machine learning algorithms to make judgments. Even with this tiny improvement, the CNN would still outperform the dermatologists.

AI in Pigmentary Skin Lesions

Several elements of psoriasis have been studied using artificial intelligence. Various computer-aided diagnostic techniques for picture categorization and psoriasis clinical risk have been developed (Shrivastava et al. 2016; Shrivastava et al. 2017). Machine learning prediction models have also been developed to evaluate psoriasis response to biologics and to distinguish psoriasis from psoriatic arthritis using genetic markers (Guo et al. 2014). Correa da Rosa et al. (2017) demonstrated that gene expression profiles of psoriasis skin lesions taken during the first 4 weeks of therapy with a biological agent can be used to correctly estimate (>80% area under the ROC curve) the clinical endpoint at 12 weeks, lowering the assessment gap by 2 months.

Emam et al. (2020) examined data from 681 psoriasis patients in the Danish registry cohort to see if machine learning might assist predict long-term biologic responses in psoriasis. Patients with early diagnosis and treatment who did not have psoriatic arthritis had a 90% likelihood of keeping on therapy, according to the study. To summarize, researchers have recently used deep learning (DL) and convolutional neural networks (CNNs) to analyze medical images from various fields, including dermatology. Based on a modest collection of predictive characteristics, machine learning algorithms estimate the probability of medication cessation and treatment duration with an accuracy of more than 80%. This strategy may be used to make decisions, communicate predicted results to patients, and produce evidence-based guidelines.

The Current State of Artificial Intelligence in Oral Diseases

A medical history and physical examination are part of the diagnostic process. Oral diseases demand a comprehensive understanding of lesions, their location, and symmetry (McCarthy et al. 2011). Many techniques, such as histology or immunofluorescence testing, rely on digital picture interpretation (Halicek et al 2019a, b). The medical history, on the other hand, is typically obtained through a question-and-answer session with the patient and includes not only a general history of the specific disorder but also the patient's occupation, hobbies, routine household duties, animal contact, and diet, as well as a variety of unrelated variables such as seasonal variation of the disease, correlation with menstruation or pregnancy, con comitant disorders, medication information, and family history (Lloyd and Craig 2007; Davis and Murray 2016).

There is widespread consensus that new technologies have the potential to assist doctors and patients make much better, more efficient healthcare decisions. Developing a good diagnosis currently needs years of medical training, and even then, diagnostics is typically a difficult and time-consuming process. Deep learning algorithms, in particular, have made significant progress in autonomously identifying pathologies (Chien et al. 2008; Chiesa-Estomba et al. 2022; Chu et al. 2021; Keser et al. 2023; Chuchu et al. 2018). Machine learning techniques may learn to detect patterns in the same way that doctors do; however, one significant distinction is that computers require a large number of real-world instances, typically thousands, in order to make meaningful predictions (Kumar et al. 2016; Alabi et al. 2019; Alabi et al. 2022; Young et al. 2020; Keser et al. 2023).

AI on Oral Diseases

Artificial intelligence can be utilized in the diagnosis and treatment of oral cavity diseases, as well as in screening and categorizing suspected changed mucosa experiencing premalignant and malignant alterations. For a large population, artificial intelligence might properly forecast a genetic propensity to oral cancer (Harangi et al. 2018; Young et al. 2020; Alabi et al. 2022; İlhan et al. 2021). Presently, a surgical biopsy and histopathologic diagnosis remain the gold standard for conclusive diagnosis of all oral mucosal lesions (Alabi et al. 2022). Patients who are afraid of a "cancer" diagnosis or of the surgery itself frequently have a negative perception of intrusive procedures. Unfortunately, both can cause delays in diagnosis and, in the event of a malignant lesion, the risk of disease progression, which can have a detrimental influence on prognosis (Alabi et al. 2022; Güneri and Epstein 2014). Furthermore, access to treatment and/or a qualified physician who can perform the necessary biopsy might be difficult for many patients, particularly those at risk of developing malignant lesions. The utilization of numerous technological developments, which are currently in use in other domains of healthcare, in the precise identification of oral mucosal diseases is necessary.

The oral mucosa is the mucous membrane lining or "skin" inside of the mouth, including cheeks and lips. Healthy skin and oral mucosa have numerous similarities in terms of tissue architecture, but they also have underlying histological variances. Although the shape and functions of the skin and oral mucosa are similar, there are distinctions in homeostatic circumstances that should be considered when comparing the healing processes in both tissue types (Waasdorp et al 2021; Keser et al. 2023).

Lichen planus is an autoimmune disease that can affect the skin as well as any mucosa that lines the inside of the mouth. Oral, esophageal, vaginal, and cutaneous mucosas might all be affected. Oral lichen planus is a long-term inflammatory mucocutaneous condition with no recognized cause (Pekiner et al. 2012; Pekiner et al. 2014). Histological features include subepithelial band-like inflammatory cell infiltration, varied amounts of intraepithelial mononuclear cells concentrating on the basal keratinocytes, and epithelial basal cell degeneration and annihilation. Increased apoptosis, most frequently restricted to the basal cell compartment, has been observed in recent oral lichen planus (OLP) studies (Neppelberg et al. 2007; Santoro et al. 2004).

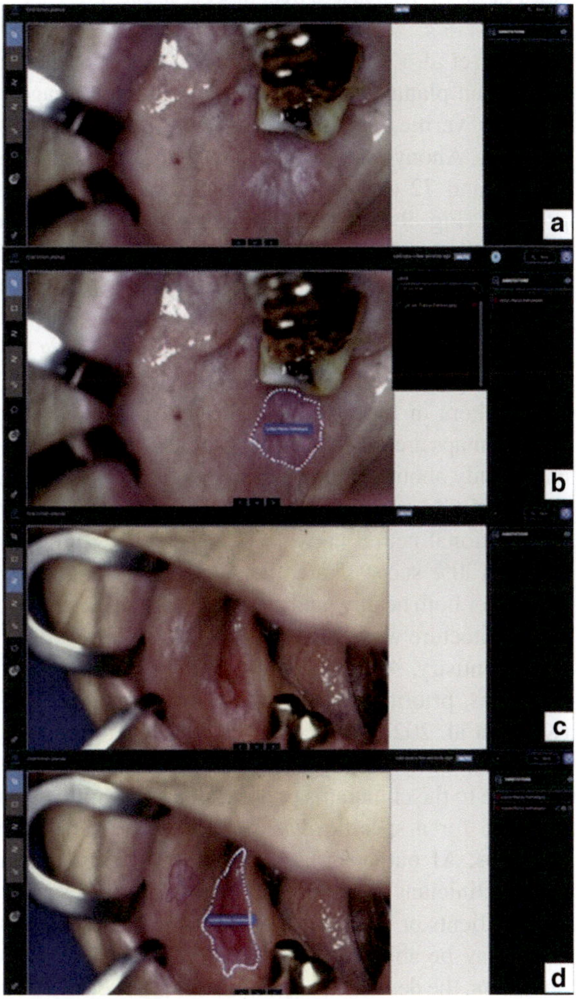

Fig. 9.7 (a–d) Representable samples showing the application of the CranioCatch (CranioCatch Eskişehir,Turkey) in detecting and labeling lesions in OLP cases. (Reproduced from Keser et al. 2023)

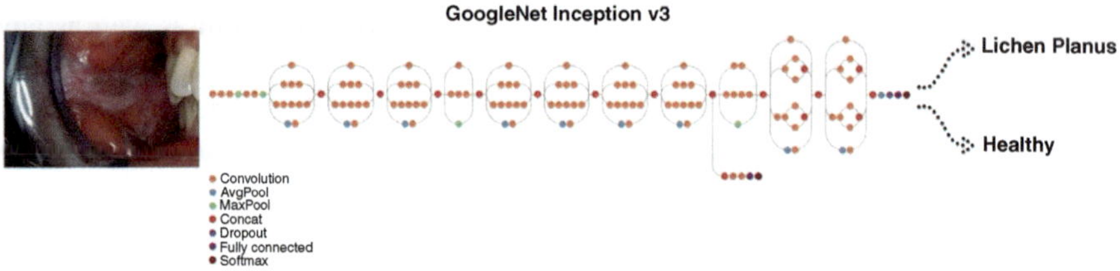

Fig. 9.8 An artificial intelligence model was developed using TensorFlow Inception V 3 architecture, which is a deep learning approach. Figure shows the whole procedure for identifying skin disease using deep learning-based techniques. The intraoral photos are entered into the system and processed in this manner. To evaluate if the disease is present, the input image is analyzed using image processing techniques such as preprocessing, feature extraction, and a machine learning-based classifier. (Reproduced from Keser et al. 2023)

Keser et al. (2023) aimed to develop a deep learning approach for identifying oral lichen planus lesions using photographic images. Patients having histopathologically verified diagnoses of oral lichen planus were involved in all of the instances. Anonymous retrospective photographic images of buccal mucosa with 65 healthy and 72 oral lichen planus lesions were identified using the CranioCatch program (Fig. 9.7a–d). All images were rechecked and verified by oral medicine and maxillofacial radiology experts. This dataset was divided into training ($n = 51$; $n = 58$), verification ($n = 7$; $n = 7$), and test ($n = 7$; $n = 7$) sets for healthy mucosa and mucosa with the oral lichen planus lesions, respectively.

The deep learning process was performed using GoogleNet Inception V3 architecture implemented with TensorFlow library. 5 × 5 filter size is changed with two 3 × 3 filters in Inception-v3. The reduction of an efficient grid size is changed. Feature maps are made by convolutions and by pooling separately. The computation cost is only about 2.5 higher than that of Inception-v1 and much more efficient than that of VGGNet, which stands for Visual Geometry Group, and it is a standard deep convolutional neural network (CNN) architecture with 42 layers' deep (Fig. 9.8). With a 100% success rate, the AI deep learning model correctly classified all test photos for both healthy and diseased mucosa. The accuracy of TensorFlow Inception V3 architecture was estimated as 1.0.

In dentistry, AI is generally used to discriminate between lesions and normal structures, prioritize risk variables, and simulate and assess prospective outcomes (Keser et al. 2023; Shan et al. 2021; Alhazmi et al. 2021; Adeoye et al. 2021). A clinician's study of symptoms, diagnostic test findings, and other criteria, which are sensitive to the clinician's poor recall and cognitive bias, forms the basis of diagnostic logic for a specific disease. When "trained" with hundreds of thousands of instances, AI outperforms even the most skilled specialist's clinical experience. Dental clinicians are currently under a lot of stress since they have to diagnose a lot more patients or instances that are more sophisticated than in the past. These clinicians may be able to overcome these obstacles with the help of AI. Like human observers, the described algorithm has high sensitivity and accuracy levels (Hayashi and Setiono 2002). This strategy can assist surgeons, radiologists, and other medical professionals, such as physical therapists, in making the most use of their time and reducing diagnostic time. The findings of artificial neural networks were compared to medical diagnostic and current classification methods to discover different treatments. Many of them discovered that neural networks are instruments for receiving reasonably optimum solutions of partial and restricted datasets since they are flexible in modeling and have logical accuracy in prediction. As a result, neural networks are capable of combining data in many forms of a system, such as data obtained through clinical examinations (Bouletreau et al. 2019; Jeon et al. 2015).

In literature, Magshoudi et al. (2013) used intelligent systems based on ANN to investigate three of the most frequent and potentially serious oral disorders: oral squamous cell carcinoma (OSCC), leukoplakia, and lichen planus. The study's population included 150 individuals, with 50 patients being considered for each condition. The results of their simulation indicated that diagnostic systems, based on artificial neural networks, give a powerful strategy in the diagnosis and prediction of oral diseases. Moreover, Idrees et al. (2021) established a machine learning artificial neural network multilayer perceptron (ANN-MLP) as a machine learning method to recognize and quantify mononuclear cells and granulocytes within inflammatory infiltrates in digitized hematoxylin and eosin microscope slides from oral lichen planus cases and validated it on a retrospective cohort of 130 cases. With scores of sensitivity of 100% and an accuracy of 94.62%, the suggested machine learning technique was capable of consistently detecting oral lichen planus patients based on the number of inflammatory cells and the number of mononuclear cells.

Concerning biochemical aspects, the possibility of interleukin 12 receptor beta 2 and tumor necrosis factor receptor superfamily member 8 as diagnostic biomarkers for oral lichen planus was investigated in another study. Support vector machine (SVM), random forest (RF), linear discriminant analysis (LDA), neural network (NN), and naive Bayes (NB) methods were used to build predictive models of IL12RB2 and TNFRSF8 expression. AUC in predictive modeling varied from 0.83 to 0.92, and their accuracy was more than 0.75 in all techniques. Focusing on the expression of inflammatory cytokine genes, ANN, SVM, and RF were all capable of discriminating oral lichen planus from other white lesions of the oral mucosa based on the expression of inflammatory cytokine genes (Jeon et al. 2015).

One of the most prevalent oral lesions is leukoplakia. It is characterized as a white plaque with a suspicious risk, omitting other illnesses or conditions that are not known to raise the risk of cancer. In a study conducted by Ferrer-Sánchez et al. (2022), deep learning was used to evaluate the likelihood of malignancy of an oral leukoplakia lesion in terms of evolution to cancer and high-risk dysplasia. A total of 261 oral leukoplakia lesions with a mean follow-up of 5.5 years were studied using standard digital photographs. A deep learning pipeline consisting of a U-Net-based segmentation of the lesion accompanied by a multitask CNN classifier was used to estimate the malignant transformation and the risk of dysplasia of the lesion. The model predicted a malignant transformation with a sensitivity of 1 and a specificity of 0.692 (Fig. 9.9). This model also obtained a specificity of 0.740 and a sensitivity of 0.928 for predicting high-risk dysplasia. The suggested deep learning model may be useful in forecasting the likely malignant progression of oral leukoplakias.

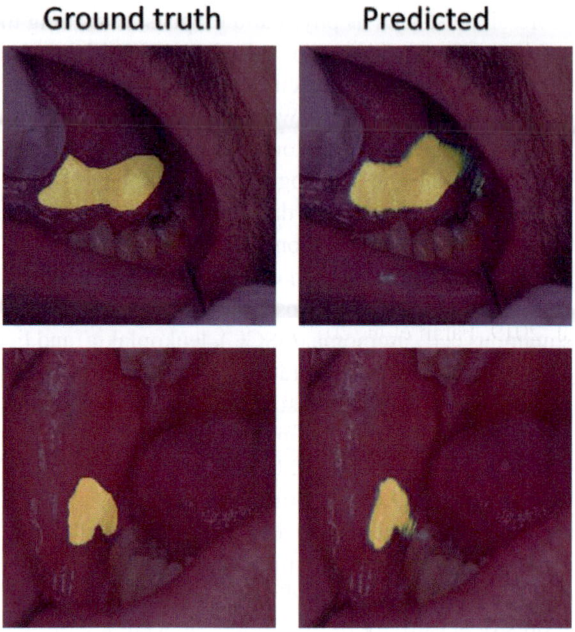

Fig. 9.9 Two examples of lesions segmented using the best U-Net model obtained. A clinical expert's segmentation (left) versus the best U-Net model prediction (right). (Reproduced from Ferrer-Sánchez et al. 2022)

AI has a wide range of functions and applications in the healthcare industry. Increased work, increased job complexity, and possible doctor tiredness may compromise diagnostic abilities, and AI components in imaging equipment would reduce this effort and boost efficiency. They can also identify oral lesions and have greater data access than humans. According to preliminary findings from the studies, deep learning has the capacity to manage this enormous task.

AI on Oral Cancer

OSCC is one of the most common malignancies in the world, with an increasing frequency in many countries. The high rate of occurrence, late diagnosis, and haphazard treatment planning continue to be major concerns. Early detection is critical for a better prognosis, treatment, and outcome (Ilhan et al. 2021; Aubreville et al. 2017; Uthoff et al. 2018; Llewellyn et al. 2004, Warnakulasuriya and Kerr 2021; Almangush et al. 2015; DuM et al. 2020; Miranda-Filho and Bray 2020). Despite recent advances in molecular pathways, late diagnosis and a precision medicine strategy for OSCC patients remain a hurdle (Coletta et al. 2020). Deep machine learning has been proposed as a way to improve precision medicine by improving early diagnosis and, as a result, lowering cancer-related mortality and morbidity (Chu et al. 2021; Ilhan et al. 2021). In recent years, this approach has reportedly achieved great progress in data extraction and interpretation of crucial information in medical imaging (Ariji et al. 2019; Ariji et al. 2020; Ariji et al. 2021; Fujima et al. 2020). As a result, it has the potential to aid in the diagnosis of oral squamous cell carcinoma at an early stage. In addition, automated image processing can help pathologists and physicians make better decisions about cancer patients.

The best method for reducing disease morbidity and death rates, increasing survival rates, and enhancing people's quality of life is early diagnosis of oral cancer. The histological diagnosis of lesions cannot be predicted just by the usual clinical examination, which includes a thorough head and neck examination, visual inspection of oral tissues, and palpation. Thus, it is necessary to create auxiliary tools that will improve clinical examination efficiency and make it easier to find and diagnose lesions associated with mouth cancer and other potentially malignant conditions (Simonato et al. 2019, Farah et al. 2019). Artificial intelligence applications paired with intraoral photos, omics technologies, and light-based imaging systems stand out as instruments that can be employed for this because of the quick and revolutionary breakthroughs in image processing and diagnostic technologies in recent years (Aubreville et al. 2017; Uthoff et al. 2018; Lylewellyn et al. 2004; Simonato et al. 2019; Farah et al. 2019). These systems are believed to be useful in a wide range of situations, including predicting the prognosis and treatment outcomes of oral cancers, detecting lymph node involvement, classifying oral mucosal lesions, and differentially diagnosing lesions with the potential for malignancy and malignant transformation.

Surgical treatment has traditionally been the basic cornerstone therapy for OSCC. For a better prognosis, therapy, and survival, early-stage diagnosis is critical (Alabi et al. 2021). This is critical in improving cancer treatment. Despite recent advances in our understanding of cancer's molecular causes, late diagnosis has impeded the pursuit of precision treatment. As a result, deep machine learning has been suggested as a method for improving early diagnosis and, as a result, lowering cancer-specific mortality and morbidity. Automated image analysis has the potential to help pathologists and physicians discover OSCC in its early stages and make educated cancer care decisions (Aubreville et al. 2017; Uthoff et al. 2018; Alabi 2019; Fu et al. 2020; Ariji et al. 2020; Kar et al. 2020).

Clinical images are increasingly being utilized in medicine to deliver deep learning solutions to automated decision support systems for disease diagnosis, prognosis, and therapy customization, as well as other activities that improve the healthcare system's efficiency (Uthoff et al. 2018; Fu et al. 2020). Deep learning has shown preliminary results in oncology research in cell type categorization and treatment outcome prediction in tumors such as breast, prostate, and oral cancer and has been utilized to identify cell types and discriminate noncancerous and malignant tissues for diagnosis in oral squamous cell carcinoma (SCC), the most frequent kind of oral cancer, mostly utilizing commonly available clinical photos (Shimizu and Nakayama 2020; Golden et al. 2017; Nagpal et al. 2020; Fu et al. 2020; Faradmal et al. 2014). It is also used in prognostic prediction in addition to diagnosis by examining metastatic lymph nodes and quantifying the quantity of tumor-infiltrating lymphocytes (Topol et al. 2019; Golden et al. 2017; Ehteşami et al. 2017; Shaban et al. 2019).

Clinical images are the most commonly used input data in cancer research to develop a deep learning model for predicting clinical outcomes. The quality of image data is a major determinant of model performance. Having high-quality data

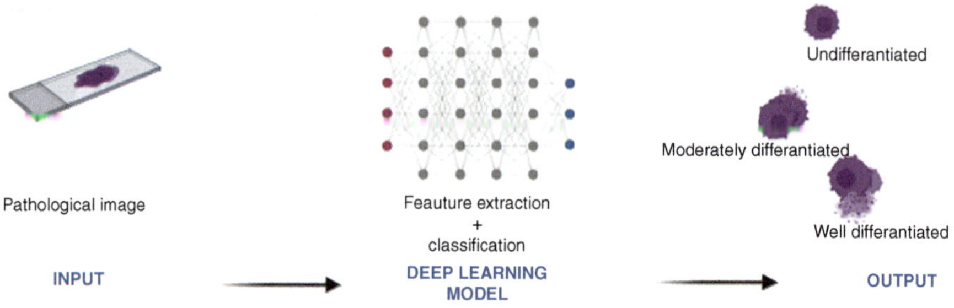

Fig. 9.10 A pathological/radiographic image (simply a histology image here as an example) is seen as a matrix in a computer. Convolutional layers, pooling layers, and fully connected layers are common components of CNNs. These several layers work together implicitly to perform feature extraction and classification. (Created with BioRender.com)

from clinical pictures, such as pathological and radiographic images taken from patients during diagnosis and/or relevant images from healthy controls, is likely the most important and time-consuming first stage in the building of a deep learning model (Uthoff et al. 2018; Fu et al. 2020; Aubreville et al. 2017; Jubair et al. 2022; Warin et al. 2021). Aside from the basic need of having excellent-quality photographs as input data for constructing a deep learning model, image data in adequate amount is also necessary to train a model with decent performance.

The actual amount of photos used should be calculated for each model individually and is dependent on a variety of criteria, such as the number of output classes and the training techniques (Esteva et al. 2019). In general, a higher number of photos would result in a more performant model. To do this, the transfer learning technique is occasionally used to transfer a huge quantity of picture information from open sources (e.g., ImageNet, which has over 14 million images). The transmitted photographs can be used to train a deep learning model before fine-tuning using project-based images (Shin et al. 2016; Pan and Yang 2009).

Another way for improving model performance is to employ image augmentation to produce an increased number of changed pictures from original photographs by random rotation, flipping, and saturation and exposure adjustments (Shorten and Khoshgoftaar et al. 2019, Chu et al. 2021). Deep learning research have employed CNN classifiers with varying architecture and complexity to assess pathological, clinical, and radiographic images (Fig. 9.10).

After staining with hematoxylin and eosin, pathological pictures of resected tissues can indicate tumor histopathology, and these tissue sections can also be subjected to immunohistochemistry for particular biomarkers to offer further information for prognosis prediction (Chu et al. 2021). The most commonly used pathological images for deep learning are digital hematoxylin and eosin-stained tissue images. Deep learning for learning histological distinctions from pathological pictures can aid in disease detection for oral cancer, particularly oral SCC, due to its capacity to categorize cell type and discriminate tumor grade. In a research, active learning was utilized to train and enhance the performance of a fully convolutional CNN classifier for discriminating cancer cells from six distinct types of non-tumor cells (stroma, lymphocytes, mucosa, keratin pearls, blood, and adipose) in hematoxylin and eosin pictures with a 96.37% accuracy (Folmsbee et al. 2018).

The main radiographic images used in deep learning for prognostic prediction are PET and CT scans (Chu et al. 2021). Given that 18F-fluorodeoxyglucose-generated PET images contain image parameters for standardized uptake values, metabolic tumor volume, heterogeneity index, and total lesion glycolysis to describe tumor characteristics, a CNN model can evaluate these images and associated/other parameters, such as clinical stage, to predict disease-free survival in patients with oral cavity SCC with 80% accuracy, sensitivity, and specificity (Fujima et al. 2020). Because CT scans have a low sensitivity for excluding extranodal extension, compared to the usage of PET images, the model will perform worse when CT images are used to a CNN model for the prediction of disease-free survival (Kann et al. 2020).

Extranodal extension in head and neck SCC is associated with poor disease-free survival; therefore, using a CNN model to analyze this variable from CT images, it is possible to predict disease-free survival in oral SCC with 66.9% sensitivity, 84% accuracy, and 89.7% specificity (Ariji et al. 2020). The detection of lymph node metastases is a potential application of deep learning and radiographic image analysis. Although these results are less accurate than those of radiologists (83.1% accuracy with AUC of 0.83, 77.5% sensitivity, and 88.8% specificity), employing CT scans for deep learning can still reach 78.2% accuracy (AUC, 0.8), 75.4% sensitivity, and 81% specificity in oral SCC (Ariji et al. 2019).

It is possible that the choice of a poor model architecture is to blame for the underperformance of this deep learning model and that improving the model's parameter could increase learning rates. In fact, a later study by the same research team showed that altering the model architecture and data preparation might increase the sensitivity of a deep learning model for detecting metastatic lymph nodes from CT images in oral SCC by up to 90%. Deep learning models can predict xerostomia, a side effect of radiation related to toxicity, with an accuracy rate of 76%, in addition to the diagnosis of metastatic lymph nodes, using CT scans of head and neck SCC (AUC, 0.84) (Ariji et al. 2021).

AI can help with early detection and reduce the mortality and morbidity linked to oral cancer. Using laser-induced autofluorescence spectra recordings, Nayak et al. (2006) employed ANN to distinguish between normal, premalignant, and tissues. The results indicated a 98.3% accuracy, 100% specificity, and 96.5% sensitivity, indicating that this method can be effectively used in real time. Using autofluorescence images and white light images, Uthoff et al. (2018) applied CNN to identify precancerous and cancerous lesions. In identifying precancerous and cancerous tumors, CNN outperformed experts. With larger datasets, the CNN model's performance can be enhanced. Based on confocal laser endomicroscopy (CLE) images, Aubreville et al. (2017) employed DL to detect oral cancer. The specificity and accuracy of this approach were both 90%. Deep neural networks were used in a comparative study by Shams et al. (2017) to forecast the emergence of oral cancer from oral possibly malignant lesions. DNN was contrasted with multilayer perception, regularized least squares, and support vector machines. In comparison with the other systems, DNN's accuracy rate was greater at 96%. Jeyaraj et al. (2019) also verified these results. Based on hyperspectral images, CNN was utilized to discriminate between cancerous and noncancerous tissues. According to the results, CNN can be used to classify and diagnose oral cancer using images without the need for professional guidance. Warin et al. (2021) created an automated classification and detection model for oral cancer screening using CNN deep learning methods. The study contained 700 clinical oral pictures from the oral and maxillofacial center that were separated into 350 photos of oral squamous cell carcinoma and 350 photos of healthy oral mucosa. DenseNet121 and faster R-CNN were used to generate the classification and detection models, respectively. The classification accuracy of the DenseNet121 model achieved 99% precision, 100% recall, 99% F1 score, 98.75% sensitivity, 100% specificity, and 99% area under the receiver operating characteristic curve. The detection accuracy of a faster R-CNN model was 76.67% precision, 82.14% recall, 79.31% F1 score, and 0.79 area under the precision recall. The DenseNet121 and faster R-CNN algorithms were shown to have adequate potential for classification and detection of malignant lesions in oral photographic images. The field of oral cancer research has seen a lot of research activity recently. Numerous research have successfully created AI models that can forecast the presence and recurrence of oral cancer (Fig. 9.11).

Deep learning (DL) algorithms and skilled radiologists have been compared in a number of studies, with varying degrees of success. The effectiveness of DL in detecting cervical node metastases using CT images was evaluated by Ariji et al. (2019). They used CT scans of 137 cervical lymph nodes with histologically proven positivity and 314 lymph nodes with histologically proven negativity from 45 patients with oral squamous cell carcinoma. The outcomes of the DL method were

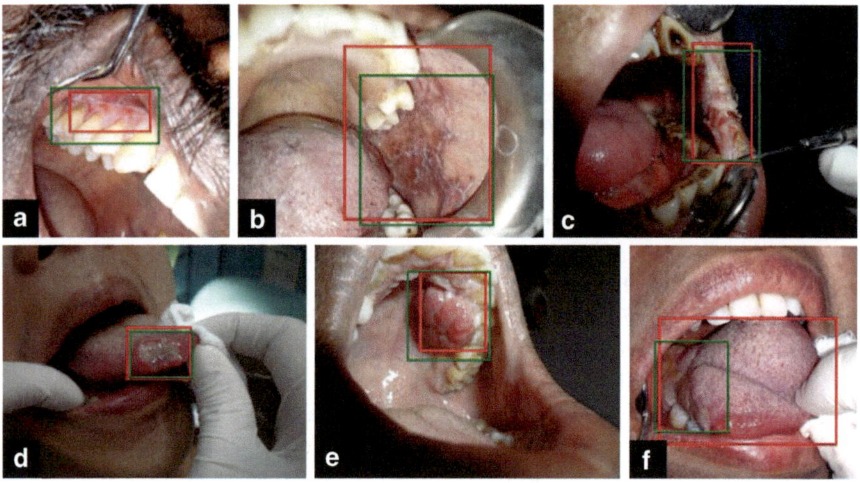

Fig. 9.11 Results of four-class object detection. (**a–d**) Correction detections, (**e**, **f**) wrong and missed detections. The composite annotation bounding boxes are green and the predicted bounding boxes are red. (Reproduced from Welikala et al. 2020)

contrasted with those of two qualified radiologists. The DL network had radiologists' level of accuracy. Additionally, the extranodal expansion of cervical lymph node metastases was identified by the researchers using DL. A total of 703 CT scans taken from 51 individuals, 20 of whom had extranodal extension, were used as training data and 80 as test data. The DL system's performance was noticeably better than the radiologist's, indicating that it can be used as a diagnostic tool to find extranodal metastases (Ariji et al. 2020).

Tanriver et al. (2021) suggested a two-stage end-to-end methodology for diagnosing oral lesions by serially merging object detection and classification tasks (Fig. 9.12). YOLOv5l is utilized in their suggested pipeline to detect lesion regions in the whole picture, and EfficientNet-b4 is used to categorize the found lesion region into three categories. The chosen networks performed well in terms of accuracy and inference time, making them ideal for use in real-time applications. The performance of the cutting-edge YOLOv5 architecture as a single-stage object detector was investigated for the identification of oral lesions. For the test set, the YOLOv5l model performed the best of all versions, with an average precision (AP) of 0.644 and an average precision at IOU = 0.5 (AP50) of 0.951.

Artificial intelligence algorithms can curate various data sources to provide judgments, evaluate risk, and recommend patients to professionals for cancer treatment (Zheng et al. 2014). The diagnostic and prognostic efficacy of artificial intelligence has been demonstrated in studies on premalignant lesions, lymph nodes, salivary gland tumors, and squamous cell carcinoma (Table 9.2). These initiatives could lower mortality rates by promoting early detection and efficient therapy approaches. Large data volumes and resources are needed for data analysis on these platforms in order to deliver an accurate and economical diagnosis. These models must be improved to obtain the highest accuracy, specificity, and sensitivity before they can be safely integrated into routine clinical operations.

AI-based clinical decision support systems developed for the differential diagnosis of oral mucosal lesions can be used in cancer screening, classification of suspicious mucosal changes, tissue diagnostics, and evaluation of lymph node involvement. Logistic regression, support vector machine (SVM), decision trees,

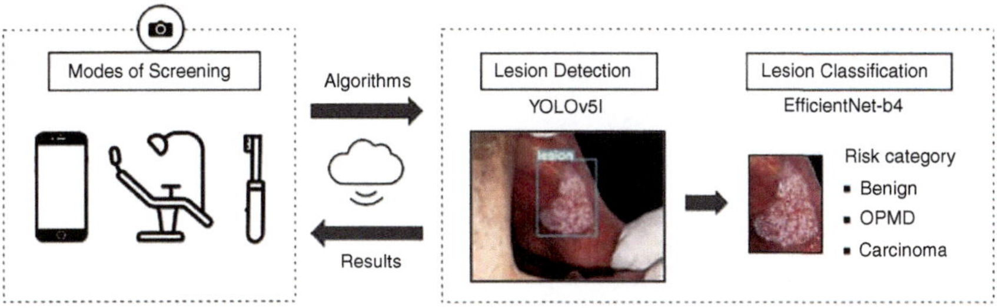

Fig. 9.12 Proposed two-stage workflow for screening for oral cancer. In the first step, it detects oral lesions using photographic images, and in the second stage, deep learning algorithms are used to classify the detection region. The YOLOv5l and EfficientNet-b4 models were chosen for the workflow because they performed well in terms of accuracy and inference time. (Reproduced from Tanriver et al. 2021)

Table 9.2 A review of studies on the application of artificial intelligence in cancer diagnosis

Study/aim	Location	Number of cases/ images	Machine learning methods	Data types used in the deep learning	Results	Algorithm performance	Conclusion
Aubreville et al. (2017) To detect oral cancer	Germany	7894	CNN	Anatomical images	The deep learning method was able to detect on image	Sensitivity: 0.86 Specificity: 0.90 Accuracy: 88.3% AUC: 0.96	The deep learning offered automatic detection of oral cancer for effective management of the cancer
Uthoff et al. (2018) To distinguish between precancerous and cancerous lesions early	USA	170	CNN	Intraoral images	Automatic and affordable smartphone based system for oral screening distinction	Sensitivity: 0.85 Specificity: 0.88	Effective management of oral cancer through early detection
Fu et al. (2020) To identify patients with OCSCC	China	44,409	CNN	Clinical images	This automated approach provides rapid and noninvasive detection of OCSCC	Sensitivity: 0.896 Specificity: 0.806 AUC: 0.935	The performance of the deep learning is comparable to an expert and better than medical student
Jubair et al. (2022) To classify clinical image into either benign and malignant or oral potentially malignant disorder (OPMD)	Jordan and Greece	716	CNN	Clinical image	The deep learning offer an effective and low-budget means of oral cancer screening	80.5% sensitivity and 51.3% specificity AUC 0.74	77.6% sensitivity and 51.3% specificity; AUC 0.70, 95 raters, including 62 board-certified dermatologists
Warin et al. (2021) To detect oral cancer	Thailand	700	DenseNet121 and faster R-CNN,	Clinical image	Algorithms were proven to offer the acceptable potential for classification and detection of cancerous lesions in oral photographic images	DenseNet121 Sensitivity: 98.75%; F1 score: 99% Faster R-CNN Precision: 76.67% F1 score: 79.31%	DenseNet121 and the faster R-CNN algorithm give acceptable results for the classification and detection of oral cancer in oral photography

Ariji et al. (2020) To detect metastasis of cervical lymph nodes	Japan	441	CNN	CT images	The diagnostic performance of the CNN model is similar to that of radiologists	Accuracy: 78.2% Sensitivity: 75.4% Specificity: 81.1%	The system may be valuable for diagnostic support
Jeyaraj et al. (2019) To detect oral cancer	India	600	CNN	Hyperspectral images	The proposed method can be deployed for the automatic classification	Accuracy of 91.4% for benign tissue and 94.5% for normal tissue	The quality of diagnosis is increased by proposed regression-based partitioned CNN learning algorithm
Gupta et al. (2019) Cell type classification	India	2688	CNN	H&E	Deep learning system although not in real time but produced promising results	Accuracy: 89.3%	Deep learning system has achieved higher accuracies almost as the experienced specialist concerned oral pathologist

Abbreviations: *AUC* area under the receiver operating characteristic curve, *H&E* hematoxylin and eosin, *CNN* convolutional neural network and Bayesian networks are among the most commonly used ML algorithms in oral cancer studies (Ilhan et al. 2021). ML-based algorithms are used to predict malignant transformation of OPMDs, lymph node metastasis of oral cancers, treatment response, and disease prognosis (Schwendicke et al. 2020). In a systematic review investigating its efficacy, accuracy rates ranged from 89% to 97% for malignant transformation, 78% to 91% for cervical lymph node metastasis, 64% to 100% for treatment response, and 71% to 99% for prognosis (Patil et al. 2022). In addition to clinically observable mucosal changes, OPMD and early oral SCC lesions are usually asymptomatic or cause mild symptoms. However, the presence of signs and symptoms that may be associated with malignancy or an increased risk of malignancy may lead to a late diagnosis of the lesion if misinterpreted by the physician or the patient. Therefore, cancer screening in the general population is considered an important opportunity for early diagnosis (İlhan et al. 2020).

The use of AI applications in cancer screening increases the possibility of early diagnosis, thanks to the elimination of observer-related fatigue and the detection of a change in a single pixel in a short time, unlike conventional methods and accelerated workflow. In a case-control study comparing different AI models with specialist physicians, sociodemographic findings, smoking and alcohol habits, and genomic data of 84 oral cancer and 87 healthy individuals were used as input variables. It was found that both AI models outperformed specialist physicians in the assessment of oral cancer development risk (Rosma et al. 2010). Similarly, Wang et al. (2020) developed a personalized ML algorithm aimed at predicting the risk of malignant transformation of OPMDs using data from 266 patients with suspected oral lesions. It has been reported that the presented model can distinguish between low- and high-risk lesions with high sensitivity and specificity values and predict the risk of oral cancer development.

Many studies in the literature have been designed to "prove" that AI-based systems can be used as a suitable adjunctive diagnostic tool for oral cancer lesions. The majority of the studies are retrospective, and limited data from a small number of patients were used. This research design causes "overlearning," and the results obtained from the existing dataset cannot be replicated in different datasets. However, many studies evaluating AI-based systems as a diagnostic tool in oral oncology and other branches of medical oncology have demonstrated the reproducibility of these systems. Its generalizability has not been tested. To maximize the learning power of AI-based systems, large-scale databases and the accumulation of large amounts of appropriately labeled data are needed (Pai and Pai 2021). Patient privacy should be considered while creating these databases, and data security should be ensured.

It has been shown that deep learning with the use of readily available clinical images from hematoxylin and eosin-stained pathological sections and CT-based radiography has the potential to assist clinical decision-making with regard to cancer diagnosis, prognosis prediction, and treatment assistance in oral cancer research, particularly that related to SCC. Deep learning models can be built for use by physicians to enhance decision-making after being carefully validated for accuracy in various patient cohorts.

Conclusions

Various artificial intelligence (AI) methods, particular algorithms, and predictive models are starting to have a significant influence on increasing diagnostic accuracy for benign and malignant lesions as image analysis and diagnostic technology in dermatology. For the automatic identification and categorization of oral benign and malignant lesions, AI-based technologies in combination with intraoral photographic pictures or optical imaging approaches are being investigated. Reproducible advanced systems and a huge number of data are needed in order for these technologies, which are still in the beginning or under development, to find wide use in cancer screening and predicting the cancer risk. The validation and verification of AI-based systems still require the development of algorithms that can be used in well-designed clinical studies and bigger populations. Particularly in environments with limited resources, the innovative techniques and technologies have enormous potential to enhance results. By giving a real-time risk assessment, such methods can be utilized to forecast oral cancer risk as a supplement to population screening.

While AI is having an increasing impact on medicine, it is vital to remember that the software is designed to be a tool to assist the physician and that the physician is ultimately accountable for diagnosis and treatment. Although Al is unlikely to replace physicians in the near future, medical professionals who use AI will replace those who do not. Our future is dependent on collaboration with intelligent machines and algorithms.

References

Abbas Q, Emre Celebi M, Garcia IF, Ahmad W. Melanoma recognition framework based on expert definition of ABCD for dermoscopic images. Skin Res Technol. 2013;19(1):93–102.

Adeoye J, Koohi-Moghadam M, Lo AWI, Tsang RK, Chow VLY, Zheng LW, et al. Deep learning predicts the malignant-transformation-free survival of oral potentially malignant disorders. Cancers (Basel). 2021;13:13.

Alabi RO, Elmusrati M, Sawazaki-Calone I, et al. Machine learning application for prediction of locoregional recurrences in early oral tongue cancer: a web-based prognostic tool. Virchows Arch. 2019;475(4):489–97.

Alabi RO, Bello IO, Youssef O, Elmusrati M, Mäkitie AA, Almangush A. Utilizing deep machine learning for prognostication of oral squamous cell carcinoma—a systematic review. Front Oral Health. 2021;2:686863.

Alabi RO, Almangush A, Elmusrati M, Mäkitie AA. Deep machine learning for oral cancer: from precise diagnosis to precision medicine. Front Oral Health. 2022;2:794248.

Alhazmi A, Alhazmi Y, Makrami A, et al. Application of artificial intelligence and machine learning for prediction of oral cancer risk. J Oral Pathol Med. 2021;50:444–50. https://doi.org/10.1111/jop.13157.

Almangush A, Bello IO, Coletta RD, Mäkitie AA, Mäkinen LK, Kauppila JH, et al. For early-stage oral tongue cancer, depth of invasion and worst pattern of invasion are the strongest pathological predictors for locoregional recurrence and mortality. Virchows Arch. 2015;467:39–46. https://doi.org/10.1007/s00428-015-1758-z.

Ariji Y, Fukuda M, Kise Y, et al. Contrast-enhanced computed tomography image assessment of cervical lymph node metastasis in patients with oral cancer by using a deep learning system of artificial intelligence. Oral Surg Oral Med Oral Pathol Oral Radiol. 2019;127(5):458–63. https://doi.org/10.1016/j.oooo.2018.10.002.

Ariji Y, Sugita Y, Nagao T, et al. CT evaluation of extranodal extension of cervical lymph node metastases in patients with oral squamous cell carcinoma using deep learning classification. Oral Radiol. 2020;36(2):148–55. https://doi.org/10.1007/s11282-019-00391-4.

Ariji Y, Fukuda M, Nozawa M, et al. Automatic detection of cervical lymph nodes in patients with oral squamous cell carcinoma using a deep learning technique: a preliminary study. Oral Radiol. 2021;37(2):290–6. https://doi.org/10.1007/s11282-019-00391-4.

Aubreville M, Knipfer C, Oetter N, et al. Automatic classification of cancerous tissue in laserendomicroscopy images of the oral cavity using deep learning. Sci Rep. 2017;7(1):11979. https://doi.org/10.1038/s41598-017-12320-8.

Bilgin G, Çifci A. Eritematöz Skuamöz Hastalıkların Teşhisinde Makine Öğrenme Algoritmalarının Etkisi. JISTA. 2021;4(2):195–202.

Bouletreau P, Makaremi M, Ibrahim B, Louvrier A, Sigaux N. Artificial intelligence: applications in orthognathic surgery. J Stomatol Oral Maxillofac Surg. 2019;120:347–54.

Brinker TJ, Hekler A, Hauschild A, Berking C, Schilling B, Enk AH, et al. Comparing artificial intelligence algorithms to 157 German dermatologists: the melanoma classification benchmark. Eur J Cancer. 2019a;111:30–7.

Brinker TJ, Hekler A, Enk AH, Klode J, Hauschild A, Berking C, et al. A convolutional neuralnetwork trained with dermoscopic images performed on par with 145 dermatologists in a clinicalmelanoma image classification task. Eur J Cancer. 2019b;111:148–54.

Celebi ME, Kingravi H, Uddin B, Iyatomi H, Aslandogan A, Stoecker WV, et al. A methodological approach to the classification of dermoscopy images. Comput Med Imaging Graph. 2007;31(6):362–73.

Chan S, Reddy V, Myers B, Thibodeaux Q, Brownstone N. Liao W machine learning in dermatology: current applications, opportunities, and limitations. Dermatol Ther. 2020;10:365–86.

Chartrand G, Cheng PM, Vorontsov E, Drozdzal M, Turcotte S, Pal CJ, et al. Deep learning: Aprimer for radiologists. Radiographics. 2017;37:2113–31.

Chien CW, Lee YC, Ma T, Lee TS, Lin YC, Wang W, et al. The application of artificial neural networks and decision tree model in predicting postoperative complication for gastric cancer patients. Hepato-Gastroenterology. 2008;55:1140–5.

Chiesa-Estomba CM, Graña M, Medela A, Sistiaga-Suarez JA, Lechien JR, Calvo-Henriquez C, et al. Machine learning algorithms as a computer-assisted decision tool for oral cancer prognosis and management decisions: a systematic review. ORL. 2022;84:278–88.

Chu CS, Lee NP, Ho JWK, Choi S, Thomson PJ. Deep learning for clinical image analyses in oral squamous cell carcinoma: a review. JAMA Otolaryngol Head Neck Surg. 2021;147(10):893–900.

Chuchu N, Takwoingi Y, Dinnes J, Matin RN, Bassett O, Moreau JF, et al. Smartphone applicationsfor triaging adults with skin lesions that are suspicious for melanoma. Cochrane Database Syst Rev. 2018;2018:CD013192.

Cireşan DC, Meier U, Gambardella LM, Schmidhuber J. Deep, big,simple neural nets for handwritten digit recognition. Neural Comput. 2010;22:3207–20.

Codella NC, Nguyen QB, Pankanti S, Gutman DA, Helba B, Halpern AC, et al. Deep learning ensembles for melanoma recognition in dermoscopy images. IBM J Res Dev. 2017;61(4/5):5–1.

Coletta RD, Yeudall WA, Salo T. Grand challenges in oral cancers. Front Oral Health. 2020;1:3. https://doi.org/10.3389/froh.2020.00003.

Correa da Rosa J, Kim J, Tian S, Tomalin LE, Krueger JG, Suárez-Fariñas M. Shrinking the psoriasis assessment gap: early gene expression profiling accurately predicts response to long-term treatment. J Invest Dermatol. 2017;137:305–12.

Cullell-Dalmau M, Otero-Viñas M, Manzo C. Research techniques made simple: deep learning for the classification of dermatological images. J Invest Dermatol. 2020;140:507–514.e1.

Das N, Hussain E, Mahanta LB. Automated classification of cells into multiple classes in epithelial tissue of oral squamous cell carcinoma using transfer learning and convolutional neural network. Neural Netw. 2020;128:47–60. https://doi.org/10.1016/j.neunet.2020.05.003.

Davis JL, Murray JF. History and physical examination. Murray and nadel's textbook of respiratory medicine. 2016;263–277.e2.
De A, Sarda A, Gupta S, Das S. Use of Artificial Intelligence in Dermatology. Indian journal of dermatology. 2020;65(5):352–57.
Du-Harpur X, Watt FM, Luscombe NM, Lynch MD. What is AI? Applications of artificial intelligence to dermatology. Br J Dermatol. 2020;183(3):423–30.
DuM NR, Jamieson L, Liu Z, Bi P. Incidence trends of lip, oral cavity, and pharyngeal cancers: global burden of disease 1990–2017. J Dent Res. 2020;99:143–51. https://doi.org/10.1177/0022034519894963.
Ehteshami Bejnordi B, Veta M, Johannes van Diest P, et al; the CAMELYON16 Consortium. Diagnostic assessment of deep learning algorithms for detection of lymph node metastases in women with breast cancer. JAMA. 2017;318(22):2199–210. https://doi.org/10.1001/jama.2017.14585.
Emam S, Du AX, Surmanowicz P, Thomsen SF, Greiner R, Gniadecki R. Predicting the long-term outcomes of biologics in patients with psoriasis using machine learning. Br J Dermatol. 2020;182:1305–7.
Esteva A, Kuprel B, Novoa RA, Ko J, Swetter SM, Blau HM, et al. Dermatologist-level classificationof skin cancer with deep neural networks. Nature. 2017;542:115–8.
Esteva A, Robicquet A, Ramsundar B, et al. A guide to deep learning in healthcare. Nat Med. 2019;25(1):24–9. https://doi.org/10.1038/s41591-018-0316-z.
Farah CS, Dost F, Do L. Usefulness of optical fluorescence imaging in identification and triaging of oral potentially malignant disorders: A study of VELscope in the LESIONS programme. Journal of oral pathology & medicine : official publication of the International Association of Oral Pathologists and the American Academy of Oral Pathology. 2019;48(7):581–7. https://doi.org/10.1111/jop.128960.
Faradmal J, Soltanian AR, Roshanaei G, Khodabakhshi R, Kasaeian A. Comparison of the performance of log-logistic regression and artificial neural networks for predicting breast cancer relapse. Asian Pac J Cancer Prev. 2014;15:5883–8. https://doi.org/10.7314/APJCP.2014.15.14.5883.
Faziloglu Y, Stanley RJ, Moss RH, Stoecker WV, McLean RP. Colour histogram analysis for melanoma discrimination in clinical images. Skin Res Technol. 2003;9:147–55.
Ferrer-Sánchez A, Bagan J, Vila-Francés J, Magdalena-Benedito R, Bagan-Debon L. Prediction of the risk of cancer and the grade of dysplasia in leukoplakia lesions using deep learning. Oral Oncol. 2022;132:105967. https://doi.org/10.1016/j.oraloncology.2022.105967.
Folmsbee J, Liu X, Brandwein-Weber M, Doyle S. Active deep learning: improved training efficiency of convolutional neural networks for tissue classification in oral cavity cancer. Paper presented at: 2018 IEEE 15th International Symposium on Biomedical Imaging, Washington, DC, April 4–7, 2018.
Fu Q, Chen Y, Li Z, et al. A deep learning algorithm for detection of oral cavity squamous cell carcinoma from photographic images: a retrospective study. EClinicalMedicine. 2020;27:100558. https://doi.org/10.1016/j.eclinm.2020.100558.
Fujima N, Andreu-Arasa VC, Meibom SK, et al. Deep learning analysis using FDG-PET to predict treatment outcome in patients with oral cavity squamous cell carcinoma. Eur Radiol. 2020;30(11):6322–30. https://doi.org/10.1007/s00330-020-06982-8.
Fujisawa Y, Otomo Y, Ogata Y, Nakamura Y, Fujita R, Ishitsuka Y, et al. Deep-learning-based,computer-aided classifier developed with a small dataset of clinical images surpasses board-certified dermatologists in skin tumour diagnosis. Br J Dermatol. 2019;180:373–81.
Garbe C, Keim U, Gandini S, et al. Epidemiology of cutaneous melanoma and keratinocyte cancer in white populations 1943–2036. Eur J Cancer. 2021;152:18–25.
Golden JA. Deep learning algorithms for detection of lymph node metastases from breast cancer: helping artificial intelligence be seen. JAMA. 2017;318(22):2184–6. https://doi.org/10.1001/jama.2017.14580.

Goyal M, Knackstedt T, Yan S, Hassanpour S. Artificial intelligence-based image classification methods for diagnosis of skin cancer: challenges and opportunities. Comput Biol Med. 2020;127:104065. https://doi.org/10.1016/j.compbiomed.2020.104065.

Güneri P, Epstein JB. Late stage diagnosis of oral cancer: components and possible solutions. Oral Oncol. 2014;50:1131–6.

Guo P, Luo Y, Mai G, Zhang M, Wang G, Zhao M, Gao L, Li F, Zhou F. Gene expression profile based classification models of psoriasis. Genomics. 2014;103(1):48–55.

Gupta RK, Kaur M, Manhas J. Tissue level based deep learning framework for early detection of dysplasia in oral squamous epithelium. J Multimedia Inf Syst. 2019;6(2):81–6. https://doi.org/10.33851/JMIS.2019.6.2.81.

Haenssle HA, Fink C, Schneiderbauer R, Toberer F, Buhl T, Blum A, et al. Man against machine: diagnostic performance of a deep learning convolutional neural network for dermoscopic melanoma recognition in comparison to 58 dermatologists. Ann Oncol. 2018;29(8):1836–42.

Haenssle HA, Fink C, Toberer F, Winkler J, Stolz W, Deinlein T, et al. Man against machine reloaded: performance of a market-approved convolutional neural network in classifying a broad spectrum of skin lesions in comparison with 96 dermatologists working under less artificial conditions. Ann Oncol. 2020;31(1):137–43.

Hajdu A, Harangi B, Besenczi R, Lázár I, Emri G, Hajdu L et al. Measuring regularity of network patterns by grid approximations using the LLL algorithm, 23rd International Conference on Pattern Recognition (ICPR), Cancún, Mexico; 2016: 1524–1529.

Halicek M, Little JV, Wang X, Chen AY, Fei B. Optical biopsy of head and neck cancer using hyperspectral imaging and convolutional neural networks. J Biomed Opt. 2019a;24(3):1–9. https://doi.org/10.1117/1.JBO.24.3.036007.

Halicek M, Shahedi M, Little JV, et al. Head and neck cancer detection in digitized whole-slide histology using convolutional neural networks. Sci Rep. 2019b;9(1):14043. https://doi.org/10.1038/s41598-019-50313-x.

Han SS, Kim MS, Lim W, Park GH, Park I, Chang SE. Classification of the clinical images for benignand malignant cutaneous tumors using a deep learning algorithm. J Invest Dermatol. 2018;138:1529–38.

Harangi B. Skin lesion classification with ensembles of deep convolutional neural networks. J Biomed Inform. 2018;86:25–32.

Hayashi Y, Setiono R. Combining neural network predictions for medical diagnosis. Comput Biol Med. 2002;32(4):237–46.

Hekler A, Utikal JS, Enk AH, Berking C, Klode J, Schadendorf D, et al. Pathologist-levelclassification of histopathological melanoma images with deep neural networks. Eur J Cancer. 2019;115:79–83.

Hogarty DT, Mackey DA, Hewitt AW. Current state and future prospects of artificial intelligence inophthalmology: a review. Clin Exp Ophthalmol. 2019;47:128–39.

Hogarty DT, Su JC, Phan K, Attia M, Hossny M, Nahavandi S, et al. Artificial intelligence indermatology-where we are and the way to the future: a review. Am J Clin Dermatol. 2020;21:41–7.

Huang G, Liu Z, Maaten LVD, Weinberger KQ. Densely connected networks. Paper presented at: 2017 IEEE conference on computer vision and pattern recognition (CVPR). New York: IEEE; 2017. p. 2261–9. https://doi.org/10.1109/CVPR.2017.243.

Idrees M, Farah CS, Shearston K, Kujan O. A machine learning algorithm for the reliable identification of oral lichen planus. J Oral Pathol Med. 2021;00:1–8.

Ilhan B, Lin K, Guneri P, Wilder-Smith P. Improving Oral Cancer Outcomes with Imaging and Artificial Intelligence. Journal of dental research. 2020;99(3):241–8.

Ilhan B, Guneri P, Wilder-Smith P. The contribution of artificial intelligence to reducing the diagnostic delay in oral cancer. Oral Oncol. 2021;116:105254. https://doi.org/10.1016/j.oraloncology.2021.105254.

Jeyaraj PR, Rajan E, Nadar S. Computer-assisted medical image classification for early diagnosis of oral cancer employing deep learning algorithm Journal of Cancer Research and Clinical Oncology. 2019;145(4):829–37. https://doi.org/10.1007/s00432-018-02834-7.

Jeon SH, Jeon EH, Lee JY, Kim YS, Yoon HJ, Hong SP, Lee JH. The potential of interleukin 12 receptor beta 2 (IL12RB2) and tumor necrosis factor receptor superfamily member 8 (TNFRSF8) gene as diagnostic biomarkers of oral lichen planus (OLP). Acta Odontol Scand. 2015;73:588–94.

Jones OT, Matin RN, van der Schaar M, Prathivadi Bhayankaram K, Ranmuthu CKI, Islam MS, et al. Artificial intelligence and machine learning algorithms for early detection of skin cancer in community and primary care settings: a systematic review. Lancet Digit Health. 2022;4(6):e466–76.

Jutzi TB, Krieghoff-Henning EI, Holland-Letz T, et al. Artificial intelligence in skin cancer diagnostics: the patients' perspective. Front Med (Lausanne). 2020;7:233.

Jubair Omar F, Dimitrios Ak, Samara M, Yusser AM, Hassona YS. A novel lightweight deep convolutional neural network for early detection of oral cancer Abstract Oral Diseases 2022;28(4):1123–30. https://doi.org/10.1111/odi.v28.410.1111/odi.13825.

Kann BH, Hicks DF, Payabvash S, Mahajan A, Du J, Gupta V, et al. Multi-institutional validation of deep learning for pretreatment ıdentification of extranodal extension in head and neck squamous cell carcinoma. J Clin Oncol. 2020;38:1304–411.

Kar A, Wreesmann VB, Shwetha V, Thakur S, Rao VUS, Arakeri G, et al. Improvement of oral cancer screening quality and reach: the promise of artificial intelligence. J Oral Pathol Med. 2020;49:72.

Karimkhani C, Boyers LN, Dellavalle RP, Weinstock MA. It's time for "keratinocyte carcinoma" to replace the term "nonmelanoma skin cancer". J Am Acad Dermatol. 2015;72:186–7.

Kasmi R, Mokrani K. Classification of malignant melanoma and benign skin lesions: implementation of automatic ABCD rule. IET Image Process. 2016;10(6):448–55.

Keser G, Bayrakdar İŞ, Pekiner FN, Çelik Ö, Orhan K. A deep learning algorithm for classification of oral lichen planus lesions from photographic images: a retrospective study. J Stomatol Oral Maxillofac Surg. 2023;124(1):101264. https://doi.org/10.1016/j.jormas.2022.08.007.

Krizhevsky A, Sutskever I, Hinton GE. ImageNet classification with deep convolutional neural networks. Neural Inform Proc Syst. 2012;25:3065386.

Kumar VB, Kumar SS, Saboo V. Dermatological disease detection using image processing and machine learning, Third International Conference on Artificial Intelligence and Pattern Recognition (AIPR). 2016; 1–6. doi: https://doi.org/10.1109/ICAIPR.2016.7585217.

LeCun Y, Boser BE, Denker JS, et al. Handwritten digit recognition with a back-propagation network. In: Touretzky DS, editor. Advances in neural information processing systems 2. Burlington, MA: Morgan-Kaufmann; 1990. p. 396–404.

LeCun Y, Bengio Y, Hinton G. Deep learning. Nature. 2015;521:436–44.

Li CX, Shen CB, Xue K, Shen X, Jing Y, Wang ZY, Xu F, Meng RS, Yu JB, Cui Y. Artificial intelligence in dermatology: past, present, and future. Chin Med J. 2019;132:2017–20. https://doi.org/10.1097/CM9.0000000000000372.

Llewellyn CD, Johnson NW, Warnakulasuriya KA. Risk factors for squamous cell carcinoma of the oral cavity in young people--a comprehensive literature review. Oral oncology. 2001;37(5):401–18.

Llewellyn CD, Johnson NW, Warnakulasuriya KA. Risk factors for oral cancer in newly diagnosed patients aged 45 years and younger: a case-control study in Southern England. Journal of oral pathology & medicine : official publication of the International Association of Oral Pathologists and the American Academy of Oral Pathology. 2004;33(9):525–32.

Lloyd H, Craig S. A guide to taking a patient's history. Nursing Standard. 2007;22(13):42–8.

MacCarthy D, Flint SR, Healy C, Stassen LF. Oral and neck examination for early detection of oral cancer a practical guide. Journal of the Irish Dental Association. 2011;57(4):195–9.

Maghsoudi R, Bagheri A, Maghsoudi MT. Diagnosis prediction of lichen planus ,leukoplakia and oral squamous cell carcinoma by using an intelligent system based on artificial neural networks. J Dentomaxillofac Radiol Pathol Surg. 2013;2:1–8.

Mahmood F, Bendayan S, Ghazawi FM, Litvinov IV. Editorial: the emerging role of artificial intelligence in dermatology. Front Med. 2021;8:751649.

Marka A, Carter JB, Toto E, Hassanpour S. Automated detection of nonmelanoma skin cancer using digital images: a systematic review. BMC Med Imaging. 2019;19:21.

Maron RC, Weichenthal M, Utikal JS, Hekler A, Berking C, Hauschild A, et al. Systematic outperformance of 112 dermatologists in multiclass skin cancer image classification by convolutional neural networks. Eur J Canc. 2019;119:57–63.

Masood A, Al-Jumaily AA. Computer aided diagnostic support system for skin cancer: a review of techniques and algorithms. Int J Biomed Imaging. 2013;2013:323268.

Miller DD, Brown EW. Artificial intelligence in medical practice: the question to the answer? Am J Med. 2018;131:129–33.

Miranda-Filho A, Bray F. Global patterns and trends in cancers of the lip, tongue and mouth. Oral Oncol. 2020;102:104551. https://doi.org/10.1016/j.oraloncology.2019.104551.

Nachbar F, Stolz W, Merkle T, Cognetta AB, Vogt T, Landthaler M, Bilek P, Braun-Falco O, Plewig G. The ABCD rule of dermatoscopy. High prospective value in the diagnosis of doubtful melanocytic skin lesions. J Am Acad Dermatol. 1994;30(4):551–9. https://doi.org/10.1016/s0190-9622(94)70061-3.

Nagpal K, Foote D, Tan F, et al. Development and validation of a deep learning algorithm for Gleason grading of prostate cancer from biopsy specimens. JAMA Oncol. 2020;6(9):1372–80. https://doi.org/10.1001/jamaoncol.2020.2485.

Nasr-Esfahani E, Samavi S, Karimi N, Soroushmehr SMR, Jafari MH, Ward K, et al. Melanoma detection by analysis of clinical images using convolutional neural network. Conf Proc IEEE EngMed Biol Soc. 2016;2016:1373–6.

Nayak Sudha GS, Keerthilatha KM, Arindam P, Satadru S, Jacob R, Lawrence K, D'Almeida BR, Krishnanand C, Santhosh VB, Kartha KK, Mahato. Principal component analysis and artificial neural network analysis of oral tissue fluorescence spectra: Classification of normal premalignant and malignant pathological conditions Abstract Biopolymers. 2006;82(2):152–66. https://doi.org/10.1002/bip.v82:210.1002/bip.20473.

Neppelberg E, Loro LL, Qiordsbakken G, Johannessen AC. Altered CD 40 and E cadherin expression putative role in oral lichen planus. J Oral Pathol Med. 2007;36:153–60.

Pai VV, Pai RB. Artificial intelligence in dermatology and healthcare: an overview. Indian J Dermatol Venereol Leprol. 2021;87:457–67.

Pan SJ, Yang Q. A survey on transfer learning. IEEE Trans Knowl Data Eng. 2009;22(10):1345–59. https://doi.org/10.1109/TKDE.2009.191.

Patil S, Albogami S, Hosmani J, Mujoo S, Kamil MA, Mansour MA, Abdul HN, Bhandi S, Ahmed SSSJ. Artificial Intelligence in the Diagnosis of Oral Diseases: Applications and Pitfalls. Diagnostics (Basel, Switzerland). 2022;12(5):1029.

Pekiner FN, Demirel GY, Borahan MO, Ozbayrak S. Evaluation of cytotoxic T cell activation, chemokine receptors, and adhesion molecules in blood and serum in patients with oral lichen planus. J Oral Pathol Med. 2012;41:484–9.

Pekiner FN, Borahan MO, Özbayrak S. Evaluation of levels of cortizoli anxiety and depression in patients with oral lichen planus OLP. Clin Exp Health Sci. 2014;4:24–8.

Polesie S, Gillstedt M, Kittler H, et al. Attitudes towards artificial intelligence within dermatology: an international online survey. Br J Dermatol. 2020;183:159–61.

Quer G, Muse ED, Nikzad N, Topol EJ, Steinhubl SR. Augmenting diagnostic vision with AI. Lancet. 2017;390:221. https://doi.org/10.1016/S0140-6736(17)31764-6.

Rosma MD, Sameemii AK, Basir A, Mazlipahiv IS, Norzaidi MD. The use of artificial intelligence to identify people at risk of oral cancer: empirical evidence in Malaysian university. Int J Sci Res Edu. 2010;3:10–20.

Saba L, Biswas M, Kuppili V, Cuadrado Godia E, Suri HS, Edla DR, et al. The present and future of deep learning in radiology. Eur J Radiol. 2019;114:14–24.

Sadeghi M, Razmara M, Lee TK, Atkins MS. A novel method for detection of pigment network in dermoscopic images using graphs. Comput Med Imaging Graph. 2011;35(2):137–43.

Santoro A, Majorana A, Bardellini E, et al. Cytotoxic molecule expression and epithelial cell apoptosis in oral and cutaneous lichen planus. Am J Clin Pathol. 2004;121:758–64.

Schwendicke F, Samek W, Krois J. Artificial Intelligence in Dentistry: Chances and Challenges. Journal of Dental Research. 2020;99(7):769–4. https://doi.org/10.1177/0022034520915714.
Shaban M, Khurram SA, Fraz MM, et al. A novel digital score for abundance of tumour infiltrating lymphocytes predicts disease free survival in oral squamous cell carcinoma. Sci Rep. 2019;9(1):13341. https://doi.org/10.1038/s41598-019-49710-z.
Shams WK, Htike ZZ. Oral Cancer Prediction Using Gene Expression Profiling and Machine Learning. Int. J. Appl. Eng. Res. 2017;12:4893–98.
Shan T, Tay FR, Gu L. Application of artificial intelligence in dentistry. J Dent Res. 2021;100:232–44.
Shimizu H, Nakayama KI. Artificial intelligence in oncology. Cancer Sci. 2020;111:1452–60.
Shin HC, Roth HR, Gao M, et al. Deep convolutional neural networks for computer-aided detection: CNN architectures, dataset characteristics and transfer learning. IEEE Trans Med Imaging. 2016;35(5):1285–98. https://doi.org/10.1109/TMI.2016.2528162.
Shorten C, Khoshgoftaar TM. A survey on image data augmentation for deep learning. J Big Data. 2019;6(1):1–48. https://doi.org/10.1186/s40537-019-0197-0.
Shrivastava VK, Londhe ND, Sonawane RS, Suri JS. Computer-aided diagnosis of psoriasis skin images with HOS, texture and color features: a first comparative study of its kind. Comput Methods Programs Biomed. 2016;126:98–109.
Shrivastava VK, Londhe ND, Sonawane RS, Suri JS. A novel and robust Bayesian approach for segmentation of psoriasis lesions and its risk stratification. Comput Methods Prog Biomed. 2017;150:9–22.
Silver D, Huang A, Maddison CJ, Guez A, Sifre L, van den Driessche G, et al. Mastering the game of go with deep neural networks andtree search. Nature. 2016;529:484–9. https://doi.org/10.1038/nature16961.
Simonato LE, Tomo S, Navarro SR, Balbin Villaverde AGJ. Fluorescence visualization improves the detection of oral, potentially malignant, disorders in population screening. Photodiagnosis and photodynamic therapy. 2019:27:74–78. https://doi.org/10.1016/j.pdpdt.2019.05.017.
Stoecker WV, Gupta K, Stanley RJ, Moss RH, Shrestha B. Detection of asymmetric blotches (asymmetric structureless areas) in dermoscopy images of malignant melanoma using relative color. Skin Res Technol. 2005;11(3):179–84.
Tanriver G, Soluk Tekkesin M, Ergen O. Automated detection and classification of oral lesions using deep learning to detect oral potentially malignant disorders. Cancers (Basel). 2021;13(11):2766.
Thiem DGE, Römer P, Gielisch M, Al-Nawas B, Schlüter M, Plaß B, et al. Hyperspectral imaging and artificial intelligence to detect oral malignancy - part 1 - automated tissue classification of oral muscle, fat and mucosa using a light-weight 6-layer deep neural network. Head Face Med. 2021;17:38.
Topol EJ. High-performance medicine: the convergence of human and artificial intelligence. Nat Med. 2019;25(1):44–56. https://doi.org/10.1038/ns41591-018-0300-7.
Tschandl P, Rosendahl C, Kittler H. The HAM10000 dataset, a large collection of multi-source dermatoscopic images of common pigmented skin lesions. Sci Data. 2018;5:180161.
Tschandl P, Rosendahl C, Akay BN, Argenziano G, Blum A, Braun RP, et al. Expert-level diagnosis of nonpigmented skin cancer by combined convolutional neural networks. JAMA Dermatol. 2019a;155(1):58–65.
Tschandl P, Codella N, Akay BN, Argenziano G, Braun RP, Cabo H, et al. Comparison of the accuracy of human readers versus machinelearning algorithms for pigmented skin lesion classification: an open, web-based, international, diagnostic study. Lancet Oncol. 2019b;20:938–47. https://doi.org/10.1016/S1470-2045(19)30333-X.
Ubeyli ED. Combined neural networks for diagnosis of erythemato-squamous diseases. Expert Syst Appl. 2009;36:5107–12.
Uthoff RD, Song B, Sunny S, Patrick S, Suresh A, Kolur T, Keerthi G, Spires O, Anbarani A, Wilder-Smith P, Kuriakose M A, Birur P, Liang R. Point-of-care smartphone-based dual-modality dual-view oral cancer screening device with neural network classification for

low-resource communities PLOS ONE 2018;13(12): e0207493. https://doi.org/10.1371/journal.pone.0207493.

Waasdorp M, Krom BP, Bikker FJ, van Zuijlen PPM, Niessen FB, Gibbs S. The bigger picture: why oral mucosa heals better than skin. Biomolecules. 2021;11:1165.

Wada M, Ge Z, Gilmore SJ, Mar VJ. Use of artificial intelligence in skin cancer diagnosis and management. Med J Aust. 2020;213:256–2591.

Wang X, Yang J, Wei C, Zhou G, Wu L, Gao Q, et al. A personalized computational model predicts cancer risk level of oral potentially malignant disorders and its web application for promotion of non-invasive screening. J Oral Pathol Med. 2020;49:417–26.

Warin K, Limprasert W, Suebnukarn S, Jinaporntham S, Jantana P. Automatic classification and detection of oral cancer in photographic images using deep learning algorithms. J Oral Pathol Med. 2021;50:911–8.

Warnakulasuriya S, Kerr AR. Oral cancer screening: Past, present, and future. J Dent Res. 2021;100:1313–20.

Welch HG, Mazer BL, Adamson AS. The rapid rise in cutaneous melanoma diagnoses. N Engl J Med. 2021;384:72–9.

Welikala RA, Remagnino P, Lim JH, et al. Automated detection and classification of oral lesions using deep learning for early detection of oral cancer. IEEE Access. 2020;8:132677–93. https://doi.org/10.1109/access.2020.3010180.

Yang J, Sun X, Liang J, Rosin PL. Clinical skin lesion diagnosis using representations inspired by dermatologist criteria. In: Proceedings of the IEEE Conference on Computer Vision and Pattern Recognition; 2018:1258–1266.

Young AT, Xiong M, Pfau J, Keiser MJ, Wei ML. Artificial intelligence in dermatology: a primer. J Invest Dermatol. 2020;140(8):1504–12.

Yu L, Chen H, Dou Q, Qin J, Heng PA. Automated melanoma recognition in dermoscopy images via very deep residual networks. IEEE Trans Med Imaging. 2017;36(4):994–1004.

Zheng B, Yoon SW, Lam SS. Breast cancer diagnosis based on feature extraction using a hybrid of K-means and support vector machine algorithms. Expert Syst Appl. 2014;41:1476–82.

Impact of AI in Obstructive Sleep Apnea 10

Kaan Orhan and Seçil Aksoy

Obstructive sleep apnea (OSA) is a sleep disorder characterized by repeated episodes of partial or complete obstruction of the upper airway during sleep (Borel et al. 2012). The underlying reasons of the condition may be highly complex and encompass various physiological factors such as the control mechanism for respiration, sensory function, anatomical abnormalities that contribute to the collapse of the upper airway, and factors related to the skeletal structure, soft tissues, and pharyngeal muscles (Badr 1998; Azagra-Calero et al. 2012).

Prevalence of OSA

One of the most frequently encountered sleep-related disorders, obstructive sleep apnea (OSA), affects a significant proportion of the global population. The overall incidence of OSA varies considerably across various demographic groups and age ranges. Several comprehensive studies, utilizing large-scale samples reflective of the broader population, have been conducted and offer prevalence estimates for OSA. In the HypnoLaus Sleep Cohort study conducted by Heinzer et al., the prevalence of moderate-to-severe sleep-disordered breathing was reported to be 23.4% in female participants and 49.7% in male participants within the Swiss population (Heinzer et al. 2015). In a large South American metropolis, a 2010 epidemiological study found that 32.8% of individuals had OSA (Tufik et al. 2010). According to the Wisconsin Sleep Study Cohort, at least moderate OSA was present in 10% of men

K. Orhan
Faculty of Dentistry, Department of Dentomaxillofacial Radiology, Ankara University, Ankara, Turkey

S. Aksoy (✉)
Faculty of Dentistry, Department of Dentomaxillofacial Radiology, Near University, Nicosia, Cyprus
e-mail: secil.aksoy@neu.edu.tr

K. Orhan, R. Jagtap (eds.), *Artificial Intelligence in Dentistry*,
https://doi.org/10.1007/978-3-031-43827-1_10

and 3% of women aged between 30 and 49 years. Furthermore, in the age group of 50 to 70 years, the prevalence increased to 17% in men and 9% in women (Peppard et al. 2013).

Impact on Public Health

Obstructive sleep apnea has substantial implications for public health due to its association with a wide range of negative health outcomes. Some key impacts include the following:

Daytime Sleepiness and Impaired Cognitive Function: The impact of OSA on individuals extends beyond nighttime disturbances. OSA has significant consequences for daytime functions, particularly in terms of excessive sleepiness and impaired cognitive function. Individuals with OSA often experience reduced alertness, leading to fatigue, work limitations and absenteeism, difficulties in maintaining attention and concentration, occupational or motor vehicle injuries, and reduced quality of life (Guglielmi et al. 2015). These symptoms can hinder cognitive performance, including episodic memory, working memory, learning ability, and executive functions. Furthermore, OSA-related cognitive impairments may manifest as decreased processing speed, impaired decision-making, and reduced visuospatial abilities (Faria et al. 2021). The interplay between disrupted sleep patterns and cognitive dysfunction in OSA underscores the importance of early diagnosis and effective treatment to mitigate the adverse effects on daytime functioning and overall quality of life.

Cardiovascular Disease Risks: The recurrent partial or complete upper airway obstructions during sleep in individuals with OSA contribute to increased sympathetic nervous system activity, resulting from factors such as intermittent hypoxemia, hypercapnia, and sleep fragmentation. This heightened sympathetic activity plays a crucial role in both the acute rise in blood pressure during obstructive apneas and the development of sustained hypertension associated with intermittent hypoxemia (Gottlieb 2021). The repetitive occurrence of these physiological changes throughout the night places significant strain on the cardiovascular system. Furthermore, the intermittent hypoxia and sleep fragmentation characteristic contribute to inflammation, oxidative stress, endothelial dysfunction, and insulin resistance, thereby contributing to the development and progression of cardiovascular diseases (Salman et al. 2020). Consequently, OSA patient is strongly linked to an increased risk of hypertension, atrial fibrillation, other arrhythmias, heart failure, coronary artery disease, cerebrovascular disease, and pulmonary hypertension (Yeghiazarians et al. 2021). Recognizing and effectively managing OSA is crucial for decreasing these cardiovascular risks and improving long-term cardiovascular outcomes for individuals affected by this sleep disorder.

Metabolic Disorders and Obesity: OSA patients are also at increased risk of developing metabolic disorders such as insulin resistance, glucose intolerance, obesity, and dyslipidemia. Similar to the mechanisms observed in cardiovascular disease, intermittent hypoxia, sleep fragmentation, and sympathetic activation in OSA cause hormonal dysregulation and disturbances in energy metabolism (Drager et al. 2013). OSA may induce metabolic disturbances that lead to weight gain, difficulty losing weight, and a higher incidence of obesity among affected individuals. Furthermore, there is often a bidirectional association between OSA and obesity, with obesity increasing the risk for OSA while OSA worsens metabolic dysfunction. This detrimental cycle intensifies OSA-related metabolic problems, perpetuating their impact on overall health.

Mood Disorders and Reduced Quality of Life: The impact of OSA extends beyond its physiological consequences and encompasses a profound influence on mood disorders and overall quality of life. Individuals with OSA may commonly experience mood disturbances such as depression, anxiety, and irritability. A review study conducted by Gupta and Simpson reported that there is evidence suggesting a potential association between OSA and certain psychiatric disorders, specifically major depressive disorder (MDD) and posttraumatic stress disorder (PTSD). However, studies in this subject exhibit significant heterogeneity and a high risk of bias. On the other hand, the available evidence is insufficient to support an increased prevalence of OSA in other psychotic disorders except PTSD (Gupta and Simpson 2015).

OSA has significant implications for public health, impacting multiple aspects of well-being. The collective impact of OSA on public health is substantial, leading to significant healthcare costs and decreased productivity. The comprehensive understanding and management of OSA are crucial for minimizing its impact on public health, improving outcomes, and enhancing the overall health and quality of life for individuals affected by this condition. The integration of AI technologies in OSA care holds promise for improving diagnosis, treatment, and overall patient outcomes.

Traditional Approaches in OSA Diagnosis and Treatment

Sleep Studies (Polysomnography)

Polysomnography (PSG) is a comprehensive diagnostic procedure that involves the simultaneous recording and analysis of neurophysiological, respiratory, cardiovascular, and other relevant physiological parameters to provide a detailed assessment of sleep patterns and disturbances, including OSA. It is a noninvasive procedure that involves monitoring various physiological parameters during sleep to assess sleep architecture and detect abnormalities. PSG measures multiple physiologic variables simultaneously, using electroencephalography (EEG), electrooculography (EOG), electromyography (EMG), electrocardiography (ECG), nasal airflow and respiratory effort, pulse oximetry, and sometimes limb movements (Rundo and Downey 3rd. 2019).

During a PSG, the patient is typically monitored overnight in a sleep laboratory, where they are tethered to electrodes and sensors that record the aforementioned signals. These recordings provide detailed information about sleep stages, the presence of apneas, hypopneas, arousals, and other sleep-related events. The analysis of

PSG results allows for the determination of the Apnea-Hypopnea Index (AHI), which represents the average number of apneas and hypopneas per hour of sleep (Berry et al. 2012). The AHI is used to classify the severity of OSA as mild (Tufik et al. 2010; Peppard et al. 2013; Guglielmi et al. 2015; Faria et al. 2021; Gottlieb 2021; Salman et al. 2020; Yeghiazarians et al. 2021; Drager et al. 2013; Gupta and Simpson 2015; Rundo and Downey 3rd. 2019; Berry et al. 2012), moderate (Berry et al. 2012; Chiu et al. 2017; Motin et al. 2019; Long et al. 2014; Al-Angari and Sahakian 2012; Almazaydeh et al. 2012; Maniaci et al. 2023; Vaquerizo-Villar et al. 2022; Bozkurt et al. 2017; Benedetti et al. 2022; Bernardini et al. 2021; Orhan et al. 2022; Tsuiki et al. 2021; Ryu et al. 2021; Scioscia et al. 2022), or severe (more than 30) (Chiu et al. 2017). Additionally, PSG can provide insights into other sleep disorders, such as periodic limb movement disorder and parasomnias.

Challenges and Limitations

Although PSG is considered the gold standard for diagnosing OSA, it has some drawbacks. The primary limitation of PSG is the potential inconvenience and disruption it poses to subjects, which can adversely affect their ability to achieve normal and natural sleep. PSG requires the application of multiple sensors and electrodes to the body, which may cause discomfort, restrict movement, and introduce artifacts that disrupt the sleep experience (Motin et al. 2019). The unfamiliar environment of the sleep laboratory, noise, and the presence of monitoring equipment can further contribute to sleep disturbances and alter sleep architecture. These factors may lead to incomplete or atypical sleep patterns, potentially affecting the accuracy and representativeness of the PSG data. Despite these challenges, efforts are being made to improve patient comfort and develop alternative home-based sleep monitoring methods to enhance the overall experience and acceptance of sleep studies in clinical practice.

PSG poses challenges in terms of cost and time requirements, as it involves multiple factors to ensure a comprehensive evaluation of OSA. The analysis of PSG data necessitates the expertise of sleep specialists for accurate interpretation and diagnosis (Motin et al. 2019). Furthermore, PSG typically requires access to a specialized sleep laboratory equipped with the necessary facilities and resources for conducting sleep studies. This availability constraint, along with the need to schedule and coordinate appointments, can lead to delays in the diagnosis and management of OSA.

Despite these challenges, PSG remains a valuable tool in diagnosing OSA and assessing its severity. The continuous advancement of technology has led to the development of portable sleep study devices and home sleep apnea testing (HSAT), which offer alternatives to in-laboratory PSG, improving accessibility and patient comfort, integrating additional monitoring parameters, such as actigraphy and respiratory effort, and utilizing machine learning algorithms for automated analysis when PSG is not available (Long et al. 2014).

AI Applications in OSA Diagnosis

The accurate and timely diagnosis of OSA is crucial for effective management and improving patient outcomes. Recent advancements in artificial intelligence (AI) have shown promise in revolutionizing OSA diagnosis.

Automated Screening Using AI Algorithms: Automated screening utilizing AI algorithms has emerged as a highly promising method for efficient diagnosis of OSA. By analyzing extensive patient data, including physiological signals and clinical information, AI algorithms can effectively identify individuals with a high risk of OSA. Recently, various machine learning algorithms, including support vector machines and deep learning models, have been found successful in accurately classifying OSA severity and predicting treatment outcomes. The utilization of these AI-based screening tools holds great potential for streamlining the diagnostic process, alleviating the workload of sleep clinics, and improving patient accessibility to comprehensive OSA evaluations. In their study, Al-Angari and Sahakian employed a support vector machine classifier to automatically identify obstructive sleep apnea (OSA). They observed that respiratory features displayed the highest sensitivity when classifying on a minute level, whereas oxygen saturation exhibited the highest specificity. In terms of subject classification, the use of a polynomial kernel substantially enhanced the accuracy of oxygen saturation, resulting in a notable accuracy of 95% for both oxygen saturation and the combined feature (Al-Angari and Sahakian 2012). Another study investigated a new classification algorithm that analyzes electrocardiogram (ECG) data in brief time segments. The findings revealed impressive accuracy levels of the automated classification system, with a success rate of 96.5% or greater in identifying sleep disorder epochs (Almazaydeh et al. 2012).

Machine Learning Techniques for Pattern Recognition: Machine learning techniques have exhibited substantial promise in discerning patterns and deriving valuable insights from intricate datasets in the field of OSA diagnosis. Through training on extensive datasets encompassing polysomnography recordings, demographic data, and clinical variables, machine learning models possess the ability to recognize distinctive patterns linked to the severity of OSA, comorbid conditions, and treatment outcomes. These models offer the potential to identify individuals at a heightened risk level, facilitate the formulation of personalized treatment strategies, and contribute to the advancement of precision medicine approaches in OSA management. Clinical-based algorithms utilizing artificial intelligence can be employed to assess patients exhibiting symptoms associated with OSA, aiding in the identification of individuals at high risk of severe OSA within the OSA framework (Maniaci et al. 2023). Vaquerizo-Villar et al. conducted a study that revealed the potential of utilizing CNN analysis of blood oxygen saturation (SpO2) recordings for the automated diagnosis of obstructive sleep apnea (OSA) in at-home oximetry tests (Vaquerizo-Villar et al. 2022). The utilization of machine learning techniques enables the estimation of probabilities pertaining to the absence of obstructive sleep apnea (OSA), as well as its mild, moderate, and severe forms. Employing such approaches has the potential to enhance the precision of initial OSA screening, thereby enabling the referral of suspected moderate or severe OSA patients exclusively to sleep laboratories for costly diagnostic tests. This could lead to a more efficient allocation of resources and reduce unnecessary testing for individuals with a lower likelihood of significant OSA severity (Bozkurt et al. 2017). Benedetti et al. used a wearable device and machine learning algorithms which demonstrated excellent performance, surpassing the limitations of questionnaires by utilizing objectively gathered data. Additionally, the widespread availability of commercial devices incorporating the algorithms allows for broad usage among the general population. Given these advantages, the application of machine learning algorithms to analyze data from smartbands leads to the compelling possibility of conducting large-scale screening for obstructive sleep apnea syndrome. This machine learning algorithms have the potential to serve as a population-wide screening tool for OSAS, offering significant benefits over traditional questionnaires (Benedetti et al. 2022). In their research, Bernardini et al. employed commonly recorded vital signs such as ECG and oxygen saturation to detect cases of obstructive sleep apnea syndrome. Their model demonstrated high precision in accurately identifying OSAS cases within the dataset and effectively determining the severity of the condition (Bernardini et al. 2021).

Image Analysis and Signal Processing: Image analysis and signal processing techniques have also been leveraged to improve OSA diagnosis. For instance, analysis of upper airway images obtained from techniques such as magnetic resonance imaging (MRI) and cone-beam computed tomography (CBCT) can provide valuable insights into anatomical abnormalities associated with OSA (Figs. 10.1, 10.2, and 10.3). Signal processing techniques, such as time-frequency analysis and spectral analysis, enable the extraction of relevant features from physiological signals

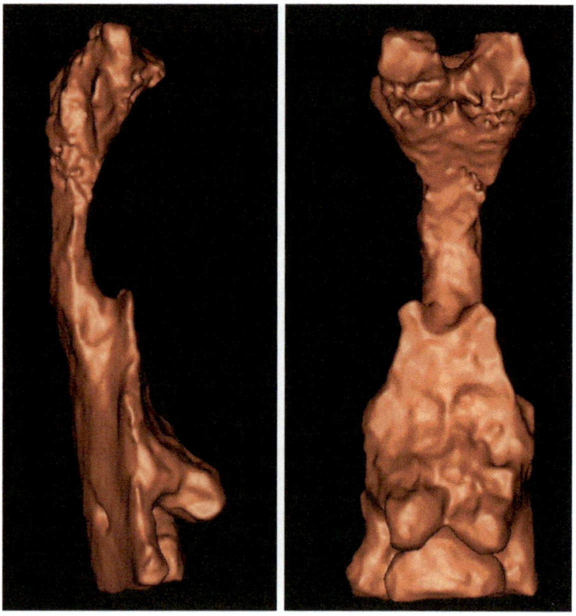

Fig. 10.1 3D AI segmentation of the pharyngeal airway from the sagittal and coronal view

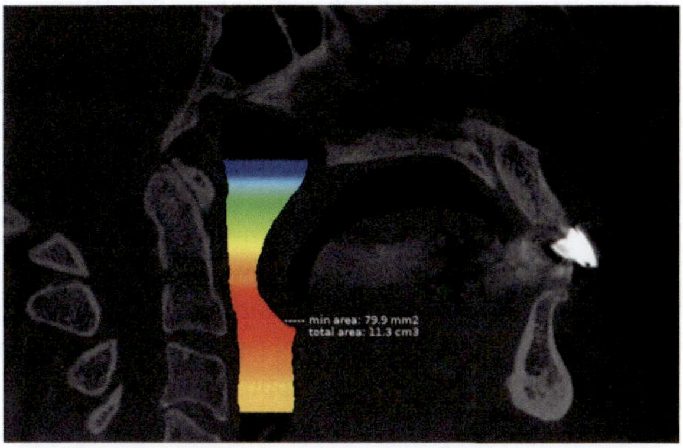

Fig. 10.2 Sagittal view of the upper airway and minimum constricted area

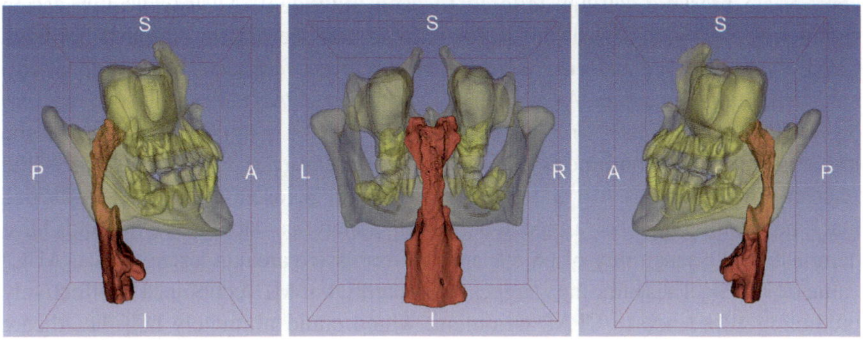

Fig. 10.3 3D volumetric assessment of pharyngeal airway AI segmentation

recorded during sleep studies. These image analysis and signal processing methods, when combined with AI algorithms, can enhance the understanding of OSA pathophysiology and assist in accurate diagnosis and treatment planning. Orhan et al. used an AI-based automated segmentation tool to assess the 3D pharyngeal airway in OSA, and their findings indicated no statistically significant disparities between the manual method and the AI system (Orhan et al. 2022). Another study utilized machine learning techniques to identify individuals with severe obstructive sleep apnea using 2D images. The findings indicated that a deep convolutional neural network (CNN) exhibited high accuracy in correctly detecting severe OSA patients. These results emphasize the potential of employing artificial intelligence systems for the identification and diagnosis of severe OSA (Tsuiki et al. 2021). Ryu et al. employed deep learning, computational fluid dynamics (CFD), and machine learning techniques to automatically segment upper airway morphology. Through this approach, they developed a predictive model capable of identifying flow characteristics associated with upper airway collapse. This auto-segmentation algorithm eliminated the time-consuming manual extraction of upper airway morphological factors, streamlining the diagnostic process. By utilizing regression and classification models, the researchers successfully analyzed flow characteristics and provided patient diagnoses within a short timeframe of 10 min. This efficient and convenient real-time diagnosis approach holds promise for clinicians seeking effective and expedited assessments in the field of upper airway disorders (Ryu et al. 2021).

AI-Driven Personalized Treatment Strategies

AI modeling in OSA treatment provide clinicians with valuable insights and decision support tools to optimize treatment strategies and personalize patient care. By analyzing a wide range of factors and patterns within patient data, these models can help identify which treatment approaches are likely to yield the best outcomes for individual patients.

CPAP therapy is a common treatment for OSA, but its effectiveness relies on appropriate pressure settings tailored to each individual. AI-driven optimization techniques use machine learning algorithms to analyze patient data and optimize CPAP therapy. By considering factors such as patient feedback, physiological signals, and compliance data, AI algorithms can adjust CPAP pressure levels, enhancing treatment outcomes and adherence. One of the primary obstacles in the implementation of continuous positive airway pressure (CPAP) treatment is the issue of low adherence. To address this challenge, Scioscia et al. have developed machine learning methods aimed at predicting adherence rates. These methods have demonstrated a sensitivity of 68.6% and an impressive area under the curve (AUC) value of 72.9%. These findings suggest the potential of ML techniques in effectively predicting adherence to CPAP treatment, which could ultimately help healthcare professionals identify patients who may require additional support to improve their adherence rates (Scioscia et al. 2022). The complexity of identifying factors that influence long-term adherence to continuous positive airway pressure (CPAP) treatment can be addressed through the use of machine learning (ML) techniques.

The implementation of a machine learning-based intelligent monitoring system for CPAP treatment has shown promising results in improving daily compliance, ensuring excellent patient satisfaction, and maintaining cost-effectiveness. Machine learning (ML) techniques facilitate the identification of patients with low adherence to CPAP treatment, enabling the provision of additional support and alternative treatment options (Turino et al. 2021).

Adaptive algorithms offer real-time monitoring and adjustment of treatment parameters to improve therapy effectiveness. These algorithms continuously analyze patient data, including physiological signals and behavioral patterns, to make dynamic treatment adjustments. In the study conducted by Chen et al., they explored the utilization of the information storage function of a smart positive pressure ventilator, which can be accessed via a local medical terminal. This comprehensive system incorporates various components such as data collection, data processing, and a medical interface design. By transmitting real-time respiratory data packets from the CPAP ventilator to the terminal, the researchers were able to analyze the information effectively. Notably, the alarm message processing function played a crucial role in monitoring the patient's breathing status, extracting pertinent alarm-related details, and generating alarms when necessary. The implementation of this telemedicine system holds a promising potential in enhancing the quality of life for individuals diagnosed with obstructive sleep apnea syndrome (Chen et al. 2021).

References

Al-Angari HM, Sahakian AV. Automated recognition of obstructive sleep apnea syndrome using support vector machine classifier. IEEE Trans Inf Technol Biomed. 2012;16(3):463–8.

Almazaydeh L, Elleithy K, Faezipour M. Obstructive sleep apnea detection using SVM-based classification of ECG signal features. Annu Int Conf IEEE Eng Med Biol Soc. 2012;2012:4938–41.

Azagra-Calero E, Espinar-Escalona E, Barrera-Mora JM, LlamasCarreras JM, Solano-Reina E. Obstructive sleep apnea syndrome (OSAS). Review of the literature. Med Oral Patol Oral Cir Bucal. 2012;17:925–9.

Badr MS. Pathophysiology of upper airway obstruction during sleep. Clin Chest Med. 1998;19:21–32.

Benedetti D, Olcese U, Bruno S, et al. Obstructive sleep apnoea syndrome screening through wrist-worn smartbands: a machine-learning approach. Nat Sci Sleep. 2022;14:941–56.

Bernardini A, Brunello A, Gigli GL, Montanari A, Saccomanno N. AIOSA: an approach to the automatic identification of obstructive sleep apnea events based on deep learning. Artif Intell Med. 2021;118:102133.

Berry RB, Budhiraja R, Gottlieb DJ, et al. Rules for scoring respiratory events in sleep: update of the 2007 AASM manual for the scoring of sleep and associated events. Deliberations of the sleep apnea definitions task force of the American Academy of sleep medicine. J Clin Sleep Med. 2012;8(5):597–619.

Borel JC, Gakwaya S, Masse JF, Melo-Silva CA, Sériès F. Impact of CPAP interface and mandibular advancement device on upper airway mechanical properties assessed with phrenic nerve stimulation in sleep apnea patients. Respir Physiol Neurobiol. 2012;183:170–6.

Bozkurt S, Bostanci A, Turhan M. Can statistical machine learning algorithms help for classification of obstructive sleep apnea severity to optimal utilization of polysomnography resources? Methods Inf Med. 2017;56(4):308–18.

Chen Z, Zhao Z, Zhang Z. Obstructive sleep apnea syndrome treated using a positive pressure ventilator based on artificial intelligence processor. J Healthc Eng. 2021;2021:5683433.

Chiu HY, Chen PY, Chuang LP, et al. Diagnostic accuracy of the Berlin questionnaire, STOP-BANG, STOP, and Epworth sleepiness scale in detecting obstructive sleep apnea: a bivariate meta-analysis. Sleep Med Rev. 2017;36:57–70.

Drager LF, Togeiro SM, Polotsky VY, Lorenzi-Filho G. Obstructive sleep apnea: a cardiometabolic risk in obesity and the metabolic syndrome. J Am Coll Cardiol. 2013;62(7):569–76.

Faria A, Allen AH, Fox N, Ayas N, Laher I. The public health burden of obstructive sleep apnea. Sleep Sci. 2021;14(3):257–65.

Gottlieb DJ. Sleep apnea and cardiovascular disease. Curr Diab Rep. 2021;21(12):64.

Guglielmi O, Jurado-Gámez B, Gude F, Buela-Casal G. Occupational health of patients with obstructive sleep apnea syndrome: a systematic review. Sleep Breath. 2015;19(1):35–44.

Gupta MA, Simpson FC. Obstructive sleep apnea and psychiatric disorders: a systematic review. J Clin Sleep Med. 2015;11(2):165–75.

Heinzer R, Vat S, Marques-Vidal P, et al. Prevalence of sleep-disordered breathing in the general population: the HypnoLaus study. Lancet Respir Med. 2015;3(4):310–8.

Long X, Fonseca P, Foussier J, Haakma R, Aarts RM. Sleep and wake classification with actigraphy and respiratory effort using dynamic warping. IEEE J Biomed Health Inform. 2014;18(4):1272–84.

Maniaci A, Riela PM, Iannella G, et al. Machine learning identification of obstructive sleep apnea severity through the patient clinical features: a retrospective study. Life (Basel). 2023;13(3):702.

Motin MA, Kumar Karmakar C, Penzel T, Palaniswami M. Sleep-wake classification using statistical features extracted from photoplethysmographic signals. Annu Int Conf IEEE Eng Med Biol Soc. 2019;2019:5564–7.

Orhan K, Shamshiev M, Ezhov M, et al. AI-based automatic segmentation of craniomaxillofacial anatomy from CBCT scans for automatic detection of pharyngeal airway evaluations in OSA patients. Sci Rep. 2022;12(1):11863.

Peppard PE, Young T, Barnet JH, Palta M, Hagen EW, Hla KM. Increased prevalence of sleep-disordered breathing in adults. Am J Epidemiol. 2013;177(9):1006–14.

Rundo JV, Downey R 3rd. Polysomnography. Handb Clin Neurol. 2019;160:381–92.

Ryu S, Kim JH, Yu H, et al. Diagnosis of obstructive sleep apnea with prediction of flow characteristics according to airway morphology automatically extracted from medical images: computational fluid dynamics and artificial intelligence approach. Comput Methods Prog Biomed. 2021;208:106243.

Salman LA, Shulman R, Cohen JB. Obstructive sleep apnea, hypertension, and cardiovascular risk: epidemiology, pathophysiology, and management. Curr Cardiol Rep. 2020;22(2):6.

Scioscia G, Tondo P, Foschino Barbaro MP, et al. Machine learning-based prediction of adherence to continuous positive airway pressure (CPAP) in obstructive sleep apnea (OSA). Inform Health Soc Care. 2022;47(3):274–82.

Tsuiki S, Nagaoka T, Fukuda T, et al. Machine learning for image-based detection of patients with obstructive sleep apnea: an exploratory study. Sleep Breath. 2021;25(4):2297–305.

Tufik S, Santos-Silva R, Taddei JA, Bittencourt LR. Obstructive sleep apnea syndrome in the Sao Paulo epidemiologic sleep study. Sleep Med. 2010;11(5):441–6.

Turino C, Benítez ID, Rafael-Palou X, et al. Management and treatment of patients with obstructive sleep apnea using an intelligent monitoring system based on machine learning aiming to improve continuous positive airway pressure treatment compliance: randomized controlled trial. J Med Internet Res. 2021;23(10):e24072.

Vaquerizo-Villar F, Álvarez D, Gutiérrez-Tobal GC, Arroyo-Domingo CA, Del Campo F, Hornero R. Deep-learning model based on convolutional neural networks to classify apnea-hypopnea events from the oximetry signal. Adv Exp Med Biol. 2022;1384:255–64.

Yeghiazarians Y, Jneid H, Tietjens JR, et al. Obstructive sleep apnea and cardiovascular disease: a scientific statement from the American Heart Association. Circulation. 2021;144(3):e56–67.

Artificial Intelligence in Temporomandibular Joint Disorders

11

Rohan Jagtap, Ibrahim Sevki Bayrakdar, and Kaan Orhan

Introduction

The temporomandibular joint (TMJ) is one of the most complex joints that connects the mandibular condyle protrusion to the temporal bone and allows movements such as rotation and sliding (Alomar et al. 2007; Buescher 2007; Hatcher 2022). It is located on the left and right sides of the mandible and resembles knee articulation. TMJ consists of a disc, bone, fibrous capsule, fluid, synovial membrane, and ligaments, and the articular surface covered with fibrocartilage (Alomar et al. 2007; Buescher 2007; Hatcher 2022). Disorders related to this joint are very common, affecting approximately one-third of adults who experience various symptoms such as jaw pain, joint noise, neck and shoulder pain, limited mouth opening, tinnitus, ear pain, and headaches (Wadhokar and Patil 2022). TMJ diseases (TMDs) have a multifactorial etiology, including biological, physical, psychological, behavioral, and psychosocial factors, as well as genetic, hormonal, and systemic disease factors (Alqurayshah et al. 2023; Suvinen et al. 2005). Therefore, diagnosing TMDs

R. Jagtap (✉)
Division of Oral and Maxillofacial Radiology, Department of Care Planning and Restorative Sciences, University of Mississippi Medical Center, Jackson, MS, USA

Department of Radiology, School of Medicine, University of Mississippi Medical Center, Jackson, MS, USA

I. S. Bayrakdar
Division of Oral and Maxillofacial Radiology, Department of Care Planning and Restorative Sciences, University of Mississippi Medical Center, Jackson, MS, USA

Department of Oral and Maxillofacial Radiology, School of Dentistry, Center of Research and Application for Computer-Aided Diagnosis and Treatment in Health, Eskisehir Osmangazi University, ESOGÜ Meşelik Yerleşkesi, Eskisehir, Turkey

K. Orhan
Faculty of Dentistry, Department of Dentomaxillofacial Radiology, Ankara University, Ankara, Turkey

K. Orhan, R. Jagtap (eds.), *Artificial Intelligence in Dentistry*,
https://doi.org/10.1007/978-3-031-43827-1_11

requires a comprehensive assessment of the patient's findings and symptoms obtained from clinical, radiological, and biological examinations, considering the behavioral and psychosocial aspects of patients (Kostrzewa-Janicka et al. 2013; Helenius et al. 2005; List and Jensen 2017). TMDs are mostly observed in the 20–40 age range and are more common in women (Gauer and Semidey 2015). Accurate diagnosis and treatment are critical to prevent potential complications (McFadden and Rishiraj 2001). The chronicity of these disorders, which affect the joints and surrounding muscles, may lead to frequent headaches, depression, anxiety, and a decrease in the individual's quality of life (Ferneini 2021).

The TMJ enables individuals to perform essential functions such as chewing, speaking, and yawning, necessary for their daily routine (Ahmed and Abuaffan 2016). Diseases associated with this joint can disrupt these routine daily activities and cause suffering for the patient (Scrivani et al. 2018). In the clinical examination of patients presenting with TMJ complaints, physicians assess the quality and symmetry of lower jaw movements and take various measurements (Ahmed and Abuaffan 2016). Additionally, patients are recommended to undergo radiographic imaging with two-dimensional (2D) or three-dimensional (3D) techniques, such as computed tomography (CT) and cone-beam CT (CBCT) (Crow et al. 2005; Almeida et al. 2019). While these imaging methods provide insight into the disease, they do not allow for a soft tissue examination (Almeida et al. 2019). Some experts suggest that examining arthrography, computed tomography, and magnetic resonance imaging (MRI) together can offer a more accurate diagnosis (Westesson 1993; Larheim 1995; Manfredini et al. 2007). However, there is still some confusion among practitioners regarding the method of choice for diagnosing these joint diseases (Brooks et al. 1997). In summary, for the correct diagnosis of TMD, different clinical parameters of the patient and diagnostic data obtained from various imaging techniques should be examined comprehensively.

Panoramic radiography is one of the routine imaging methods used in dental practice. Some studies indicate that condyles can be easily visualized using this radiography technique and can be useful in TMJ examinations (Kurita et al. 2001, 2003). However, it does not allow for the visualization of the disc, joint space, and fossa and has limited use as it does not show the internal irregularities of the joint (Kurita et al. 2001, 2003). Techniques such as arthrography or MRI may be preferred for TMJ soft tissue analysis or to examine intra-articular inflammatory changes and joint effusion (Larheim 1995; Westesson 1984). On the other hand, 3D imaging methods have been shown to be superior to both magnetic resonance imaging and conventional two-dimensional imaging methods, especially in bone-related situations (Honey et al. 2007; Larheim et al. 2015). Despite these advancements, physicians should have sufficient knowledge, skills, and experience in using and interpreting these methods (Zakirov et al. 2018; Westbrook 2017; Salins and Butani 2019), bringing computer-assisted technologies to mind, which can aid physicians in these diagnostic processes (Fatima et al. 2022; Bas et al. 2012).

With the advancement of technology, many applications in the field of health and dentistry have been digitized, particularly in radiographic image interpretation, reporting, and preliminary treatment planning, aiming to develop systems that assist physicians (De Angelis et al. 2022; Barragán-Montero et al. 2021). Artificial intelligence (AI) systems are technologies that imitate human intelligence, capable of learning, thinking, interpreting, and predicting (Khanagar et al. 2021; Ramlakhan et al. 2022). They provide a decision-support mechanism to physicians in stages such as diagnosis and treatment decisions, preventing errors and oversights that may occur due to fatigue, intensity, emotional stress, and lack of experience in physicians (Park et al. 2020; Schwalbe and Wahl 2020; Kurt Bayrakdar et al. 2021; Schwendicke et al. 2020). Consequently, there is a growing interest in utilizing AI technologies in various health-related fields (Davenport and Kalakota 2019). In dentistry, many studies have demonstrated the usability of these systems for purposes such as the automatic determination of certain conditions and diseases and treatment planning (Hiraiwa et al. 2019; Orhan et al. 2020, 2021; Lahoud et al. 2021; Kwak et al. 2020; Devito et al. 2008). Although TMDs are a common problem in society, they pose one of the most challenging diagnoses for dentists. In light of this information, an AI system that can provide a diagnosis with high success rates would be of great value in the clinical practice of physicians. Numerous studies have been conducted for this purpose in literature (Bianchi et al. 2020, 2021; Lee et al. 2020; Choi et al. 2021; Zhang et al. 2020; Brosset et al. 2020; Almăşan et al. 2023; Jha et al. 2022). The objective of this chapter is to present the uses and benefits of AI in TMDs based on the current literature.

Automatic Segmentation of Temporomandibular Joint Anatomical Structures

Temporomandibular Joint (TMJ) is one of the most complex joints in the human body (Chang et al. 2018). Defining and 3D modeling TMJ anatomical structures in radiological images are significantly important for the diagnosis and management of TMJ diseases (Barghan et al. 2012). The segmentation of TMJ structures is difficult as they have complex anatomy and consist of small structures (Sagl et al. 2022; Iwaszenko et al. 2021) (Fig. 11.1). Deep-learning (DL)-based AI algorithms are capable of segmenting medical images (Wong et al. 2020). Integrating AI-based segmentation tools into clinical practice could ease the 3D evaluation of TMJs for diagnosis and long-term patient follow-up (Fig. 11.2). With this perspective, several studies in the literature have focused on the automatic segmentation of TMJ structures on radiological images (Ito et al. 2022; Nozawa et al. 2022; Vinayahalingam et al. 2023).

In a study conducted by Ito et al. (2022), deep-learning models were developed, including a convolutional neural network encoder-decoder called 3DiscNet (Detection for Displaced articular DISC using convolutional neural NETwork), U-Net, and SegNet-Basic, for the fully automatic segmentation of the articular disc of the temporomandibular joint on magnetic resonance images. Both 3DiscNet and SegNet-Basic demonstrated relatively good performance in the segmentation task. This study suggests that the deep-learning approach has the potential to be used for the assessment of temporomandibular disorders in clinical practice.

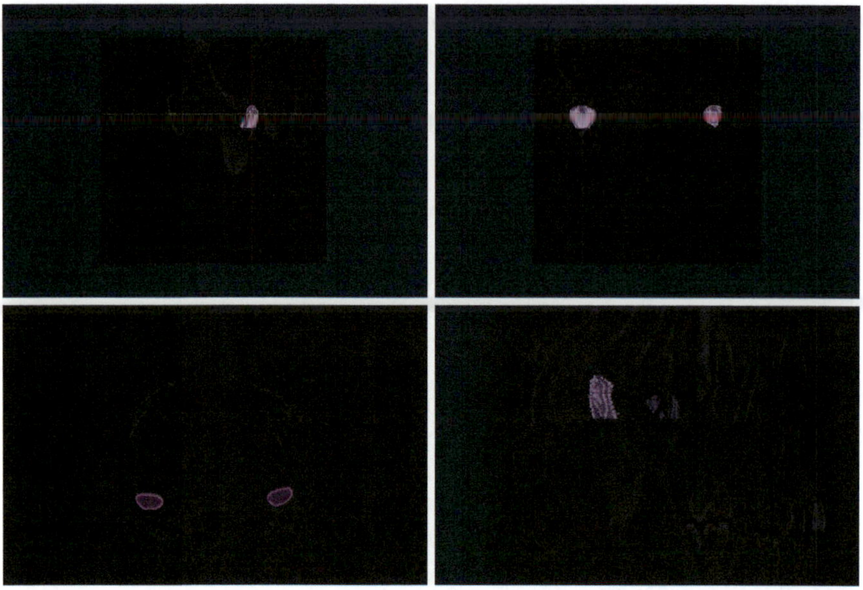

Fig. 11.1 Automatic segmentation of the mandibular condyle using AI tool. (Courtesy by CranioCatch AI software)

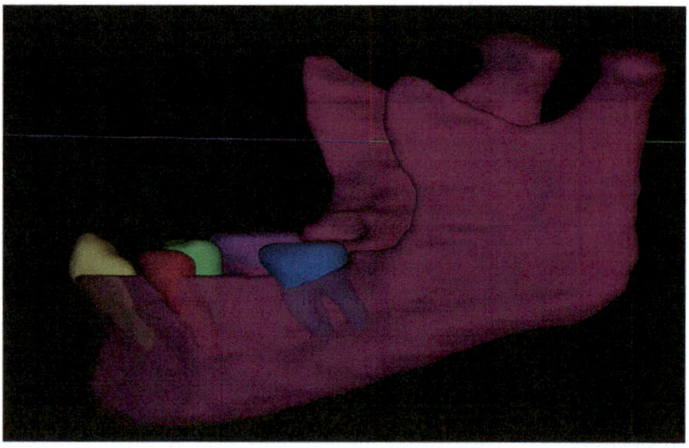

Fig. 11.2 3D.stl model of the mandible, created by automatic segmentation using an AI tool. (Courtesy by CranioCatch AI software)

Nozawa et al. (2022) introduced a deep-learning model designed for the automatic segmentation of the temporomandibular joint (TMJ) disc on magnetic resonance (MR) images. The model demonstrated a recall (sensitivity) performance of above 80% for detecting the position of anterior disc displacement on both internal and external test data. Based on their findings, the researchers concluded that this deep-learning-based segmentation model could be valuable in determining disc positions on MR images, particularly in the closed-mouth position.

In a study by Vinayahalingam et al. (2023), a DL-based automatic segmentation tool was created using a 3D U-Net algorithm for accurate 3D reconstruction of the temporomandibular joint (TMJ). The tool employed a three-step deep-learning approach, including region of interest (ROI) determination, bone segmentation, and TMJ classification, to segment the condyles and glenoid fossae on cone-beam computed tomography (CBCT) datasets. The AI segmentation achieved an intersection over union (IoU) of 0.955 and 0.935 for the condyles and glenoid fossae, respectively. Comparatively, the IoU of the two independent observers for manual condyle segmentation were 0.895 and 0.928, respectively. AI segmentation proved to be about 105 times faster than manual segmentation, demonstrating high accuracy, speed, and consistency in segmenting the mandibular condyles and glenoid fossae.

In another study by Li et al. (2022), two AI algorithms were developed using U-Net++ and nnU-Net models to segment the mandibular condyle, articular eminence, and TMJ disc in MRI images. The AI models exhibited performance close to that of experts in the segmentation of TMJ structures.

Diagnosis of Temporomandibular Joint Osteoarthritis

Osteoarthritis (OA) is a joint disease that leads to the chronic destruction of soft and hard tissues, causing various degenerative changes around the affected joints, including cartilage damage, bone remodeling, synovitis, and joint discomfort (Yue and Berman 2022; Mathiessen et al. 2016). Temporomandibular joint osteoarthritis (TMJ-OA) is one of the most prevalent degenerative joint disorders (Derwich et al. 2021; He et al. 2021) (Fig. 11.3). It is characterized by degenerative bone changes on the mandibular condyle, fossa, and articular eminence, such as resorption, erosion, sclerosis, flattening, osteophyte formation, and subchondral cyst (Alzahrani et al. 2020; Lee et al. 2017; Deshpande et al. 2015). Early diagnosis of TMJ-OA is challenging, as it may not show signs before severe degeneration (Lee et al. 2019), making it crucial for proper management. Radiologic evaluation of TMJ-OA is of significant importance, and AI has the potential to aid in this evaluation. Numerous studies have been conducted to assess AI performance in diagnosing TMJ-OA based on radiographs.

Jung et al. (2023) developed a diagnostic support tool using pre-trained ResNet152 and EfficientNet-B7 as a transfer learning model for classifying panoramic radiographs of the TMJ into normal and TMJ-OA cases. The classification accuracies of ResNet-152 and EfficientNet-B7 were 0.87 and 0.88, respectively. The trained models focused on specific areas in osteoarthritis images where erosion or osteophytes were observed. The AI models enhanced the diagnostic success of TMJ-OA on panoramic radiographs, making it an effective screening tool for diagnosing TMJ-OA.

Choi et al. (2021) developed an AI model using Karas' ResNet model to classify panoramic images into three categories according to the presence of TMJ-OA: normal, indeterminate TMJ-OA, and TMJ-OA. However, when AI was developed with three categories, the model's performance was found unsatisfactory compared to an oral and maxillofacial radiologist's performance of diagnosing OA using panoramic radiographs confirmed by CBCT images. To improve performance, the indeterminate TMJ-OA images were reclassified as normal, TMJ-OA, or excluded. After this

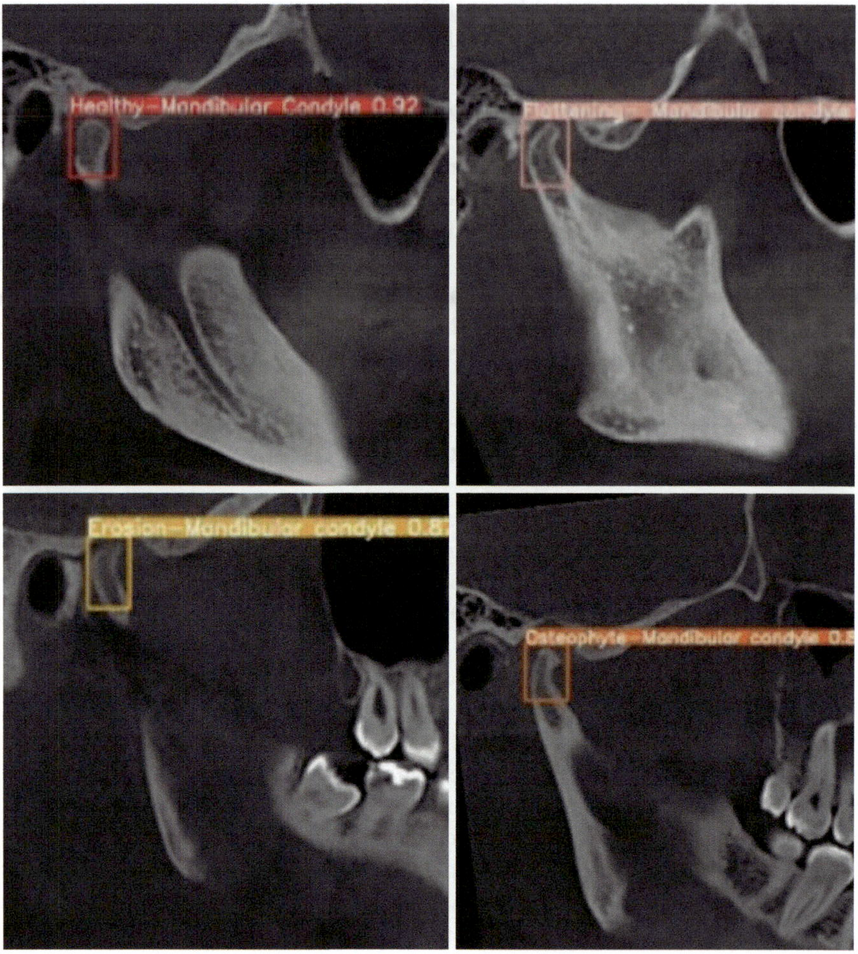

Fig. 11.3 Automatic classification of temporomandibular joint osteoarthritis (TMJ-OA) on cone-beam computed tomography (CBCT) images. (Courtesy by CranioCatch AI software)

adjustment, the AI showed similar performance compared to experts in diagnosing TMJ-OA, emphasizing its role in the primary diagnosis of TMJ-OA from panoramic radiographs.

In another study, Lee et al. (2020) developed an AI-based diagnostic tool to automatically detect TMJ-OA, including irregular contour, osseous defects, loss of cortication, and flattening of the condylar head, from cone-beam computed tomography (CBCT) images. They used a single-shot detection object detection model for classification into two categories: TMJ-OA or not. The average accuracy was found to be 0.86, and they concluded that it may be used as a clinical decision-support system for diagnosing TMJ-OA.

Eşer et al. (2023) created an AI model using the YOLOv5 architecture for TMJ segmentation and classification of TMJ-OA on sagittal images of CBCT. The accuracy value for segmentation and classification was found to be 0.9953 and 0.7678, respectively.

de Dumast et al. (2018) developed a web-based neural network-based system to classify TMJ-OA from 3D surface mesh images of mandibular condyles retrieved from CBCT scans. They used the ShapeVariationAnalyzer (SVA) method as a deep neural network classifier for 3D condylar morphology. The DSCI system trained and tested the neural network, indicating five stages of structural degenerative changes in condylar morphology in the TMJ, with 91% close agreement between the clinician consensus and the SVA classifier.

Automatic Detection of Disc Displacement and Perforation of Temporomandibular Joint

TMJ disc displacement is an abnormal relationship among the articular disc, mandibular condyle, and mandibular fossa. The determination of the disc structure and position is indispensable for evaluating TMJ disorders. MRI is considered the gold standard for the examination of the TMJ and verifying disc location. However, the interpretation of MRI images and determining the joint disc can be challenging. AI has shown promising results in determining the joint disc and evaluating its position (Larheim 1995; Tamimi et al. 2019).

In a study by Lin et al. (2022), an algorithm was developed for the automatic detection of anterior disc displacement (ADD) of the temporomandibular joint (TMJ) on sagittal MRI images before orthodontic treatment. They used the ResNet architecture and the "ImageNet" database with five-fold cross-validation, oversampling, and data augmentation techniques for model development. The maximum open-mouth position model showed excellent performance with 99% accuracy and 97% AUC. Closed-mouth position models showed 86.3% accuracy and 92.2% AUC for diagnostic Criteria 1 and 83.9% accuracy and 88.5% AUC for diagnostic Criteria 2. The CNN-based AI model demonstrated high accuracy in detecting ADD of TMJ, showing potential for use before orthodontic treatment to improve treatment outcomes.

Radke et al. (2003) conducted a study using an ANN-based expert system to determine non-reducing disc displacement from frontal chewing data. The system detected the presence and type of non-reducing disc displacement from frontal chewing data in patients with TMD at an acceptable level of error.

Kao et al. (2023) offered a novel AI diagnostic tool for automatically extracting discriminative features and detecting temporomandibular joint disc displacement (TMJDD) on MRI images. They used the U-Net algorithm to detect the joint cavity between the temporal bone and the mandibular condyle, using four convolutional neural networks, including InceptionResNetV2, InceptionV3, DenseNet169, and VGG16, for classification. InceptionV3 and DenseNet169 were found to be the best models, achieving an accuracy value of 0.85. Automated detection of TMJDD from sagittal MRI images was considered a promising technique to support clinicians in diagnosing patients with TMJDD.

Lee et al. (2022a) developed a VGG16 algorithm-based automatic deep-learning detection model of anterior disc displacement (ADD) from sagittal magnetic resonance imaging (MRI) of patients with temporomandibular joint disorder (TMD). The VGG16 model was trained using three methods: from-scratch, fine-tuning, and freeze. The fine-tuning model demonstrated a perfect estimation performance with an AUC value of 87.75% and an accuracy value of about 77%. ADD information was successfully learned in the CNN features without using pre-trained weights. The CNN model showed higher estimation specificity compared to human experts, and the ensemble of three fine-tuning models displayed improved accuracy from 77 to 83%.

Yoon et al. (2023) proposed an AI-based clinical decision-support system for diagnosing TMJ ADD using MR images. The system was built upon two deep-learning models, including a region of interest (ROI) detection model that contained the temporal bone, disc, and condyle within the entire sagittal MRI image and a classification model that could classify TMJ as normal, ADD without reduction, and ADD with reduction within the detected ROI by the first model. RetinaNet was used with weights trained on the ImageNet dataset, and resnet50 was adopted as the backbone network for developing the ROI detection model. A multi-input convolutional neural network was used as the classification model. The ROI detection model achieved a 0.819 mAP value at 0.75 intersection over union (IoU) thresholds in the internal test. In both internal and external tests, the ADD classification model obtained AUROC values of 0.985 and 0.960, sensitivity values of 0.950 and 0.926, and specificity values of 0.919 and 0.892, respectively. This study concluded that the AI-based clinical decision-support system provides clinicians with estimated results and can be integrated with the patient's clinical examination findings for the final diagnosis.

Lee et al. (2022b) presented the pix2pix generative adversarial network (GAN) model for T2-weighted image (WI) synthesis from proton density (PD)-WI in TMJ MRIs. The proposed model showed perfect agreement with the gold standard for disc position and effusion.

Kim et al. developed a deep-learning-based algorithm to estimate temporomandibular joint (TMJ) disc perforation based on the findings of magnetic resonance imaging (MRI). The presence of TMJ disc perforation was confirmed during surgery, and two groups were created: the perforated and non-perforated disc groups. Experienced clinicians evaluated the TMJ MRI images of each group for feature extraction. Random forest and multilayer perceptron (MLP) models were used to develop an estimation model for TMJ disc perforation. MLP showed superior performance with a 0.940 AUC. The application of DL methods to the estimation of TMJ disc perforation is helpful compared to conventional methods.

Prediction of Temporomandibular Joint Disorders: Clinical, Biological, and Radiologic Radiomics Markers

Temporomandibular joint disorder (TMD) is an inclusive term that explains dysfunction of the TMJ and related masticatory muscles, as well as pain. Clinical, radiological, and biological findings are used for the diagnosis and management of TMD. Machine learning algorithms have been employed in studies, utilizing extracted data from a combination of clinical, biological, and radiomic markers, to support a definitive diagnosis of TMJ. These studies have obtained promising results (Almăşan et al. 2023; Farook and Dudley 2023).

Diniz de Lima et al. (2022) presented a study on the detection of temporomandibular joint disorder (TMD) using infrared thermography (IT) images with ML classifiers, including K-nearest neighbors (KNN), support vector machine (SVM), and multilayer perceptron (MLP). Three machine learning (ML) attribute extraction methods were employed: radiomic, semantic, and radiomic-semantic. IT lateral projection images were used, and the masseter and temporal muscles were selected as regions of interest (ROI) for attribute extraction. For radiomic attribute extraction, 20 texture attributes were evaluated using the co-occurrence matrix at a standardized angulation of 0°. The semantic features consisted of the ROI mean temperature and pain intensity data. To evaluate radiomic-semantic associations, a single dataset comprising 28 features was used. The study concluded that semantic and radiomic-semantic-associated ML feature extraction methods, along with the MLP classifier, should be preferred for TMD detection using IT images and pain scale data. Machine learning demonstrates promising results for the detection of TMD on IT images.

Fang et al. (2023) presented a machine-learning-based multidimensional nomogram using 36 cephalometric parameters extracted from lateral cephalogram to scan degenerative temporomandibular disorders (TMDs). The cephalometric parameters were utilized to develop an estimated machine learning algorithm. A multivariable logistic regression approach was employed to build an integrated model, incorporating ceph scores and clinical features, such as age, gender, limited mouth opening, and crepitus. This integrated model demonstrated excellent performance with an AUC value of 0.893, indicating its potential to assist in the diagnosis of degenerative TMDs in clinical practice.

Bianchi et al. (2020) evaluated the diagnostic performance of four machine learning models, including Logistic Regression, Random Forest, LightGBM, and XGBoost, to analyze 52 clinical, biological, and high-resolution CBCT radiomics markers from TMJ-OA patients and controls. The XGBoost + LightGBM model achieved an accuracy of 0.823, AUC of 0.870, and F1-score of 0.823, enabling the correct diagnosis of early stages of TMJ-OA using some of these markers. These markers included Headaches; Range of mouth opening without pain; Energy, Haralick Correlation, Entropy, and interactions of TGF-β1 in Saliva and Headaches; VE-cadherin in Serum and Angiogenin in Saliva; VE-cadherin in Saliva and Headaches; PA1 in Saliva and Headaches; PA1 in Saliva and Range of mouth opening without pain; Gender and Muscle Soreness; Short Run Low Grey Level Emphasis and Headaches; Inverse Difference Moment; and Trabecular Separation.

Mackie et al. (2022) attempted to enhance the performance of ML algorithms in detecting TMJ-OA by combining quantitative biomarkers of bone texture and morphometric features of the articular fossa and joint space. They found that while there were no significant differences in the articular fossa radiomic biomarkers between TMJ-OA and normal patients, those with TMJ-OA had a significantly smaller superior condyle to fossa distance. The inclusion of radiomic biomarkers of the articular fossa improved the success of ML models in identifying TMJ-OA, particularly with its interaction effects.

The LightGBM model obtained an AUC of 0.842 in diagnosing patients with TMJ-OA, with Headaches and Range of Mouth Opening Without Pain graded as the best features. Noteworthy interactions included VE-cadherin in Serum and Angiogenin in Saliva, TGF-β1 in Saliva and Headaches, Gender and Muscle Soreness, PA1 in Saliva and Range of Mouth Opening Without Pain, Lateral Condyle Grey Level Non-Uniformity and Lateral Fossa Short Run Emphasis, TGF-β1 in Serum and Lateral Fossa Trabeculae number, MMP3 in Serum and VEGF in Serum, Headaches and Lateral Fossa Trabecular spacing, Headaches and PA1 in Saliva, and Headaches and BDNF in Saliva. These preliminary findings suggest that imaging features of the mandibular condyle may hold more value regarding main effects, whereas the imaging features of the mandibular fossa may play a greater role in interaction effects.

Lee et al. (2021) aimed to use AI to identify major biological and psychosocial risk factors for temporomandibular disorders (TMDs), including stress, socioeconomic status, and working conditions. Six AI methods were employed to determine the factors related to TMDs, including regression, decision trees, naïve Bayes, random forest, support vector machines, and an artificial neural network. The best mean accuracy was achieved using logistic regression, random forest, support vector machines, and artificial neural networks. Additionally, the best AUC value was obtained using an artificial neural network and logistic regression for self-reported TMD and doctor-reported TMD, respectively. The authors concluded that a predictive algorithm could serve as a decision-support system in the diagnosis of TMDs, utilizing 37 independent variables related to demographic factors, socioeconomic status, stress, working conditions, biological factors, and comorbidities.

Zhang et al. (2021) used the privileged information (LUPI) paradigm for diagnosing TMJ-OA. They developed three LUPI classifiers with non-LUPI analogues for TMJ-OA diagnosis. Six clinical features, including age of the patient, headaches in the last 6 months, muscle soreness in the last 6 months, vertical range unassisted without pain (mm), vertical range unassisted maximum (mm), and vertical range assisted maximum (mm), were extracted. Additionally, 23 texture and bone morphology features were extracted from the lateral condyle, and an additional 23 features were obtained from the mandibular fossa. Furthermore, 25 protein features were collected from saliva, resulting in a dataset comprising 77 features, including 6 clinical, 46 imaging, and 25 protein features, from a total of 92 patients. Support vector machine (SVM), random vector functional link network (RVFL), and iterated privileged learning model (IPL) were used to develop LUPI Algorithms. The KRVFL+ model using privileged protein features showed the best classification performance with an AUC of 0.80 and an accuracy of 75.6%. The authors concluded that LUPI-based algorithms using privileged protein data can enhance the final diagnostic performance of TMJ-OA classification.

Le et al. (2021) developed a machine learning-based diagnostic tool named TMJOAI for classifying TMJ using 52 clinical, biological, and jaw condyle radiomic markers. These markers included 2 demographic values, 13 protein level values from serum, 12 protein level values from saliva, 5 clinical features evaluating pain, and 20 imaging features from the lateral region of the trabecular bone of the condyle, demonstrating the grey-level values of the region of interest. Additionally, 32 mandibular fossa radiomic features were tested to create more powerful radiomic markers. Five different ML algorithms, including Random Forest, XGBoost, LightGBM, Ridge, and Logistic Regression, were employed. The best prediction performance was achieved with the XGBoost and LightGBM models.

Reda et al. (2023) conducted a preliminary case study to support the early diagnosis of temporomandibular disorders using AI. They presented the experience of a commercially available AI service for assisting non-expert dentists in early TMD recognition. The AI-based system consisted of two modules: one for ensuring probable diagnoses in terms of the list of symptoms and another for the question and answer tool. Seven available clinical cases were reviewed for the evaluation of performance. The study demonstrated that AI is a beneficial tool to enhance the detection of TMDs by assisting in primary diagnosis and proved the concept that AI-based systems can aid non-specialists in the early detection of TMDs.

Kreiner and Viloria (2022) developed a novel multilayer perceptron neural network to diagnose orofacial pain and TMD. Four clinical experts collaborated to create clinical scenarios and their corresponding accurate diagnoses, which served as the gold standard. The clinical situations encompassed six diagnostic categories, including acute pain of dental origin, orofacial pain of neuropathic origin (paroxysmal trigeminal neuralgia), post-traumatic trigeminal neuropathic pain, referred facial and dental pain of cardiac origin, TMJ dysfunction (disc displacement with and/or without reduction), and facial neurovascular pain (migraine). Eleven clinical cases were prepared, covering these categories, and presented to twelve general dental clinicians. The clinicians' diagnoses were compared to those made by the AI neural network. The AI's diagnostic accuracy was found to be superior, especially in cases with non-dental and referred orofacial pains. The authors concluded that ANN-based AI algorithms can assist medical and general dental clinicians in diagnosing various types of orofacial pain and dysfunction, including TMD, neuropathic, neurovascular, and referred cardiac pain, potentially playing a life-saving role.

Bas et al. (2012) utilized ANN for the estimation of two subgroups of temporomandibular joint (TMJ) internal derangements (IDs) and normal joints, using characteristic clinical signs and symptoms of the diseases. TMJs of each patient were diagnosed as normal, ADD with reduction, or ADD without reduction. A back-propagation neural network was employed to develop the classification model. The authors concluded that the application of ANNs for diagnosing subtypes of TMJ IDs may be a useful supportive diagnostic method.

References

Ahmed L, Abuaffan A. Prevalence of temporomandibular joint disorders among Sudanese university students. J Oral Hyg Health. 2016;4(2). https://doi.org/10.4172/2332-0702.1000202.

Almăşan O, Leucuţa DC, Hedeşiu M, Mureşanu S, Popa ŞL. Temporomandibular joint osteoarthritis diagnosis employing artificial intelligence: systematic review and meta-analysis. J Clin Med. 2023;12(3):942.

Almeida FT, Pacheco-Pereira C, Flores-Mir C, Le LH, Jaremko JL, Major PW. Diagnostic ultrasound assessment of temporomandibular joints: a systematic review and meta-analysis. Dentomaxillofac Radiol. 2019;48(2):20180144.

Alomar X, Medrano J, Cabratosa J, Clavero JA, Lorente M, Serra I, et al. Anatomy of the temporomandibular joint. Semin Ultrasound CT MR. 2007;28(3):170–83.

Alqurayshah HHH, Al Omar SMS, Al Omar NMS, Alyami AMS, Alhazmi AA, Al Salem SM, et al. Stress and musculoskeletal disorders: TMJ disorder as an example. Ann Clin Anal Med. 2023;10(1).

Alzahrani A, Yadav S, Gandhi V, Lurie AG, Tadinada A. Incidental findings of temporomandibular joint osteoarthritis and its variability based on age and sex. Imaging Sci Dent. 2020;50(3):245–53.

Barghan S, Tetradis S, Mallya S. Application of cone beam computed tomography for assessment of the temporomandibular joints. Aust Dent J. 2012;57(Suppl 1):109–18.

Barragán-Montero A, Javaid U, Valdés G, Nguyen D, Desbordes P, Macq B, et al. Artificial intelligence and machine learning for medical imaging: a technology review. Phys Med. 2021;83:242–56.

Bas B, Ozgonenel O, Ozden B, Bekcioglu B, Bulut E, Kurt M. Use of artificial neural network in differentiation of subgroups of temporomandibular internal derangements: a preliminary study. J Oral Maxillofac Surg. 2012;70(1):51–9.

Bianchi J, de Oliveira Ruellas AC, Gonçalves JR, Paniagua B, Prieto JC, Styner M, et al. Osteoarthritis of the temporomandibular joint can be diagnosed earlier using biomarkers and machine learning. Sci Rep. 2020;10(1):8012.

Bianchi J, Ruellas A, Prieto JC, Li T, Soroushmehr R, Najarian K, et al. Decision support systems in temporomandibular joint osteoarthritis: a review of data science and artificial intelligence applications. Semin Orthod. 2021;27(2):78–86.

Brooks SL, Brand JW, Gibbs SJ, Hollender L, Lurie AG, Omnell KA, et al. Imaging of the temporomandibular joint: a position paper of the American Academy of Oral and Maxillofacial Radiology. Oral Surg Oral Med Oral Pathol Oral Radiol Endod. 1997;83(5):609–18.

Brosset S, Dumont M, Bianchi J, Ruellas A, Cevidanes L, Yatabe M, et al. 3D auto-segmentation of mandibular condyles. Annu Int Conf IEEE Eng Med Biol Soc. 2020;2020:1270–3.

Buescher JJ. Temporomandibular joint disorders. Am Fam Physician. 2007;76(10):1477–82.

Chang CL, Wang DH, Yang MC, Hsu WE, Hsu ML. Functional disorders of the temporomandibular joints: internal derangement of the temporomandibular joint. Kaohsiung J Med Sci. 2018;34(4):223–30.

Choi E, Kim D, Lee JY, Park HK. Artificial intelligence in detecting temporomandibular joint osteoarthritis on orthopantomogram. Sci Rep. 2021;11(1):10246.

Crow HC, Parks E, Campbell JH, Stucki DS, Daggy J. The utility of panoramic radiography in temporomandibular joint assessment. Dentomaxillofac Radiol. 2005;34(2):91–5.

Davenport T, Kalakota R. The potential for artificial intelligence in healthcare. Future Healthc J. 2019;6(2):94–8.

De Angelis F, Pranno N, Franchina A, Di Carlo S, Brauner E, Ferri A, et al. Artificial intelligence: a new diagnostic software in dentistry: a preliminary performance diagnostic study. Int J Environ Res Public Health. 2022;19(3):1728.

de Dumast P, Mirabel C, Cevidanes L, Ruellas A, Yatabe M, Ioshida M, et al. A web-based system for neural network based classification in temporomandibular joint osteoarthritis. Comput Med Imaging Graph. 2018;67:45–54.

Derwich M, Mitus-Kenig M, Pawlowska E. Orally administered NSAIDs-general characteristics and usage in the treatment of temporomandibular joint osteoarthritis—a narrative review. Pharmaceuticals (Basel). 2021;14(3):219.

Deshpande P, Patil K, Guledgud MV, D'souza RS. Diagnostic imaging in TMJ osteoarthritis: a case report and overview. Int J Dent Sci Res. 2015;3:56–9.

Devito KL, de Souza BF, Felippe Filho WN. An artificial multilayer perceptron neural network for diagnosis of proximal dental caries. Oral Surg Oral Med Oral Pathol Oral Radiol Endod. 2008;106(6):879–84.

Diniz de Lima E, Souza Paulino JA, de Farias L, Freitas AP, Viana Ferreira JE, Barbosa JDS, Bezerra Silva DF, et al. Artificial intelligence and infrared thermography as auxiliary tools in the diagnosis of temporomandibular disorder. Dentomaxillofac Radiol. 2022;51(2):20210318.

Eşer G, Duman ŞB, Bayrakdar İŞ, Çelik Ö. Classification of temporomandibular joint osteoarthritis on cone-beam computed tomography images using artificial intelligence system. J Oral Rehabil. 2023;50(9):758–66.

Fang X, Xiong X, Lin J, Wu Y, Xiang J, Wang J. Machine-learning-based detection of degenerative temporomandibular joint diseases using lateral cephalograms. Am J Orthod Dentofac Orthop. 2023;163(2):260–71.e5.

Farook TH, Dudley J. Automation and deep (machine) learning in temporomandibular joint disorder radiomics: a systematic review. J Oral Rehabil. 2023;50(6):501–21.

Fatima A, Shafi I, Afzal H, Díez IT, Lourdes DRM, Breñosa J, et al. Advancements in dentistry with artificial intelligence: current clinical applications and future perspectives. Healthcare (Basel). 2022;10(11):2188.

Ferneini EM. Temporomandibular joint disorders (TMD). J Oral Maxillofac Surg. 2021;79(10):2171–2.

Gauer RL, Semidey MJ. Diagnosis and treatment of temporomandibular disorders. Am Fam Physician. 2015;91(6):378–86.

Hatcher DC. Anatomy of the mandible, temporomandibular joint, and dentition. Neuroimaging Clin N Am. 2022;32(4):749–61.

He D, Wang J, Li Y, Wu G, Zhu G, Chen L. Low-intensity pulsed ultrasound promotes aggrecan expression via ZNT-9 in temporomandibular joint chondrocytes. Gene. 2021;768:145318.

Helenius LM, Hallikainen D, Helenius I, Meurman JH, Könönen M, Leirisalo-Repo M, et al. Clinical and radiographic findings of the temporomandibular joint in patients with various rheumatic diseases. A case-control study. Oral Surg Oral Med Oral Pathol Oral Radiol Endod. 2005;99(4):455–63.

Hiraiwa T, Ariji Y, Fukuda M, Kise Y, Nakata K, Katsumata A, et al. A deep-learning artificial intelligence system for assessment of root morphology of the mandibular first molar on panoramic radiography. Dentomaxillofac Radiol. 2019;48(3):20180218.

Honey OB, Scarfe WC, Hilgers MJ, Klueber K, Silveira AM, Haskell BS, et al. Accuracy of cone-beam computed tomography imaging of the temporomandibular joint: comparisons with panoramic radiology and linear tomography. Am J Orthod Dentofac Orthop. 2007;132(4):429–38.

Ito S, Mine Y, Yoshimi Y, Takeda S, Tanaka A, Onishi A, et al. Automated segmentation of articular disc of the temporomandibular joint on magnetic resonance images using deep learning. Sci Rep. 2022;12(1):221.

Iwaszenko S, Munk J, Baron S, Smoliński A. New method for analysis of the temporomandibular joint using cone beam computed tomography. Sensors (Basel). 2021;21(9):3070.

Jha N, Lee KS, Kim YJ. Diagnosis of temporomandibular disorders using artificial intelligence technologies: a systematic review and meta-analysis. PLoS One. 2022;17(8):e0272715.

Jung W, Lee KE, Suh BJ, Seok H, Lee DW. Deep learning for osteoarthritis classification in temporomandibular joint. Oral Dis. 2023;29(3):1050–9.

Kao ZK, Chiu NT, Wu HH, Chang WC, Wang DH, Kung YY, et al. Classifying temporomandibular disorder with artificial intelligent architecture using magnetic resonance imaging. Ann Biomed Eng. 2023;51(3):517–26.

Khanagar SB, Al-Ehaideb A, Maganur PC, Vishwanathaiah S, Patil S, Baeshen HA, et al. Developments, application, and performance of artificial intelligence in dentistry—a systematic review. J Dent Sci. 2021;16(1):508–22.

Kostrzewa-Janicka J, Mierzwinska-Nastalska E, Jurkowski P, Okonski P, Nedzi-Gora M. Assessment of temporomandibular joint disease. Adv Exp Med Biol. 2013;788:207–11.

Kreiner M, Viloria J. A novel artificial neural network for the diagnosis of orofacial pain and temporomandibular disorders. J Oral Rehabil. 2022;49(9):884–9.

Kurita H, Ohtsuka A, Kobayashi H, Kurashina K. Resorption of the lateral pole of the mandibular condyle in temporomandibular disc displacement. Dentomaxillofac Radiol. 2001;30(2):88–91.

Kurita H, Ohtsuka A, Kobayashi H, Kurashina K. Relationship between increased horizontal condylar angle and resorption of the posterosuperior region of the lateral pole of the mandibular condyle in temporomandibular joint internal derangement. Dentomaxillofac Radiol. 2003;32(1):26–9.

Kurt Bayrakdar S, Orhan K, Bayrakdar IS, Bilgir E, Ezhov M, Gusarev M, et al. A deep learning approach for dental implant planning in cone-beam computed tomography images. BMC Med Imaging. 2021;21(1):86.

Kwak GH, Kwak EJ, Song JM, Park HR, Jung YH, Cho BH, et al. Automatic mandibular canal detection using a deep convolutional neural network. Sci Rep. 2020;10(1):5711.

Lahoud P, EzEldeen M, Beznik T, Willems H, Leite A, Van Gerven A, et al. Artificial intelligence for fast and accurate 3-dimensional tooth segmentation on cone-beam computed tomography. J Endod. 2021;47(5):827–35.

Larheim TA. Current trends in temporomandibular joint imaging. Oral Surg Oral Med Oral Pathol Oral Radiol Endod. 1995;80(5):555–76.

Larheim TA, Abrahamsson AK, Kristensen M, Arvidsson LZ. Temporomandibular joint diagnostics using CBCT. Dentomaxillofac Radiol. 2015;44(1):20140235.

Le C, Deleat-Besson R, Turkestani NA, Cevidanes L, Bianchi J, Zhang W, et al. TMJOAI: an artificial web-based intelligence tool for early diagnosis of the temporomandibular joint osteoarthritis. Clin Image Based Proced Distrib Collab Learn Artif Intell Combat COVID 19 Secur Priv Preserv Mach Learn (2021). 2021;12969:78–87.

Lee PP, Stanton AR, Hollender LG. Greater mandibular horizontal condylar angle is associated with temporomandibular joint osteoarthritis. Oral Surg Oral Med Oral Pathol Oral Radiol. 2017;123(4):502–7.

Lee YH, Hong IK, Chun YH. Prediction of painful temporomandibular joint osteoarthritis in juvenile patients using bone scintigraphy. Clin Exp Dent Res. 2019;5(3):225–35.

Lee KS, Kwak HJ, Oh JM, Jha N, Kim YJ, Kim W, et al. Automated detection of TMJ osteoarthritis based on artificial intelligence. J Dent Res. 2020;99(12):1363–7.

Lee KS, Jha N, Kim YJ. Risk factor assessments of temporomandibular disorders via machine learning. Sci Rep. 2021;11(1):19802.

Lee YH, Won JH, Kim S, Auh QS, Noh YK. Advantages of deep learning with convolutional neural network in detecting disc displacement of the temporomandibular joint in magnetic resonance imaging. Sci Rep. 2022a;12(1):11352.

Lee C, Ha EG, Choi YJ, Jeon KJ, Han SS. Synthesis of T2-weighted images from proton density images using a generative adversarial network in a temporomandibular joint magnetic resonance imaging protocol. Imaging Sci Dent. 2022b;52(4):393–8.

Li M, Punithakumar K, Major PW, Le LH, Nguyen KT, Pacheco-Pereira C, et al. Temporomandibular joint segmentation in MRI images using deep learning. J Dent. 2022;127:104345.

Lin B, Cheng M, Wang S, Li F, Zhou Q. Automatic detection of anteriorly displaced temporomandibular joint discs on magnetic resonance images using a deep learning algorithm. Dentomaxillofac Radiol. 2022;51(3):20210341.

List T, Jensen RH. Temporomandibular disorders: old ideas and new concepts. Cephalalgia. 2017;37(7):692–704.
Mackie T, Al Turkestani N, Bianchi J, Li T, Ruellas A, Gurgel M, et al. Quantitative bone imaging biomarkers and joint space analysis of the articular fossa in temporomandibular joint osteoarthritis using artificial intelligence models. Front Dent Med. 2022;3:1007011.
Manfredini D, Bucci MB, Nardini LG. The diagnostic process for temporomandibular disorders. Stomatologija. 2007;9(2):35–9.
Mathiessen A, Cimmino MA, Hammer HB, Haugen IK, Iagnocco A, Conaghan PG. Imaging of osteoarthritis (OA): what is new? Best Pract Res Clin Rheumatol. 2016;30(4):653–69.
McFadden LR, Rishiraj B. Treatment of temporomandibular joint ankylosis: a case report. J Can Dent Assoc. 2001;67(11):659–63.
Nozawa M, Ito H, Ariji Y, Fukuda M, Igarashi C, Nishiyama M, et al. Automatic segmentation of the temporomandibular joint disc on magnetic resonance images using a deep learning technique. Dentomaxillofac Radiol. 2022;51(1):20210185.
Orhan K, Bayrakdar IS, Ezhov M, Kravtsov A, Özyürek T. Evaluation of artificial intelligence for detecting periapical pathosis on cone-beam computed tomography scans. Int Endod J. 2020;53(5):680–9.
Orhan K, Bilgir E, Bayrakdar IS, Ezhov M, Gusarev M, Shumilov E. Evaluation of artificial intelligence for detecting impacted third molars on cone-beam computed tomography scans. J Stomatol Oral Maxillofac Surg. 2021;122(4):333–7.
Park CW, Seo SW, Kang N, Ko B, Choi BW, Park CM, et al. Artificial intelligence in health care: current applications and issues. J Korean Med Sci. 2020;35(42):e379.
Radke JC, Ketcham R, Glassman B, Kull R. Artificial neural network learns to differentiate normal TMJs and nonreducing displaced disks after training on incisor-point chewing movements. Cranio. 2003;21(4):259–64.
Ramlakhan S, Saatchi R, Sabir L, Singh Y, Hughes R, Shobayo O, et al. Understanding and interpreting artificial intelligence, machine learning and deep learning in emergency medicine. Emerg Med J. 2022;39(5):380–5.
Reda B, Contardo L, Prenassi M, Guerra E, Derchi G, Marceglia S. Artificial intelligence to support early diagnosis of temporomandibular disorders: a preliminary case study. J Oral Rehabil. 2023;50(1):31–8.
Sagl B, Schmid-Schwap M, Piehslinger E, Kundi M, Stavness I. Effect of facet inclination and location on TMJ loading during bruxism: an in-silico study. J Adv Res. 2022;35:25–32.
Salins M, Butani P, editors. A comprehensive review of the intra-articular anatomy of the ankle joint on magnetic resonance (MR) arthrography-the basics2019: European Congress of Radiology-ECR; 2019.
Schwalbe N, Wahl B. Artificial intelligence and the future of global health. Lancet. 2020;395(10236):1579–86.
Schwendicke F, Samek W, Krois J. Artificial intelligence in dentistry: chances and challenges. J Dent Res. 2020;99(7):769–74.
Scrivani SJ, Khawaja SN, Bavia PF. Nonsurgical management of pediatric temporomandibular joint dysfunction. Oral Maxillofac Surg Clin North Am. 2018;30(1):35–45.
Suvinen TI, Reade PC, Kemppainen P, Könönen M, Dworkin SF. Review of aetiological concepts of temporomandibular pain disorders: towards a biopsychosocial model for integration of physical disorder factors with psychological and psychosocial illness impact factors. Eur J Pain. 2005;9(6):613–33.
Tamimi D, Kocasarac HD, Mardini S. Imaging of the temporomandibular joint. Semin Roentgenol. 2019;54(3):282–301.
Vinayahalingam S, Berends B, Baan F, Moin DA, van Luijn R, Bergé S, et al. Deep learning for automated segmentation of the temporomandibular joint. J Dent. 2023;132:104475.
Wadhokar OC, Patil DS. Current trends in the management of temporomandibular joint dysfunction: a review. Cureus. 2022;14(9):e29314.
Westbrook C. Opening the debate on MRI practitioner education—is there a need for change? Radiography. 2017;23:S70–S4.

Westesson PL. Arthrography of the temporomandibular joint. J Prosthet Dent. 1984;51(4):535–43.

Westesson PL. Reliability and validity of imaging diagnosis of temporomandibular joint disorder. Adv Dent Res. 1993;7(2):137–51.

Wong KK, Fortino G, Abbott D. Deep learning-based cardiovascular image diagnosis: a promising challenge. Futur Gener Comput Syst. 2020;110:802–11.

Yoon K, Kim JY, Kim SJ, Huh JK, Kim JW, Choi J. Explainable deep learning-based clinical decision support engine for MRI-based automated diagnosis of temporomandibular joint anterior disk displacement. Comput Methods Prog Biomed. 2023;233:107465.

Yue L, Berman J. What is osteoarthritis? JAMA. 2022;327(13):1300.

Zakirov A, Ezhov M, Gusarev M, Alexandrovsky V, Shumilov E. Dental pathology detection in 3D cone-beam CT. arXiv preprint. 2018. arXiv:181010309.

Zhang K, Li J, Ma R, Li G, editors. An end-to-end segmentation network for the temporomandibular joints CBCT image based on 3D U-Net. 2020 13th international congress on image and signal processing, biomedical engineering and informatics (CISP-BMEI); 2020: IEEE.

Zhang W, Bianchi J, Turkestani NA, Le C, Deleat-Besson R, Ruellas A, et al. Temporomandibular joint osteoarthritis diagnosis using privileged learning of protein markers. Annu Int Conf IEEE Eng Med Biol Soc. 2021;2021:1810–3.

Artificial Intelligence for 3D Printing and Bioprinting

12

Isil Yazgan, Utku Serhat Derici, Burak Barıs Altunay, Osama Ali Hindy, and Pinar Yilgor Huri

3D Printing for Medical Applications

3D printing, also known as additive manufacturing, is the transformation of digital designs in the computer environment into physical objects. This is revealed by using design programs or by the 3D scanning method. The 3D printing method, which is used in many fields such as the defense industry, aviation, and architecture (Dawood et al. 2015), started to be used in the medical field in the 1990s (Strub et al. 2006). In particular, preliminary studies have been carried out for the tailor-made production of craniofacial implants.

For the use of 3D printers, which are becoming increasingly widespread in the medical field, first of all, it is necessary to detect the defective area of the patient by using medical imaging methods such as X-ray, CT, or MRI in order to make personalized designs (Aimar et al. 2019). The resulting images are then labeled by the segmentation process. The purpose of this process is to isolate the desired region and develop a 3D model in the computer environment. One of the most important aspects of 3D printing is computer-aided design (CAD) programs (Miyazaki and Hotta 2011). With the help of CAD programs, the necessary designs are made for the creation of 3D objects. After the 3D model is developed, it is converted to STL files (Satyanarayana and Prakash 2015) so that it can be printed. Although it differs according to the types of printers, in general, after the parameters such as speed and pressure are adjusted and the relevant optimization processes are performed, the printing of the file starts. As a result, personalized 3D objects emerge using the data obtained from the patient (Fig. 12.1).

Many different technologies have been introduced since the development of 3D printers. Many of these technologies can be given as examples, such as Stereolithography (SLA), Fused Deposition Modelling (FDM), Selective Laser

I. Yazgan · U. S. Derici · B. B. Altunay · O. A. Hindy · P. Yilgor Huri (✉)
Department of Biomedical Engineering, Ankara University, Ankara, Turkey
e-mail: phuri@ankara.edu.tr

K. Orhan, R. Jagtap (eds.), *Artificial Intelligence in Dentistry*,
https://doi.org/10.1007/978-3-031-43827-1_12

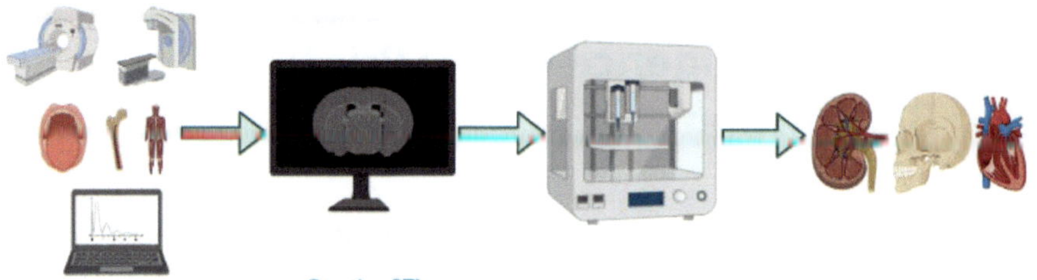

Fig. 12.1 Schematic representation of the 3D printing process. (Designed with Biorender)

Sintering (SLS), and Selective Laser Melting (SLM) (Chen and Gariel 2012). Each technology has various advantages and disadvantages according to its uses in the medical field, the materials used for printing, and the time required for printing.

3D printing, which is rapidly developing and continues to develop in the medical field, is used in many different fields such as cardiology, urology, orthopedics, plastic surgery, and gastroenterology (Aimar et al. 2019). In addition to these, its use in dentistry is increasing rapidly. In dentistry, 3D printing is useful and preferred in terms of making personalized designs, choosing the materials to be used, and processing images in different geometries taken from the patient (Dawood et al. 2015). However, health-related protocols should be followed and sterilization processes should be considered.

Bioprinting for Engineering Functional Tissues and Organs

3D printers are frequently used in fields such as tissue engineering and regenerative medicine. Based on these studies, the term bioprinting was born. Bioprinting can be defined as cellular printing by integrating cells suitable for the developed materials (Derby 2012). In this way, structures with heterogeneous cell distribution suitable for tissue forms can be formed. With the use of cell-containing biomaterials, also known as "bioinks," it has become possible to produce living, functional tissues and organs in the laboratory environment (Murphy and Atala 2014). Based on this, the difference between the terms 3D printing and 3D bioprinting is that in 3D printing, biological structures are not used during printing, while in 3D bioprinting there is cellular printing (Vijayavenkataraman et al. 2018).

As in 3D printing, imaging methods such as X-ray, CT, and MRI are used, and 3D model designs are created in the computer environment. For this, there are design approaches such as biomimicry and self-assembly (Murphy and Atala 2014). After the design is completed, the main technologies used for bioprinting are inkjet bioprinting, extrusion bioprinting, and laser bioprinting. In inkjet bioprinting, the cell-attached material is flowed in the form of droplets. They accumulate in the desired area in accordance with the models designed using computer programs.

Drops show flow according to the set pressure and speed (Xu et al. 2008). Since changes can be made in droplets in this type of printing, complex structures can be printed more easily. Filaments are used in extrusion bioprinting. There is a continuous flow of filaments and therefore the materials used must be fluid. The deposited structure must be strong and the solubility is low compared to the others (Melchels et al. 2012). Laser bioprinting requires a laser beam, a ribbon, and a film containing materials. The laser is absorbed on the ribbon, and the films are located on this ribbon. The advantage of laser bioprinting is that there is no clogging because there is no spraying. However, cell viability is low compared to other varieties because laser energy is used (Xia et al. 2018).

The materials used in bioprinting must also have some properties because the material must be compatible with biological structures as well as being printable and mechanically durable. In this respect, there is not much material diversity and this is a limitation of this method. Materials such as alginate, chitosan, polyethylene glycol, and gelatin are used in bioprinting. Another point that is as important as the materials is the selection of the appropriate cell. Since there are cells with different functions in tissues, the cells used must be able to differentiate into other structures. They should have high strength during printing. Cell proliferation should be neither too low nor too high. If it is low, the tissue cannot perform its function; if it is too high, apoptosis occurs. The cells recommended to be used in this direction are mesenchymal or induced pluripotent stem cells (Murphy and Atala 2014) (Fig. 12.2).

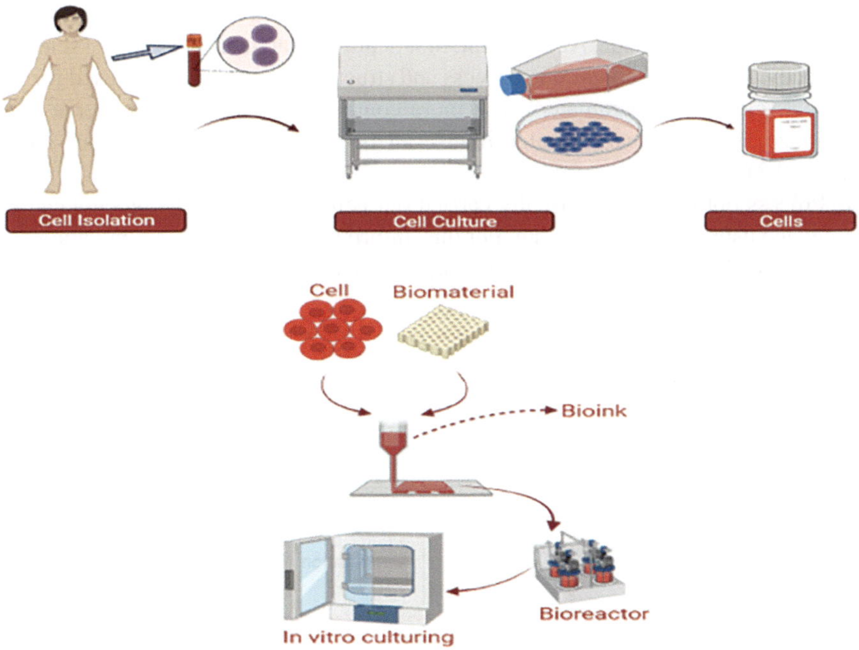

Fig. 12.2 Demonstration of the bioprinting process. (Designed with Biorender)

Many tissue and organ experiments such as aortic valve (Hockaday et al. 2012), human skin (Lee et al. 2014), bionic ear (Mannoor et al. 2013), neural cell structures (Xu et al. 2006), and blood vessel-like structures (Skardal et al. 2010) have been made with bioprinting. However, although bioprinting is promising, the range of materials should be expanded. Parameters such as speed and resolution of the printers used should be improved. Nevertheless, many studies on cell-material compatibility and cell durability are required.

Process Optimization for 3D Printing Applications

3D printing needs to be optimized in terms of being more functional and less costly and requiring less energy. At the same time, optimization is a necessary step for a more accurate assessment of the material properties to be used and the requirements for the application.

During the optimization in 3D printing, variables such as the structural properties of the material to be used in the printing, the volume, shape, and dimensions of the object to be printed, temperature changes during the printing of the printer, pressure, and environmental conditions should be taken into account (Rojek et al. 2021).

Process Optimization with AI

Process optimization is usually performed when working with a new material or when a new print is made. At this point, first of all, the parameters should be selected correctly. A database containing process and structure properties can be used for the correct selection of parameters. The more complex the object, the harder it is to optimize. Machine learning algorithms can be used for this (Goh et al. 2021) (Fig. 12.3).

Process optimization is usually carried out before printing. The process can be predicted using machine learning. For this, information on process optimization can be obtained by entering the properties such as the density, melting temperature, and

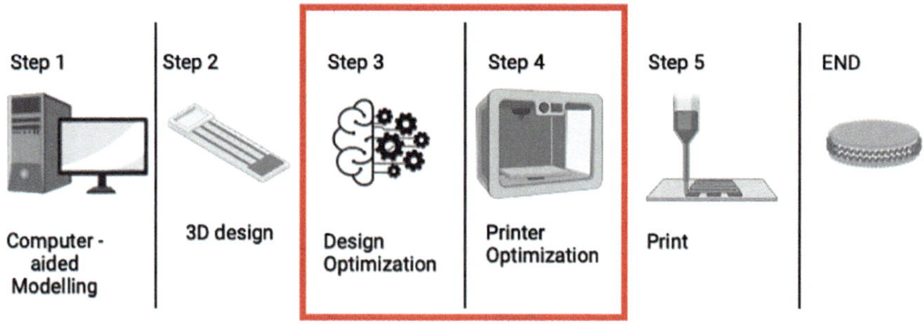

Fig. 12.3 The 3D printing process showing the steps that require optimization protocols. (Designed with Biorender)

freezing temperature of the material to be used and the properties such as the volume, thickness, length, and shape of the object to be printed. Variables such as needle tip size, printing speed, pressure, printing temperature, cost, and time can be estimated before printing. As a result of these estimations, less costly and better-quality 3D prints with less deformation can be obtained (Yu and Jiang 2020) (Fig. 12.4). The same results apply to 3D bioprinting. In the 3D cell bioprinting process, with the help of machine learning, values such as cell damage and the number of cells per area can be predicted during the process.

In addition, researchers and algorithm developers can develop existing algorithms together with the cloud system. In this way, process optimization can give more stable and accurate results day by day. Usually, four techniques of machine learning can be used for optimization. These can be called supervised learning, unsupervised learning, semi-supervised learning, and reinforced learning. In addition to these techniques, the deep learning method can also be used (Fig. 12.5).

Supervised learning: Algorithms are supervised first and then the boundaries that determine the clusters of supervised algorithms are determined. By modeling the relationship between labeled outputs and input properties with supervised learning algorithms, input properties for the desired output can be predicted.

Unsupervised learning: Unsupervised learning algorithms extract the input data features for the desired output and classify them with the help of taught rules. This technique is often used to highlight unseen relationships between input and output data.

Semi-supervised learning: The semi-supervised learning technique, which is a combination of supervised and unsupervised learning, has advantages and disadvantages compared to the other two techniques. Therefore, it can be used in

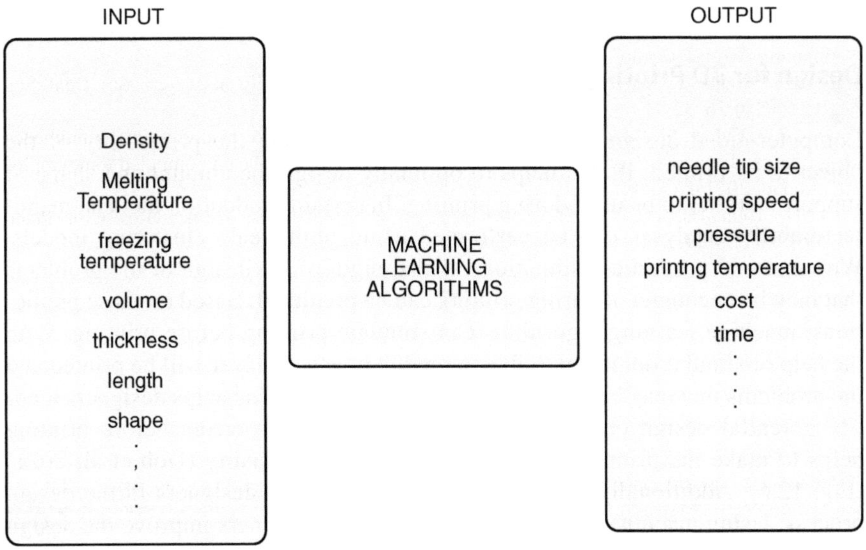

Fig. 12.4 Optimization protocols are required prior to the 3D printing application

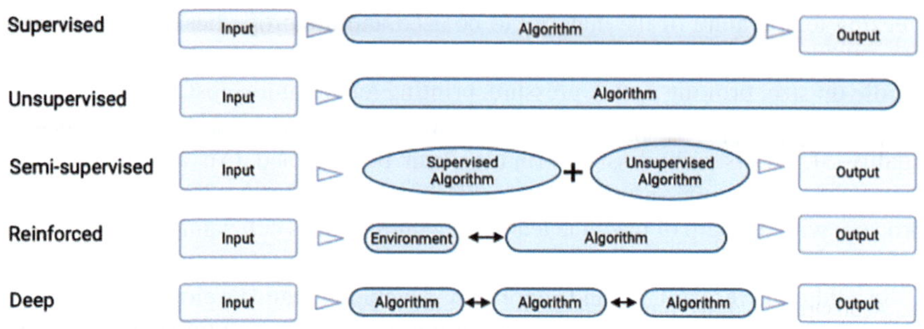

Fig. 12.5 Schematic representation of machine learning methods

complex and large volumes of data. It is more advantageous than unsupervised learning since there will be some labeled data. At the same time, it is more advantageous in terms of less cost and easier teaching compared to supervised learning.

Reinforced learning: Reinforced learning learns in a similar way to supervised learning. However, by interacting with the environment and previous algorithms, reinforced learning is acting more and more accurately and stable, interacting with the environment rather than too much labeled data, providing certain feedback. This feedback reinforces the behavior of the algorithm. With these technical feedbacks, which can learn more slowly and by observing, more and more optimal solutions can be produced (Goh et al. 2021).

Deep learning: Deep learning is a technique that uses a set of algorithms with multiple hidden layers applied to a new dataset (Malekpour and Chen 2022). Deep learning usually has three steps, namely preprocessing, feature extraction, and classification, and it works in that order.

Design for 3D Printing

Computer-aided design can be thought of as ensuring the printability of the object to be printed. It also helps to optimally design the amount and shape of support material to be used during printing. In certain production models, manufacturability analyses can be performed using multi-scale clustering models. With material properties estimations, the strength of the design or the problems that may be encountered during printing can be predicted. Based on these predictions, machine learning algorithms can simulate printing before printing. With the help of simulation, it is possible to predict how each layer will be printed and the problems that may be encountered during printing. This helps designers identify potential design errors before printing. Correcting errors before printing helps to make the print less imperfect and of higher quality (Goh et al. 2021) (Fig. 12.6). Additionally, it assists more inexperienced designers in the design process. Using machine learning techniques helps designers improve the design

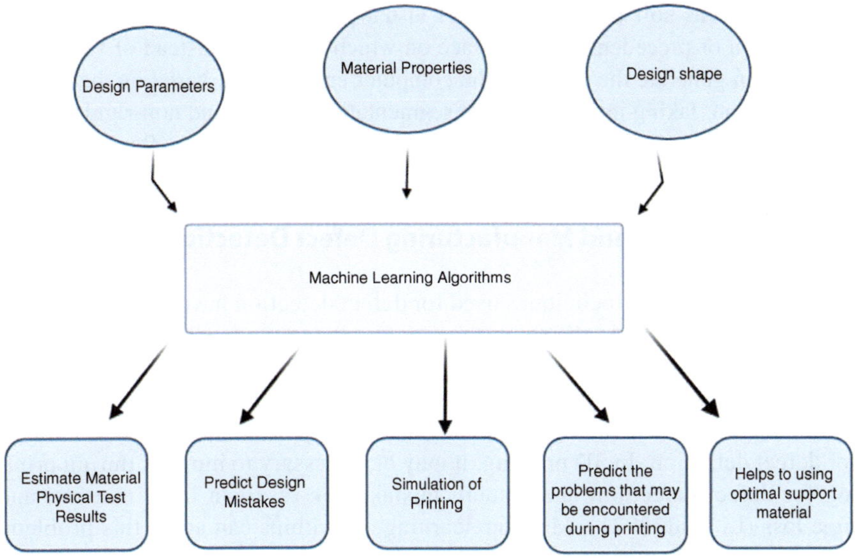

Fig. 12.6 Estimation of 3D design variables with machine learning algorithms

by making feature predictions of models. In addition, it is possible to estimate the physical tests to be made after printing. With material properties and design inputs, physical tests of the material can be estimated. This provides advantages in terms of time and cost.

Machine learning algorithms can also be used for 3D bioprinting. It is essential to design and analyze material properties for 3D bioprinting. Examples include scaffolds and cell adhesion properties in tissue engineering. Predicting the growth of cells according to material properties and designing scaffolds can be facilitated by machine learning algorithms (Yu and Jiang 2020).

Robotic sensing systems can also be used for 3D printing. Surface area, surface shape, and surface deformations on human organs and tissues can be detected by robotic perception systems and designed with artificial intelligence. These systems can be divided into low-level visual perception and high-level visual perception.

Low-level visual perception: Image processing algorithms are used to detect features such as low-level visual perception, colors, and textures, similar to human visual perception. The image can be reconstructed on the computer based on triangulation and projection techniques. These techniques form the basis of techniques such as stereovision and structured light scanning from motion. However, low-level visual perception may not perform properly and stably on wet or reflective surfaces.

High-level visual perception: High-level visual perception, similar to the perception of the brain and nervous system, can model and predict deformation on surfaces such as soft tissue. High-level visual perception, which can predict the continuation or precedent of the surface on which it is seen, instead of visual perception, can generate the image in the computer environment based on the estimation algorithm, taking into account the segmentation of rigid and non-rigid regions, and geometric constraints arising from rigid body transformations (Zhu et al. 2021).

Image Processing and Manufacturing Defect Detection

Artificial intelligence techniques used for defect detection have recently become popular and reliable. At the same time, defect detection has become an important part of real-time data collection and quality control systems. Many different techniques such as vision-based ultrasound, acoustic emission, laser scanning, electromagnetic, and radiographic and thermographic techniques can be used for defect detection. In 3D printing, it may be necessary to monitor during printing for defect detection, and a small mistake can result in large material and time loss (Li et al. 2021). Machine learning algorithms can avoid this problem. Errors and disadvantages such as poor surface quality, cracks, pores, and distortions can be detected with machine learning algorithms. Acoustic data can be obtained using computer-aided scans, visual data, and sound sensors (Farhan Khan et al. 2021).

With monitoring devices such as sensors, digital cameras, and 3D scanners at every stage of the printing process, a defect in the printing can be detected quickly. Careful monitoring of each layer of the print ensures that if there is a defect, the print can be stopped. This prevents the loss of time and material since printing will not continue after the defect (Li et al. 2021) (Fig. 12.7).

Defect detection can be done using computer scan-assisted machine learning algorithms by labeling abnormal and nominal conditions. In line with the research, it has been seen that machine learning algorithms in defect detection give more accurate and higher-quality results than an operator's manual detection (Gobert et al. 2018).

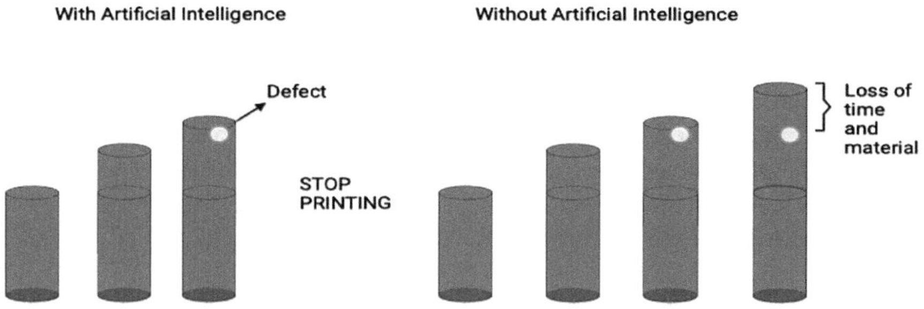

Fig. 12.7 Defect detection within images for the production of 3D models for 3D printing

Use of AI for 3D Printing of Surgical Guides

In recent years development of artificial intelligence (AI) technology has accelerated and gained worldwide recognition for its utility. AI technologies such as machine learning and deep learning can automate image reading, repetitive operations, and the reporting process, resulting in increased clinical workflow efficiency (Banerjee et al. 2022). Artificial intelligence technologies allow radiologists to observe and compare relevant cases, learn from other professionals, improve overall diagnostic accuracy, and enhance individual radiologist competence.

Over the last decade, use of 3D printing technology has increased in a variety of fields such as aerospace, automotive, and healthcare (Liu et al. 2018). Medical use of 3D printing is generally patient specific and can be divided into sub-categories such as 3D-printed implants, improving surgical instruments by 3D printing, and preoperative planning (Kang et al. 2016). For preoperative planning, clinicians generally use computed tomography (CT) and magnetic resonance imaging (MRI) images to understand patients' conditions accurately before operations. 3D printing allows a transformation from 2D to 3D; thus, imaging data can be transformed from virtual to actual models with high accuracy. By 3D printing, a three-dimensional anatomical model allows surgeons to establish and simulate a surgical plan before entering the operating room. In this way, surgeons have a good grasp of the patient's anatomical model before the operation and can determine the medical equipment and devices to be used before entering the operating room. However, the biggest challenge in the preoperative use of 3D printing is the precise segmentation of the patient's radiological data. Segmentation is the process of separating and categorizing images into comparable attributes. To find regions of interest (ROI) image processing is used according to image gray level, contrast, and texture (Sharma et al. 2010). This is one of the most critical, but also the most time-consuming, steps in generating a 3D image. Machine learning might be able to help automate the segmentation process. The time it takes a radiologist to perform segmentation might be cut in half or removed entirely if AI tools are fully developed to use in this field.

Use of AI in Medical Models

Creating models from ROIs using DICOM (Digital Imaging and Communications in Medicine) images is one of the most common uses of 3D printing in radiology. However, the DICOM image format is not a file format that can be used by 3D printers. Individual items are defined by surfaces that enclose a region of space in 3D printers. Standard Tessellation Language (STL) is a file format that is used for defining these surfaces. These surfaces, defined in STL format, are made up of triangles and fit into each other like pieces of a puzzle (Mitsouras et al. 2015). In this way, the image obtained with medical imaging techniques is converted into a format that 3D printers can understand. To create a 3D-printed model, radiologists' separate structures on DICOM images based on tissues and pathophysiology to create objects of interest. These desired regions can be 3D printed once they are defined in STL format. In comparison to typical 3D visualization, this radiologist-centered procedure of translating DICOM format into STL format is a unique new requirement. Image acquisition, image postprocessing, and 3D printing are three aspects of the process required to create a medical 3D model.

Image Acquisition

Obtaining an image is a very important step in creating a 3D object, since the quality of the data received by imaging will directly affect the quality of the object to be produced with the 3D printer. Volumetric image datasets with sufficient contrast and resolution obtained at this stage can be used to create 3D medical models. Clinical image acquisition can currently be done with ultra-high spatial resolution (400–600 microns) and high-quality contrast (Mahesh 2002). Even though CT and MRI are both effective data acquisition modalities, CT is the most utilized imaging modality for rapid prototyping due to its wide variety of applications and ease of image processing (Rengier et al. 2010). The high contrast, signal-to-noise ratio, and spatial resolution increase structural differentiation while reducing partial volume effects, which may restrict 3D printing (Mitsouras et al. 2015). Other imaging modalities that can be employed for data collecting include cone beam computed tomography, positron emission tomography, single photon emission computed tomography, and ultrasonography (Rengier et al. 2010). The cross-section size of the acquired images is also important for the accuracy of the model. Image portions should be reconstructed using isotropic voxels with a size of 1.25 mm or smaller (Mahesh 2002). Thicker sections reduce model accuracy, whereas very tiny sections (e.g., 0.25 mm) necessitate significant segmentation and STL refining, especially in the presence of an image artifact. Finally, acquired data is stored in the universal DICOM format, regardless of imaging modality.

Image Postprocessing

In radiology, postprocessing emerged to visualize volumetric data in any plane and then render that volume on a 2D display (Mitsouras et al. 2015). The manipulation of DICOM images to be used in 3D printing includes accurate segmentation of the targeted tissue and transfer of the generated ROI to STL format without any loss. The approaches used at this stage are new to radiologists and often require the use of specialized tools and programs used in engineering applications. Therefore, the segmented STL model should be carefully examined and verified by a radiologist.

ROI segmentation can be done manually or automatically (e.g., thresholding, edge detection, region growth). More advanced techniques, such as dynamic adjustment of the thresholding range, are usually required. A segmented region's "wrapping" can also be utilized to construct a solid model by filling genuine anatomic spaces, such as those in cancellous bone (Harrysson et al. 2007). Another useful tool is region growth. This tool is used to determine whether the segmented voxels to be

3D printed belong to the same or different components. Typically, region expanding lessens the burden of the next stage, which is human editing of the 3D ROIs that surround segmented voxels; this includes manually altering ROI boundaries as well as manually erasing, merging, and changing sections. Many software programs generate a 3D STL file of post-segmentation ROI using algorithms such as interpolation and pattern recognition to preserve anatomical features (Mitsouras et al. 2015). Radiologists pick voxels that encompass a 3D surface using ROIs. If the segmented surface is not smooth, conversion to STL can employ any number of triangle facets to fit these surfaces; too few will compromise anatomic features in the 3D-printed model, while too many will result in excessive roughness in the object.

After all these processes, computer-aided design (CAD) or computer-aided manufacturing (CAM) software for 3D part manipulation, as well as operator expertise, is required for accurate 3D printing. Finally, data is sent to a 3D printer after all corrections are complete.

Artificial Intelligence Tools for Segmentation

Artificial intelligence approaches are used in automatic segmentation algorithms. There are two types of techniques that can be used for this in machine learning: supervised and unsupervised. Supervised segmentation necessitates operator interaction throughout the process, whereas unsupervised approaches typically necessitate operator involvement only once segmentation is complete. Unsupervised approaches are favored to ensure reproducibility; however, operator engagement is still necessary for mistake correction if the outcome is poor (Olabarriaga and Smeulders 2001).

Supervised Methods

Supervised algorithms are based on artificial neural networks (ANNs). ANNs consist of structures called artificial neurons, which can solve certain problems with many interconnected processing components working together. Advantages of ANNs are adaptive learning ability, the power to solve complex problems with training data, self-organization capability, and the ability to perform in real time due to parallel configuration with the information provided by the training data (Vijayakumar et al. 2007).

ANNs can be used for segmentation and classification in both supervised and unsupervised methods. Although various neural network-based algorithms have been developed for texture-based segmentation and high classification accuracy, most of these texture classifier algorithms require extensive supervision and training. Their performance is impacted by presence of noise and is sensitive to training parameters (van Engeland et al. 2006). In some cases, supervised image segmentation and classification approaches can be challenging because selecting and labeling the proper training data is expensive, complex, and very time consuming. Any ANN-based method requires training data, and classifiers must be trained before they can be applied to segmentation and classification tasks to ensure accuracy. Moreover, the entire process of picking the training dataset and training must be completed for other datasets, as well as analysis of different images of varied type and format (Gletsos et al. 2003).

Unsupervised Methods

Most unsupervised algorithms are cluster-based and do not require training. The purpose of clustering is to generate decision boundaries from unlabeled training data (Jain et al. 2000). In multidimensional feature space, clustering is the process of finding natural grouping clusters. However, this is problematic because multidimensional feature space can contain clusters of various shapes and sizes. Image segmentation can be thought of as a clustering process in which pixels are grouped into attribute regions based on the texture feature vector calculated around the pixel local neighborhood (Bandyopadhyay 2005).

K-means and fuzzy C-means are two popular clustering techniques (Bezdek et al. 1993). The k-means technique produces hard segmentation results, but the fuzzy C-means approach produces soft segmentation that can be converted to hard segmentation by ensuring that pixels belong to clusters with the highest membership coefficients. Fuzzy clustering is a useful method for categorizing a set of data points into numerous clusters with varying degrees of membership. Most of the neural network-based techniques that perform texture-based segmentation and high-accuracy classification require substantial supervision and training. In addition, their success depends on the training method and the training data used. Finally, the high accuracy, reliability, stability, repeatability, robustness, and minimum operator dependency of these automated tools, which segment using artificial intelligence, will expand the use of these tools in the medical field (Sharma et al. 2010).

3D Printing

For the transition from 2D to 3D, all 3D printers use files containing data encoded in STL format. There are many factors to consider when choosing the 3D platform on which the model prepared on the computer will be produced. Key 3D printing parameters include print time, availability, printer and material costs, material selection, biocompatibility, sterilization capability, material temperature and moisture resistance, transparency, molding, and casting properties. Most technologies use materials classified as class VI or 10993 by the United States Pharmacopeial Convention, which correspond to levels of minimum in vivo biologic reactivity (U.S. Food and Drug Administration. Use of International Standard ISO-10993).

In order to print a part without any errors, mesh surfaces of design must be free of holes. Therefore, steps for verification and fixing are essential. Removal of excessive (noise) shells, intersecting elements, and holes in the model are important to get a successful final build. After choosing the 3D printing platform (selective laser sintering, stereolithography, fused deposition modeling, etc.), it is important to adjust wall thickness and resolution parameters to get an accurate print. If the created model has smaller structures than 3D printer resolution, printing will result in missing components or shapes. There is a good amount of software available to analyze and adjust these settings automatically or manually to avoid printer-related errors. Finally, build orientation needs to be performed uniquely for the 3D print platform.

Model Precision: In general, the difference between the segmented model and the 3D printed model is 0–1 mm (1–3%) (Ibrahim et al. 2009; Taft et al. 2011). This difference is clinically negligible. Differences can be minimized by thinning the section thickness during image acquisition and reducing the z-axis print layer thickness of the 3D printer. Since 3D model generation from a medical image is the result of a multi-stage process, an error may occur when processing a dataset and this error can be propagated due to the segmentation method. These errors may include excessive smoothing of the anatomy, destruction of some anatomical structures in the desired region, and scaling problems between the types of software used. In addition, errors can be caused by image acquisition, postprocessing (Huotilainen et al. 2014), and the 3D printing process (Choi et al. 2002; Hazeveld et al. 2014). Losses during image segmentation and conversion to STL format and resolution differences of 3D printer modalities and materials can be the biggest causes of errors, so they should be carefully analyzed (Salmi et al. 2013).

There are two solutions to avoid errors that may occur in these processes. First, through careful segmentation of the image obtained from the patient by a specialist (ideally a radiologist) or with the semi-automatic segmentation method, the radiologist supervises the process and prevents possible segmentation-related losses/errors. Second, the development of artificial intelligence-supported tools and software needs to be accelerated, and programs with high accuracy and stability are expected to prevent data loss in this area.

3D Printing and Artificial Intelligence in Dentistry

3D printing technology was introduced in the dental field around two decades ago. Its applications are still increasing, and the last decade has seen rapid growth in 3D image analysis and printing methods, resulting in various digital dentistry applications. Nowadays, the applications of 3D printing have numerous advantages in biomedical engineering, with applications in the field of dentistry that range from endodontics, orthodontics, and prosthodontics to oral implantology, periodontology, and oral and maxillofacial surgery. The most common applications include creating working models for surgery and diagnosis, in addition to a variety of implantable devices, which can be helpful for dentists and patients (Nesic et al. 2020). The applications of 3D printing can help in providing patients with less costly, less invasive, more personalized services and more predictable processes (Fig. 12.8).

The presence of the CAD/CAM technology and the development of digital image acquirement have allowed the development of a fully digitalized dental treatment. Nowadays, instead of using plastic imprints, intra-oral scanning has been utilized to create CAM digital-physical models. Moreover, for the complex structures of some

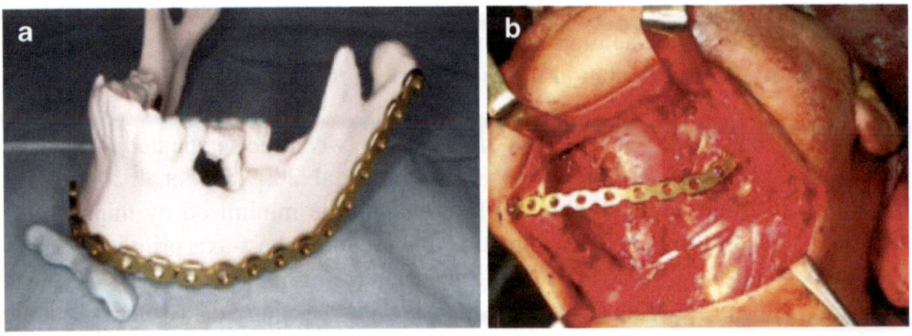

Fig. 12.8 (**a**) Three-dimensional (3D) medical rapid prototyping model produced by using powder bed and inkjet head 3D printing with the attached pre-bent reconstruction plate. (**b**) The pre-bent reconstruction plate based on the model is fixed on the residual bone. (Images from the study of Tian et al. 2021)

products, 3D printing has the ability to produce complex geometric forms by using numerous material types and by depending on the digital data given, and thus precisely fulfill the personalized necessities in the dental field.

Presurgical Virtual Planning and Dental Surgical Guides

The addition of 3D imaging data and the combination of haptics and artificial intelligence technology led to the presence of dental haptic simulators and created virtual oral anatomy that expedited the simulation of dental procedures. In contrast, the technology of haptics is mainly based on the sense of touch and its interaction with the virtual environment (Nesic et al. 2020). Therefore, the convergence of 3D printing technology with haptic instruments resulted in the development of patient-specific instrumentation, such as surgical guide instruments that reduce the time and cost of surgeries in addition to reducing the risk of infection. In addition, the use of surgical guide devices has increased accuracy during surgery (Fig. 12.9).

Through the 3D digital treatment simulation, the modified design of stainless steel arch-wires and surgical splints has allowed for an accurate production as well as the prediction of the jaw and dental movements. This method has rapidly improved the aesthetics of tooth braces, decreased the treatment time, and reinforced decompensatory tooth movements (Tian et al. 2021). Moreover, numerous commercial software programs and applications have been established to ease 3D virtual treatment planning. Examples of the surgical planning software include InVivo6® (Anatomage, San Jose, CA, USA), Virtual Surgical Planning (VSP®) Technology (3D Systems; Littleton, CO, USA), and ProPlan CMF™ (Materialise, Leuven, Belgium). The main role of the software is to integrate the intra-oral occlusal scans and the CT data to create a complete 3D model (Nesic et al. 2020). The surgical osteotomies and dental movements can be simulated interactively between the orthodontist, engineer, and surgeon. Hence, the final clinical plan is used to create a final splint that is formed via 3D printing. The orthodontist generates the

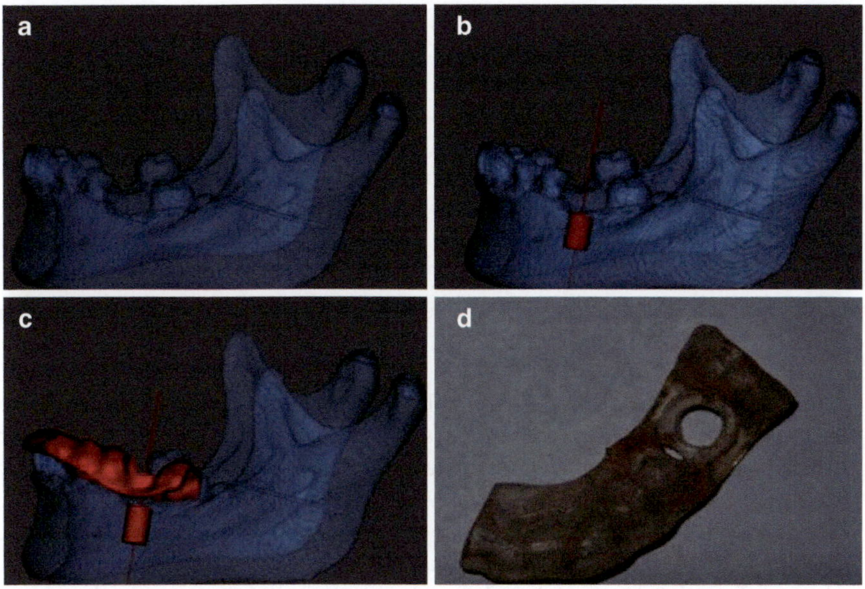

Fig. 12.9 The design and construction procedure of the surgical guide. (**a**) Digital model of the mandible obtained by scanning. (**b**) Identify the implant position in the design software. (**c**) Design surgical guide. (**d**) Print surgical guide using stereolithography (SLA). (Images from the study of Tian et al. 2021)

pathway and the sequence for the tooth movements as well as the virtual set-up of the final occlusion. The sequenced aligners or models can be produced with a relatively cheap 3D printer in a dental laboratory or even in the orthodontist's workplace. An easy transfer of digital data allows the design of anatomically perfectly shaped structures that can be customized for each patient. Thus, the rapid developments of 3D printing technology lead to new and exciting approaches in all medical fields, including dentistry.

Artificial Intelligence 3D Printing for Dentistry

In recent years, 3D printing has developed to reach the cellular level, where 3D bioprinting has a great potential to generate numerous tissues. For instance, after being only represented in the experimental applications, the application of 3D printing in oral soft tissue biomaterials has been reflected in clinical applications as well. The most common dental field that machine learning has a great impact on is the automated interpretation of dental imaging (Pethani 2021). Therefore, to develop the CAD/CAM process, machine learning is mainly utilized since its applications include all the main features of final 3D printed products, including their manufacturing process, efficiency, and printing design (Tandon et al. 2020).

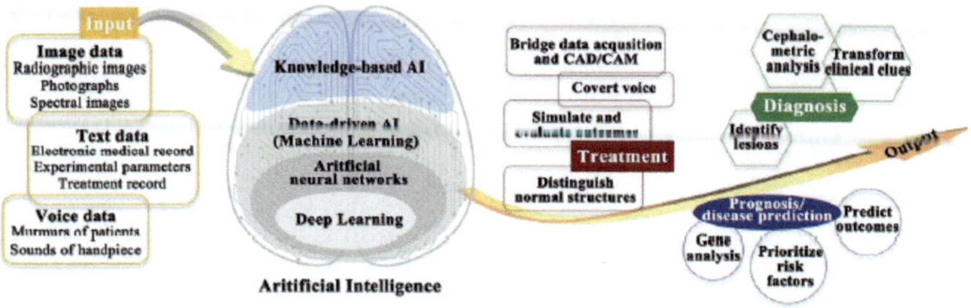

Fig. 12.10 A schematic representation of the hierarchy and major dental applications of AI (Shan et al. 2021)

The distinctive abilities of AI technology and dentists create great chances to enhance and develop patient care. AI systems work based on two main types for healthcare and medical applications: virtual and physical. The virtual models work based on software-based approaches, which help in clinical decision-making, whereas the physical components include automated or complex robots (Wang et al. 2014). In dentistry, the virtual AI models are the most commonly used algorithms in order to differentiate between disorders and normal structures, recognize the type of bone, show the risk factors, and make accurate surgical guides for implant replacements. In contrast, the integration of AI in 3D printing assists production at the prefabrication level. For instance, AI software can help in predicting the possible failure of 3D printing and in identifying the problem behind this failure. Therefore, the combination of AI algorithms and 3D printing software makes the 3D printer function more efficiently and helps to identify any quality problems (Shan et al. 2021). Hence, with the AI technology combined with the 3D printing software, dentists can design the best prostheses considering various aspects including facial measurements, ethnicity, and patient desire (Fig. 12.10).

Future Prospects

AI technology has started to appear in almost every field day by day. It is thought that using it in 3D bioprinting will collect a lot of data and speed up the optimization processes. By using artificial intelligence techniques in 3D printing and bioprinting studies, data collection will be easier, the time spent will be shortened, and a more effective way will be tried to determine the parameters. In this direction, more work is needed in this area.

Cell viability and printability are important in bioprinting. Optimization processes, which are mostly done by trial and error in studies in this field, have disadvantages in terms of both cost and time. In this context, the use of machine learning algorithms can reduce these disadvantages. Machine learning in areas such as design and optimization can be used in 3D printing. There is very little work being done using machine learning in the field of 3D printing and this needs to be increased in the future. There is a need to determine the parameters related to the studies to be carried out. It is necessary to present the data obtained from the studies for machine learning. Although it is very comprehensive, machine learning algorithm techniques are among the areas that need to be developed more in the future.

AI technology is developing rapidly with its applications in treatment, prognosis predictions, and diagnostics. It has also been shown to be an excellent technology for dentists, especially in preparing treatment plans, making clinical decisions, and increasing the efficiency of dental practice. It is clear that artificial intelligence will never completely replace the work of the dentist as technology develops, but will help more to avoid mistakes during dental practice.

References

Aimar A, Palermo A, Innocenti B. The role of 3D printing in medical applications: a state of the art. J Healthc Eng. 2019;2019:5340616. https://doi.org/10.1155/2019/5340616.

Bandyopadhyay S. Simulated annealing using a reversible jump Markov chain Monte Carlo algorithm for fuzzy clustering. IEEE Trans Knowl Data Eng. 2005;17(4):479–90. https://doi.org/10.1109/TKDE.2005.64.

Banerjee A, Haridas HK, SenGupta A, Jabalia N. Artificial intelligence in 3D printing: a revolution in health care; 2022. pp. 57–79. https://doi.org/10.1007/978-981-33-6703-6_4.

Bezdek JC, Hall LO, Clarke LP. Review of MR image segmentation techniques using pattern recognition. Med Phys. 1993;20(4):1033–48. https://doi.org/10.1118/1.597000.

Chen HJ, Gariel M. A roadmap from idea to implementation: 3D printing for pre-surgical application, 1st ed. 2012.

Choi J-Y, Choi J-H, Kim N-K, Kim Y, Lee J-K, Kim M-K, Lee J-H, Kim M-J. Analysis of errors in medical rapid prototyping models. Int J Oral Maxillofac Surg. 2002;31(1):23–32. https://doi.org/10.1054/ijom.2000.0135.

Dawood A, Marti BM, Sauret-Jackson V, Darwood A. 3D printing in dentistry. Br Dent J. 2015;219(11):521–9. https://doi.org/10.1038/sj.bdj.2015.914.

Derby B. Printing and prototyping of tissues and scaffolds. Science. 2012;338(6109):921–6. https://doi.org/10.1126/science.1226340.

Farhan Khan M, Alam A, Ateeb Siddiqui M, Saad Alam M, Rafat Y, Salik N, Al-Saidan I. Real-time defect detection in 3D printing using machine learning. Mater Today Proc. 2021;42:521–8. https://doi.org/10.1016/j.matpr.2020.10.482.

Gletsos M, Mougiakakou SG, Matsopoulos GK, Nikita KS, Nikita AS, Kelekis D. A computer-aided diagnostic system to characterize CT focal liver lesions: design and optimization of a neural network classifier. IEEE Trans Inf Technol Biomed. 2003;7(3):153–62. https://doi.org/10.1109/TITB.2003.813793.

Gobert C, Reutzel EW, Petrich J, Nassar AR, Phoha S. Application of supervised machine learning for defect detection during metallic powder bed fusion additive manufacturing using high resolution imaging. Addit Manuf. 2018;21:517–28. https://doi.org/10.1016/j.addma.2018.04.005.

Goh GD, Sing SL, Yeong WY. A review on machine learning in 3D printing: applications, potential, and challenges. Artif Intell Rev. 2021;54(1):63–94. https://doi.org/10.1007/s10462-020-09876-9.

Harrysson OLA, Hosni YA, Nayfeh JF. Custom-designed orthopedic implants evaluated using finite element analysis of patient-specific computed tomography data: femoral-component case study. BMC Musculoskelet Disord. 2007;8(1):91. https://doi.org/10.1186/1471-2474-8-91.

Hazeveld A, Huddleston Slater JJR, Ren Y. Accuracy and reproducibility of dental replica models reconstructed by different rapid prototyping techniques. Am J Orthod Dentofac Orthop. 2014;145(1):108–15. https://doi.org/10.1016/j.ajodo.2013.05.011.

Hockaday LA, Kang KH, Colangelo NW, Cheung PYC, Duan B, Malone E, Wu J, Girardi LN, Bonassar LJ, Lipson H, Chu CC, Butcher JT. Rapid 3D printing of anatomically accurate and mechanically heterogeneous aortic valve hydrogel scaffolds. Biofabrication. 2012;4(3):035005. https://doi.org/10.1088/1758-5082/4/3/035005.

Huotilainen E, Jaanimets R, Valášek J, Marcián P, Salmi M, Tuomi J, Mäkitie A, Wolff J. Inaccuracies in additive manufactured medical skull models caused by the DICOM to STL conversion process. J Craniomaxillofac Surg. 2014;42(5):e259–65. https://doi.org/10.1016/j.jcms.2013.10.001.

Ibrahim D, Broilo TL, Heitz C, de Oliveira MG, de Oliveira HW, Nobre SMW, dos Santos Filho JHG, Silva DN. Dimensional error of selective laser sintering, three-dimensional printing and PolyJet™ models in the reproduction of mandibular anatomy. J Cranio-Maxillofac Surg. 2009;37(3):167–73. https://doi.org/10.1016/j.jcms.2008.10.008.

Jain AK, Duin PW, Mao J. Statistical pattern recognition: a review. IEEE Trans Pattern Anal Mach Intell. 2000;22(1):4–37. https://doi.org/10.1109/34.824819.

Kang H-W, Lee SJ, Ko IK, Kengla C, Yoo JJ, Atala A. A 3D bioprinting system to produce human-scale tissue constructs with structural integrity. Nat Biotechnol. 2016;34(3):312–9. https://doi.org/10.1038/nbt.3413.

Lee V, Singh G, Trasatti JP, Bjornsson C, Xu X, Tran TN, Yoo S-S, Dai G, Karande P. Design and fabrication of human skin by three-dimensional bioprinting. Tissue Eng Part C Methods. 2014;20(6):473–84. https://doi.org/10.1089/ten.tec.2013.0335.

Li R, Jin M, Paquit VC. Geometrical defect detection for additive manufacturing with machine learning models. Mater Des. 2021;206:109726. https://doi.org/10.1016/j.matdes.2021.109726.

Liu J, Gaynor AT, Chen S, Kang Z, Suresh K, Takezawa A, Li L, Kato J, Tang J, Wang CCL, Cheng L, Liang X, To AC. Current and future trends in topology optimization for additive manufacturing. Struct Multidiscip Optim. 2018;57(6):2457–83. https://doi.org/10.1007/s00158-018-1994-3.

Mahesh M. The AAPM/RSNA physics tutorial for residents. Radiographics. 2002;22(4):949–62. https://doi.org/10.1148/radiographics.22.4.g02jl14949.

Malekpour A, Chen X. Printability and cell viability in extrusion-based bioprinting from experimental, computational, and machine learning views. J Funct Biomater. 2022;13(2):40. https://doi.org/10.3390/jfb13020040.

Mannoor MS, Jiang Z, James T, Kong YL, Malatesta KA, Soboyejo WO, Verma N, Gracias DH, McAlpine MC. 3D printed bionic ears. Nano Lett. 2013;13(6):2634–9. https://doi.org/10.1021/nl4007744.

Melchels FPW, Domingos MAN, Klein TJ, Malda J, Bartolo PJ, Hutmacher DW. Additive manufacturing of tissues and organs. Prog Polym Sci. 2012;37(8):1079–104. https://doi.org/10.1016/j.progpolymsci.2011.11.007.

Mitsouras D, Liacouras P, Imanzadeh A, Giannopoulos AA, Cai T, Kumamaru KK, George E, Wake N, Caterson EJ, Pomahac B, Ho VB, Grant GT, Rybicki FJ. Medical 3D printing for the radiologist. Radiographics. 2015;35(7):1965–88. https://doi.org/10.1148/rg.2015140320.

Miyazaki T, Hotta Y. CAD/CAM systems available for the fabrication of crown and bridge restorations. Aust Dent J. 2011;56:97–106. https://doi.org/10.1111/j.1834-7819.2010.01300.x.

Murphy SV, Atala A. 3D bioprinting of tissues and organs. Nat Biotechnol. 2014;32(8):773–85). Nature Publishing Group. https://doi.org/10.1038/nbt.2958.

Nesic D, Schaefer BM, Sun Y, Saulacic N, Sailer I. 3D printing approach in dentistry: the future for personalized oral soft tissue regeneration. J Clin Med. 2020;9(7):2238. https://doi.org/10.3390/jcm9072238.

Olabarriaga SD, Smeulders AWM. Interaction in the segmentation of medical images: a survey. Med Image Anal. 2001;5(2):127–42. https://doi.org/10.1016/S1361-8415(00)00041-4.

Pethani F. Promises and perils of artificial intelligence in dentistry. Aust Dent J. 2021;66(2):124–35. https://doi.org/10.1111/adj.12812.

Rengier F, Mehndiratta A, von Tengg-Kobligk H, Zechmann CM, Unterhinninghofen R, Kauczor H-U, Giesel FL. 3D printing based on imaging data: review of medical applications. Int J Comput Assist Radiol Surg. 2010;5(4):335–41. https://doi.org/10.1007/s11548-010-0476-x.

Rojek I, Mikołajewski D, Macko M, Szczepański Z, Dostatni E. Optimization of extrusion-based 3D printing process using neural networks for sustainable development. Materials. 2021;14(11):2737. https://doi.org/10.3390/ma14112737.

Salmi M, Paloheimo K-S, Tuomi J, Wolff J, Mäkitie A. Accuracy of medical models made by additive manufacturing (rapid manufacturing). J Cranio-Maxillofac Surg. 2013;41(7):603–9. https://doi.org/10.1016/j.jcms.2012.11.041.

Satyanarayana B, Prakash KJ. Component replication using 3D printing technology. Procedia Mater Sci. 2015;10:263–9. https://doi.org/10.1016/j.mspro.2015.06.049.

Shan T, Tay FR, Gu L. Application of artificial intelligence in dentistry. J Dent Res. 2021;100(3):232–44. SAGE Publications Inc. https://doi.org/10.1177/0022034520969115.

Sharma N, Ray A, Shukla K, Sharma S, Pradhan S, Srivastva A, Aggarwal L. Automated medical image segmentation techniques. J Med Phys. 2010;35(1):3. https://doi.org/10.4103/0971-6203.58777.

Skardal A, Zhang J, Prestwich GD. Bioprinting vessel-like constructs using hyaluronan hydrogels crosslinked with tetrahedral polyethylene glycol tetracrylates. Biomaterials. 2010;31(24):6173–81. https://doi.org/10.1016/j.biomaterials.2010.04.045.

Strub JR, Rekow ED, Witkowski S. Computer-aided design and fabrication of dental restorations. J Am Dent Assoc. 2006;137(9):1289–96. https://doi.org/10.14219/jada.archive.2006.0389.

Taft RM, Kondor S, Grant GT. Accuracy of rapid prototype models for head and neck reconstruction. J Prosthet Dent. 2011;106(6):399–408. https://doi.org/10.1016/S0022-3913(11)60154-6.

Tandon D, Rajawat J, Banerjee M. Present and future of artificial intelligence in dentistry. J Oral Biol Craniofac Res. 2020;10(4):391–6. https://doi.org/10.1016/j.jobcr.2020.07.015.

Tian Y, Chen C, Xu X, Wang J, Hou X, Li K, Lu X, Shi H, Lee E-S, Jiang HB. A review of 3D printing in dentistry: technologies, affecting factors, and applications. Scanning. 2021;2021:9950131. https://doi.org/10.1155/2021/9950131.

van Engeland S, Timp S, Karssemeijer N. Finding corresponding regions of interest in mediolateral oblique and craniocaudal mammographic views. Med Phys. 2006;33(9):3203–12. https://doi.org/10.1118/1.2230359.

Vijayakumar C, Damayanti G, Pant R, Sreedhar CM. Segmentation and grading of brain tumors on apparent diffusion coefficient images using self-organizing maps. Comput Med Imaging Graph. 2007;31(7):473–84. https://doi.org/10.1016/j.compmedimag.2007.04.004.

Vijayavenkataraman S, Yan W-C, Lu WF, Wang C-H, Fuh JYH. 3D bioprinting of tissues and organs for regenerative medicine. Adv Drug Deliv Rev. 2018;132:296–332. https://doi.org/10.1016/j.addr.2018.07.004.

Wang L, Wang D, Zhang Y, Ma L, Sun Y, Lv P. An automatic robotic system for three-dimensional tooth crown preparation using a picosecond laser. Lasers Surg Med. 2014;46(7):573–81. https://doi.org/10.1002/lsm.22274.

Xia Z, Jin S, Ye K. Tissue and organ 3D bioprinting. SLAS Technol. 2018;23(4):301–14. https://doi.org/10.1177/2472630318760515.

Xu T, Gregory C, Molnar P, Cui X, Jalota S, Bhaduri S, Boland T. Viability and electrophysiology of neural cell structures generated by the inkjet printing method. Biomaterials. 2006;27:3580. https://doi.org/10.1016/j.biomaterials.2006.01.048.

Xu T, Olson J, Zhao W, Atala A, Zhu J-M, Yoo JJ. Characterization of cell constructs generated with inkjet printing technology using in vivo magnetic resonance imaging. J Manuf Sci Eng. 2008;130(2):021013. https://doi.org/10.1115/1.2902857.

Yu C, Jiang J. A perspective on using machine learning in 3D bioprinting. Int J Bioprint. 2020;6(1):253. https://doi.org/10.18063/ijb.v6i1.253.

Zhu Z, Ng DWH, Park HS, McAlpine MC. 3D-printed multifunctional materials enabled by artificial-intelligence-assisted fabrication technologies. Nat Rev Mater. 2021;6(1):27–47. https://doi.org/10.1038/s41578-020-00235-2.

Artificial Intelligence in Dental Education

13

Ibrahim Sevki Bayrakdar, Kaan Orhan, and Rohan Jagtap

Introduction

Paradigm-shifting has begun in various fields of human life with the recent rapid development of information technologies, including the metaverse, Virtual Reality (VR), Augmented Reality (AR), Mixed Reality (MR), blockchain, and Artificial Intelligence (AI). These game-changing technologies have aroused great interest in the education sector and are now being explored within the scope of Artificial Intelligence in Education (AIEd) and Learning Analytics (LA).

The purpose of AIEd is to create an AI-human hybrid confirmative platform that improves student learning through various AI applications, human-computer interaction, and the learning sciences. On the other hand, LA aims to plan education and analyze, predict, optimize, and shape learning methods, principles, and environments using knowledge about students and learning environments. LA enhances students' study success by increasing motivation to participate in university courses (Gandedkar et al. 2021; Luckin et al. 2016; Ifenthaler and Yau 2019).

I. S. Bayrakdar (✉)
Division of Oral and Maxillofacial Radiology, Department of Care Planning and Restorative Sciences, University of Mississippi Medical Center, Jackson, MS, USA

Department of Oral and Maxillofacial Radiology, School of Dentistry, Center of Research and Application for Computer-Aided Diagnosis and Treatment in Health, Eskisehir Osmangazi University, ESOGÜ Meşelik Yerleşkesi, Eskisehir, Turkey

K. Orhan
Faculty of Dentistry, Department of Dentomaxillofacial Radiology, Ankara University, Ankara, Turkey

R. Jagtap
Division of Oral and Maxillofacial Radiology, Departments of Care Planning and Restorative Sciences and Radiology, School of Medicine, University of Mississippi Medical Center, Jackson, MS, USA

K. Orhan, R. Jagtap (eds.), *Artificial Intelligence in Dentistry*,
https://doi.org/10.1007/978-3-031-43827-1_13

Concurrently, as the perspective on education evolves with the breakthrough technologies, its impact is being felt in dentistry. Discussions have started about the necessity of curriculum changes and the integration of these technologies into dental education to improve accessibility, acceptability, and practicality in the contemporary age. The rapid adoption of AI and other game-changing digital technologies has presented the potential of technology-powered learning platforms to enhance the learning experience of modern dental students. Consequently, there is an increasing emphasis on the need to improve the current learning curriculum in dentistry (Gandedkar et al. 2021; Luckin et al. 2016; Ifenthaler and Yau 2019; Thurzo et al. 2023; Heo et al. 2021; Schwendicke et al. 2020; Schwendicke et al. 2023).

AI has demonstrated immense development and growth, with a rising trend in clinical use and research in dentistry. The integration of AI into clinical applications can be seen as augmented intelligence, but AI must overcome certain conventional limitations in teaching to become a significant part of dental education. The objective of this chapter is to elucidate the current state and requirements, the transformation, and the future direction of dental education through the utilization of AI-driven technological tools.

Artificial Intelligence Applications in Dental Education

Dental education encompasses a blend of theoretical, pre-clinical, and clinical training, encompassing both didactic and clinical skills instruction. The ongoing AI-driven revolution in dental education can be observed through these fundamental aspects (Islam et al. 2022; Gandedkar et al. 2021; Coşkun and Güngör 2023).

AI-Powered Theoretical Education

AI is being utilized to manage the educational process, support instructors and teaching methods, and enhance student learning assessment in theoretical education.

AI-supported education management information systems: An education management information system (EMIS) is a comprehensive collection of information and documentation services used for gathering, storing, processing, analyzing, and disseminating data for educational planning and management. There is a growing emphasis on integrating or developing AI technologies and tools that can upgrade EMIS, thereby enhancing data collection and processing. This, in turn, makes education management and provision more equitable, inclusive, open, and personalized. Furthermore, new models for delivering education and training in diverse learning institutions and settings are being introduced, facilitated by AI, to cater to different stakeholders, such as students, teaching staff, parents, and communities (Gandedkar et al. 2021; UNESCO 2019; Pedró et al. 2019).

AI-supported instructors and teaching: AI ensures opportunities to support instructors in their educational and pedagogical responsibilities. Instructors can work effectively and enhance their personal development with AI-enriched educational settings. AI applications aid in instructing human interaction and collaboration with students. The research-oriented learning model encourages students to ask questions and develop critical thinking skills. AI-driven research-oriented teaching facilitates sustainable learning for students (Gandedkar et al. 2021; UNESCO 2019; Pedró et al. 2019).

AI-supported Intelligent Tutoring Systems (ITS): The primary purpose of Intelligent Tutoring Systems (ITS) is to provide students with the means to obtain information and improve their knowledge and skills within a specialized system. ITS is designed with four interconnected modules to enable perceivable interactions, including the domain module, pedagogical module, student module, and dialogue module.

The domain module evaluates expert knowledge and skill sets based on quantification, notional mapping, and relations. The pedagogical module incorporates technology-facilitated teaching methods. The student module simulates students' characteristics, including strategy, knowledge, and learning styles, to foster an engaging learning environment. The dialogue module facilitates three-way interactive communication among the tutor, student, and computer.

The incorporation of AI in ITS, such as in the Unified Medical Language System (UMLS), provides significant improvements for students in receiving feedback (Gandedkar et al. 2021; UNESCO 2019; Pedró et al. 2019; Khanna and Dhaimade 2017; Zheng et al. 2020; Sharma et al. 2021).

AI-supported learning and learning assessment systems: AI has enormous potential to enhance the learning experience and learning assessments in dental education. The deep integration of AI in the learning process can lead to a transformation of learning experiences in dentistry.

AI-integrated learning systems allow students to engage in self-learning, draw lessons from successful use cases, and follow evidence-based practices. Instructors can utilize AI for automatic grading of students, enabling the assessment of multiple aspects of students' qualifications with extensive and remote evaluation.

AI can be employed to personalize learning experiences for dental students by analyzing their strengths and weaknesses, creating a tailored learning plan based on their individual needs (Gandedkar et al. 2021; UNESCO 2019; Pedró et al. 2019; González-Calatayud et al. 2021).

AI-supported text and image generators: Generative AI algorithms, using machine learning models, can generate text or images based on input data. An example of this is ChatGPT, an AI-powered chatbot developed by OpenAI, which generates human-like text in response to input (Fig. 13.1). Additionally, models like Midjourney AI and DALL-E2 can generate images using generative AI technology. These models have the potential to create detailed educational information, texts, schemes, and drawings for use in dental education, thereby revolutionizing communication, tutoring systems, lectures, and research for both students and instructors.

Moreover, with the adoption of such technologies, the process of writing essays, dissertations, or scientific articles may need to adapt to these changes (Gandedkar et al. 2021; Tadinada et al. 2023; UNESCO 2019; Pedró et al. 2019).

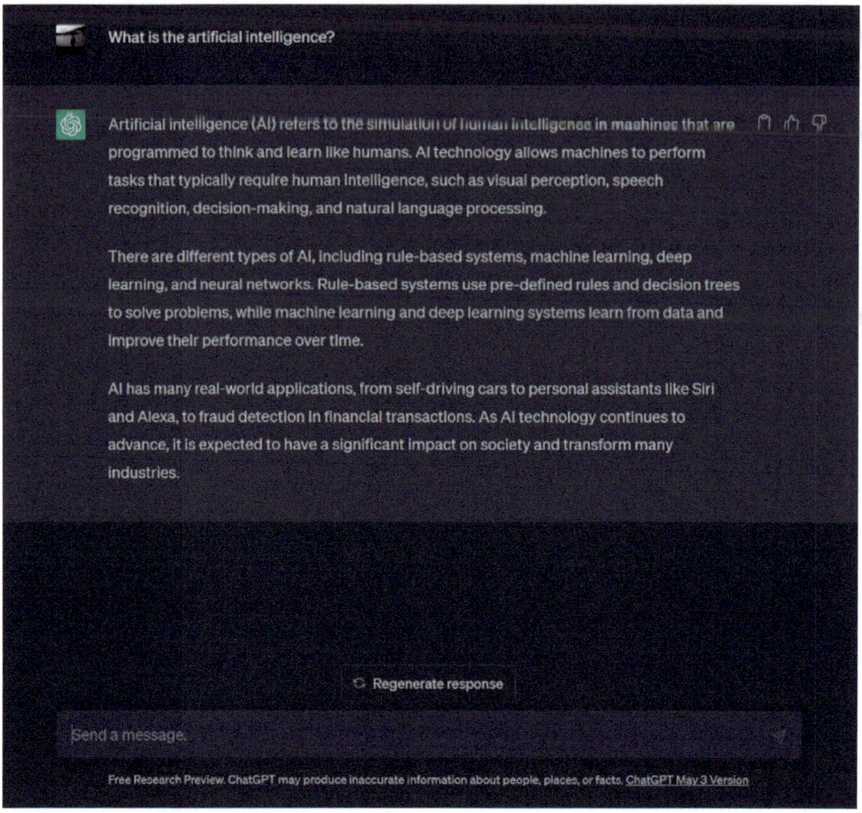

Fig. 13.1 The ChatGPT application, developed by OpenAI Inc., answered the question "What is artificial intelligence?"

AI-Powered Laboratory and Pre-clinical Teaching

Dental education should include practices to develop students' didactic and clinical skills. AI-simplified laboratory and pre-clinical teaching systems that provide virtual training environments are becoming an essential part of the modern era's education system. These systems help improve students' motor skills and efficiency, reducing the time they spend with tutors or in school. Integrating AI-powered tools into dental simulations and other hands-on activities in laboratory and pre-clinical teaching enhances the power of simulations for dental students (Duman et al. 2022; Gandedkar et al. 2021; Saghiri et al. 2022; Eaton et al. 2008; Ferro et al. 2019; Rhienmora et al. 2010; Dragan et al. 2020; Schleyer et al. 2012; Mangano et al. 2023).

Virtual reality (VR): VR is a technological process that creates virtual 3D environments, providing users with immersive experiences by combining different technologies (Fig. 13.2). AI-powered VR simulators can offer dental students a hands-on experience in a controlled and safe environment. These simulators can be used to

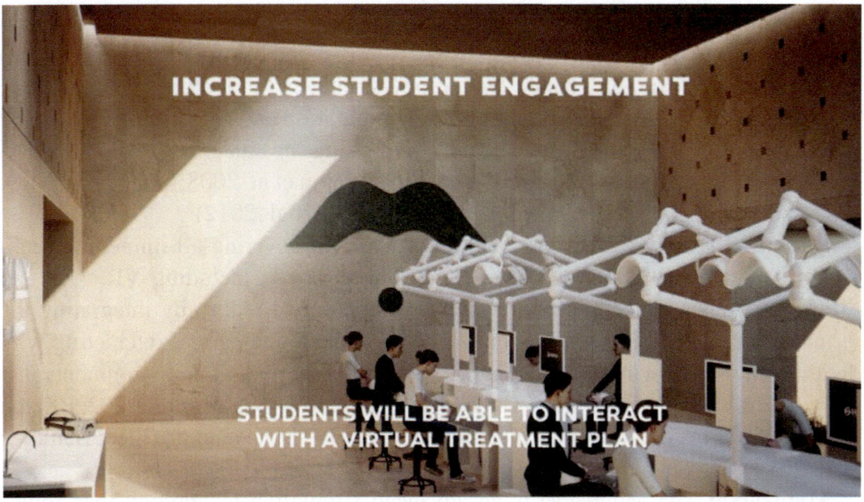

Fig. 13.2 Virtual reality environment from Dentaverse (Courtesy by Dentaverse.eth Ltd. company)

practice various procedures in dental education, including giving a nerve block, tooth extractions, suturing, cavity filling, and root canal treatments. Such applications can remarkably enhance students' techniques while also providing immediate feedback on their procedure applications.

VR has found significant use, especially in skull and teeth simulation for anatomy and variations, surgery simulation, and dental implant education. It allows students to gain experience through repeated virtual training and receive consistent feedback. AI integration can further aid in providing direction and feedback (Gandedkar et al. 2021; Saghiri et al. 2022; Eaton et al. 2008; Ferro et al. 2019; Rhienmora et al. 2010; Dragan et al. 2020; Schleyer et al. 2012).

Augmented reality (AR): AR is a technology that superimposes digital content onto the 3D real-world environment, increasing the user's perception of reality. AR technology detects the user's actual physical environments using a camera and sensors in a device like a smartphone or AR headset and overlays digital information onto the view of the real world displayed on the device's screen. This allows the user to interact with both real and virtual elements of their surrounding environment.

In dental education, AR provides students with the ability to understand and access content, displaying a 360° spatial surrounding of the real world. AR has been used for various applications, including cavity preparation, surgical navigation, and dental implant planning (Gandedkar et al. 2021; Saghiri et al. 2022; Eaton et al. 2008; Ferro et al. 2019; Rhienmora et al. 2010; Dragan et al. 2020; Schleyer et al. 2012; Mangano et al. 2023).

Mixed reality (MR): MR is a technology that blends components of both VR and AR to produce a hybrid experience, combining virtual objects with the real world in a seamless integration. In MR, virtual objects interact with the user's physical environment, providing responses and interactions with real-world objects that are different from AR, including visual, auditory, and haptic (the sense of touch) interactions. For example, haptic technology simulates the feeling of vibration or pressure in dental education. It allows tooth preparation and performing local anesthesia without a live patient, significantly improving the students' learning experience (Gandedkar et al. 2021; Saghiri et al. 2022; Eaton et al. 2008; Ferro et al. 2019; Rhienmora et al. 2010; Dragan et al. 2020; Schleyer et al. 2012).

Extended reality (XR): XR is an umbrella term covering all immersive technologies between the real world and the digital world, including VR, AR, and MR. XR is designed to extend the user's perception of reality by integrating the virtual and real worlds. It offers a novel way of experiencing and interacting with digital content, allowing users to manipulate and explore digital environments in a more natural and intuitive way (Gandedkar et al. 2021; Saghiri et al. 2022; Eaton et al. 2008; Ferro et al. 2019; Rhienmora et al. 2010; Dragan et al. 2020; Schleyer et al. 2012).

Metaverse: The Metaverse is an advanced simulation technology that allows users to interconnect with each other and a digital virtual environment. VR, AR, MR, and XR technologies are collected in one large network within the Metaverse. It imitates the natural world and can be utilized in dental education and telemedicine consultations (Figs. 13.3 and 13.4). In addition to AI, blockchain technology and smart contracts can be integrated to ease the use of the dental field in the Metaverse. The combination of knowledge from various digital technologies transforms dental education in a digital way, creating a synergy between students and instructors to enhance learning (Locurcio 2022; Rhienmora et al. 2010; Dragan et al. 2020).

AI-supported dental education software: AI is a growing field in dentistry, particularly in radiological disease detection and treatment planning. AI algorithms

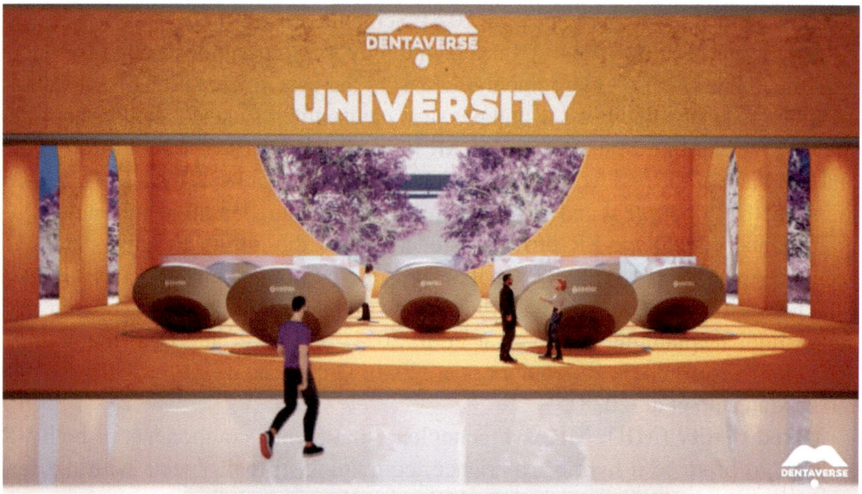

Fig. 13.3 Dentaverse Metaverse University (Courtesy by Dentaverse.eth Ltd. company)

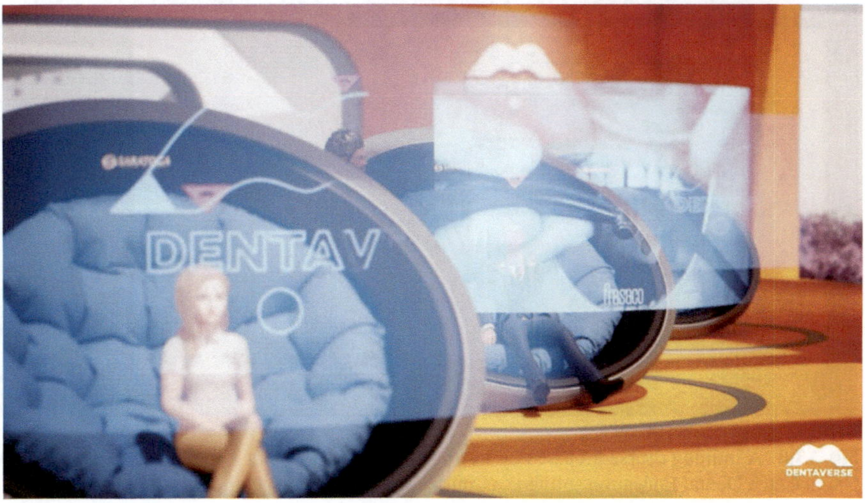

Fig. 13.4 Dentaverse Metaverse University (Courtesy by Dentaverse.eth Ltd. company)

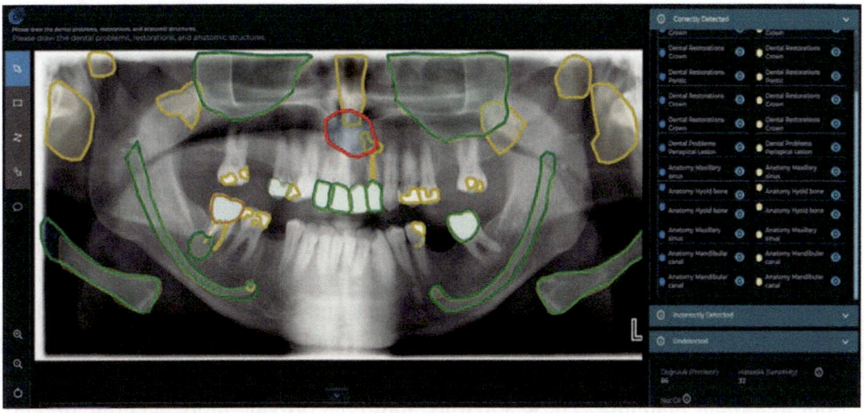

Fig. 13.5 A training course from CranioCatch Dental Education software. (Green: Correct detection performed by the student, Red: Incorrect detection performed by the students, Yellow: Right answers) (Courtesy of CranioCatch company)

can accurately segment anatomical structures and pathological changes, including caries, periapical lesions, impacted teeth, and more (Schleyer et al. 2012; Mangano et al. 2023).

AI-supported dental education software provides an AI-based platform that allows educators to prepare courses or exams. Students can draw anatomical structures and pathologies on images, and the software can assess their accuracy using AI algorithms. Instructors and students can instantly comment on the questions, and the platform can automatically grade the students' work (Figs. 13.5 and 13.6). This

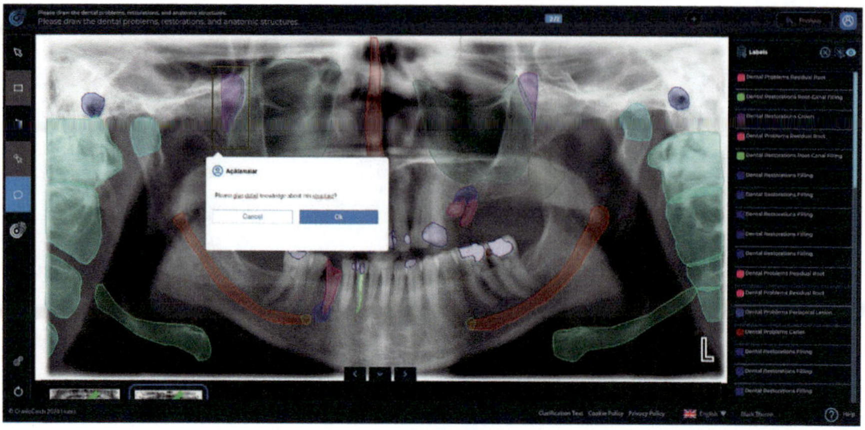

Fig. 13.6 A training course prepared by instructors and opened with instant comment tools from CranioCatch Dental Education software. (Courtesy of CranioCatch company)

creates strong communication between students and instructors, allowing students to improve their knowledge, experience, and self-confidence before clinical practice.

AI-Powered Practical/Clinical Education

AI is used to analyze patient data and create plans and simulations, providing telemonitoring of patients and improving patient care. In this way, AI can play a significant role in clinical dental education.

AI-supported dental diagnosis and treatment planning software: AI can help dentists assess dental radiographs, scans, and images, providing a second pair of eyes for more accurate diagnoses and treatment plans. AI-supported clinical decision support system software can automatically identify dental problems that might be missed due to fatigue, intense workload, or lack of experience, and offer views about treatment planning. These software solutions provide more accurate diagnosis and treatment planning, contributing to enhancing the experience and knowledge of dental students in clinical practice as well (Figs. 13.7 and 13.8).

Artificial Intelligence (AI) and Dental Education Curriculum

Due to the rapid change in technology, the integration of new technologies into dental education is inevitable to train dentists equipped with twenty-first-century skills. AI is one of these technologies changing the most of field affects in the human-being, and it starts to shift paradigms in dentistry. When the scientific literature related to dental education and AI analysis, it was seen that dental students have insufficient education and knowledge about AI. A study conducted by Yüzbaşıoğlu et al. (2021) evaluated the dental students' knowledge and attitudes toward AI and

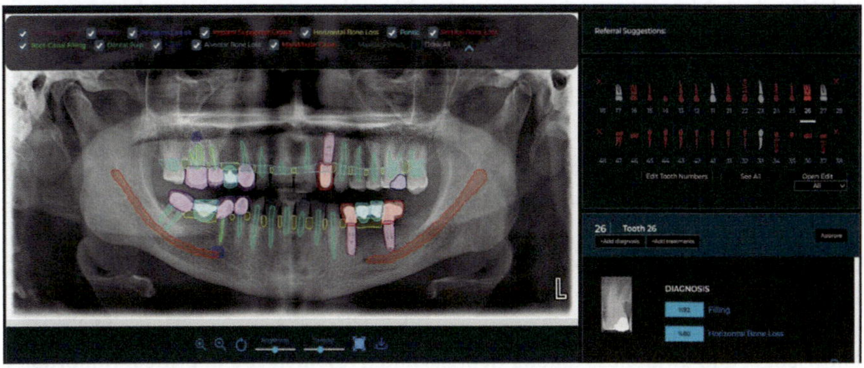

Fig. 13.7 A case evaluated by CranioCatch AI-supported dental diagnosis and treatment planning software (Courtesy by CranioCatch company)

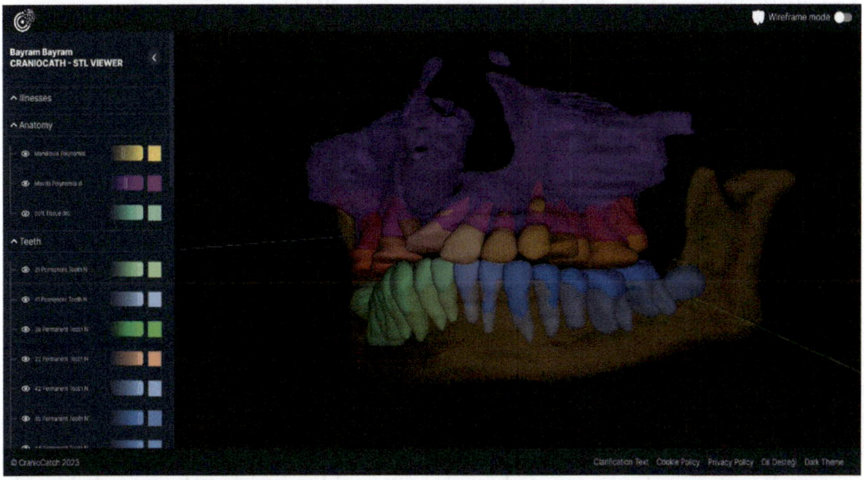

Fig. 13.8 A CBCT case automatically segmented by CranioCatch 3D.stl AI software (Courtesy by CranioCatch company)

possible applications in dentistry. In this study, a total of 1103 students replied to the survey with 21.69% response rate. About 48.40% of these students had basic information about AI technologies, and 10.6% of them had no information about AI. Of them, 85.70% thought that AI would revolutionize dentistry. Besides, 74.60% and 79.80% agreed that topics about AI should be included in undergraduate and postgraduate dental education, respectively. They concluded that although students have a lack of knowledge of AI, they wanted to enhance their knowledge and believed that AI would have a valuable influence on dental practice in the future (Thurzo et al. 2023). Another study conducted by Jeong et al. (2023) investigated Korean dental hygiene, students' perceptions, and attitudes toward AI, and purposed to determine educational needs for strong professional qualification. In this survey 800

(61.1%) dental hygiene students joined. Although participants stated lower confidence in AI's diagnosis (14.8%), they had positive beliefs in its usefulness and the potential for improvement in dentistry. They suggested that the dental hygiene curriculum strongly needs AI-related lectures in schools to prepare for the future (Schwendicke et al. 2023).

Considering the rapid changes in technology, oral and dental healthcare is undergoing substantial transformations. Additionally, teaching and learning methodologies are also dramatically evolving. With all these developments and students' demands, the necessity of changing the core curriculum of dental education and integrating dental AI is becoming evident. It is estimated that the integration of AI in clinical practice will provide numerous benefits in dentistry. Thus, AI literacy, knowledge, and awareness among dentists and hygienists are of critical importance to assess and consciously use AI tools in dental practice. By adapting AI into the core dentistry curriculum in schools, dentists' literacy, knowledge, and awareness about AI can be increased (Gandedkar et al. 2021; Luckin et al. 2016; Ifenthaler and Yau 2019; Thurzo et al. 2023; Schwendicke et al. 2023).

A new article published by Schwendicke et al. (2023) on behalf of IADR e-oral health network and the ITU/WHO focus group AI for health, entitled "Artificial intelligence for oral and dental healthcare: Core education curriculum," identified four main curricular domains:

1. What AI is, and how it works for most medical applications?
2. Where AI occurs in the oral and dental healthcare sector and what applications are or will likely be available?
3. How to evaluate medical and dental AI?
4. What further aspects dentists and oral healthcare providers should know or assess?

In this study, Schwendicke et al. aimed to define a core curriculum about AI for undergraduate and postgraduate dental education programs. AI will significantly impact dentistry, and it is essential for dentists and hygienists to be knowledgeable about AI and its potential effects in dentistry. Therefore, there is a need for revising the core dental curriculum and integrating AI into clinical and academic settings, which should be considered by dental schools and institutions.

Challenges, Opportunities, and Future Directions of AI and Related Technologies in Dental Education

Informatics technologies such as AI, VR, AR, MR, XR, Metaverse, and blockchain are evolving rapidly, making it difficult to keep up. New products equipped with these technologies are being launched for use by dental professionals and organizations on a daily basis. However, while technology progresses swiftly, the knowledge and awareness of dental professionals about these technologies do not progress at the same pace. This discrepancy arises from the difficulty of integrating these technologies into educational and clinical workflows due to their higher costs. Nevertheless, it is expected that these barriers will be resolved over time as these technologies become more affordable and accessible.

To bridge the gap, curriculum changes and the introduction of these technologies in scientific congresses, symposiums, lectures, etc., will aid in familiarizing dental professionals with these technological advancements. Dentistry is shifting toward an evidence-based and data-driven approach in diagnosis and treatment planning, which further promotes the use of digital technologies in dental education.

AI-based diagnostic tools, capable of interpreting radiographs, including 2D and 3D images, will be utilized in dental training. The combination of AI-supported tools and simulation technologies and activities will enhance learning, understanding, and self-confidence among dental students. Consequently, dentists trained with twenty-first-century skills, utilizing AI and other advanced technologies, are likely to replace traditional dentists in the near future.

References

Coşkun S, Güngör M. A comparative study of use of artificial intelligence in oral radiology education. Eur Ann Dent Sci. 2023;50(1):41–6.

Dragan IF, Walji M, Vervoorn M, Quinn B, Johnson L, Davis J, Garcia LT, Valachovic RW. ADEA-ADEE shaping the future of dental education III: the impact of scientific technologies and discoveries on oral health globally. J Dent Educ. 2020;84(1):111–6.

Duman S, Çelik Özen D, Duman ŞB. Metaverse in paediatric dentistry. Eur Arch Paediatr Dent. 2022;23(4):655–6.

Eaton KA, Reynolds PA, Grayden SK, Wilson NH. A vision of dental education in the third millennium. Br Dent J. 2008;205(5):261–71.

Ferro AS, Nicholson K, Koka S. Innovative trends in implant dentistry training and education: a narrative review. J Clin Med. 2019;8(10):1618.

Gandedkar NH, Wong MT, Darendeliler MA. Role of virtual reality (VR), augmented reality (AR) and artificial intelligence (AI) in tertiary education and research of orthodontics: an insight. Semin Orthod. 2021;27(2):69–77.

González-Calatayud V, Prendes-Espinosa P, Roig-Vila R. Artificial intelligence for student assessment: a systematic review. Appl Sci. 2021;11(12):5467.

Heo MS, Kim JE, Hwang JJ, Han SS, Kim JS, Yi WJ, Park IW. Artificial intelligence in oral and maxillofacial radiology: what is currently possible? Dentomaxillofac Radiol. 2021;50(3):20200375.

Ifenthaler D, Yau JY-K. Higher education stakeholders' views on learning analytics policy recommendations for supporting study success. Int J Learn Anal Artific Intell Educ. 2019;1:28–42.

Islam NM, Laughter L, Sadid-Zadeh R, Smith C, Dolan TA, Crain G, Squarize CH. Adopting artificial intelligence in dental education: a model for academic leadership and innovation. J Dent Educ. 2022;86(11):1545–51.

Jeong H, Han SS, Kim KE, Park IS, Choi Y, Jeon KJ. Korean dental hygiene students' perceptions and attitudes toward artificial intelligence: an online survey. J Dent Educ. 2023;87(6):804–12.

Khanna SS, Dhaimade PA. Artificial intelligence: transforming dentistry today. Indian J Basic Appl Med Res. 2017;6(3):161–7.

Locurcio LL. Dental education in the metaverse. Br Dent J. 2022;232(4):191.

Luckin R, Holmes W, Griffiths M, Forcier LB. Intelligence unleashed: an argument for AI in education. London: Pearson Education; 2016.

Mangano FG, Admakin O, Lerner H, Mangano C. Artificial intelligence and augmented reality for guided implant surgery planning: a proof of concept. J Dent. 2023;133:104485.

Pedró F, Subosa M, Rivas A, Valverde P. Artificial intelligence in education: challenges and opportunities for sustainable development, UNESCO working papers on education policy. 2019.

Rhienmora P, Haddawy P, Khanal P, Suebnukarn S, Dailey MN. A virtual reality simulator for teaching and evaluating dental procedures. Methods Inf Med. 2010;49(4):396–405.

Saghiri MA, Vakhnovetsky J, Nadershahi N. Scoping review of artificial intelligence and immersive digital tools in dental education. J Dent Educ. 2022;86(6):736–50.

Schleyer TK, Thyvalikakath TP, Spallek H, Dziabiak MP, Johnson LA. From information technology to informatics: the information revolution in dental education. J Dent Educ. 2012;76(1):142–53.

Schwendicke F, Samek W, Krois J. Artificial intelligence in dentistry: chances and challenges. J Dent Res. 2020;99(7):769–74.

Schwendicke F, Chaurasia A, Wiegand T, Uribe SE, Fontana M, Akota I, Tryfonos O, Krois J, IADR e-oral health network and the ITU/WHO focus group AI for health. Artificial intelligence for oral and dental healthcare: core education curriculum. J Dent. 2023;128:104363.

Sharma D, Malik G, Koshy G, Sharma V. Artificial intelligence: need to reboot dental education. Univ J Dent Sci. 2021;7(2):138–42.

Tadinada A, Gul G, Godwin L, Al Sakka Y, Crain G, Stanford CM, Johnson J. Utilizing an organizational development framework as a road map for creating a technology-driven agile curriculum in predoctoral dental education. J Dent Educ. 2023;87(3):394–400.

Thurzo A, Strunga M, Urban R, Surovková J, Afrashtehfar KI. Impact of artificial intelligence on dental education: a review and guide for curriculum update. Educ Sci. 2023;13(2):150.

UNESCO. Beijing consensus on artificial intelligence and education, international conference on artificial intelligence and education, planning education in the AI era: lead the leap. Beijing; 2019.

Yüzbaşıoğlu E. Attitudes and perceptions of dental students towards artificial intelligence. J Dent Educ. 2021;85(1):60–8.

Zheng L, He Z, Wei D, Keloth V, Fan JW, Lindemann L, Zhu X, Cimino JJ, Perl Y. A review of auditing techniques for the unified medical language system. J Am Med Inform Assoc. 2020;27(10):1625–38.

Advantages, Disadvantages, and Limitations of AI in Dental Health

14

Rohan Jagtap, Sevda Kurt Bayrakdar, and Kaan Orhan

Introduction

Artificial intelligence (AI) is a field of computer science that focuses on imitating human intelligence (Krittanawong et al. 2017; Khanam et al. 2019). This technology can think, learn, evaluate complex and multiple questions, and find solutions to them (Holzinger et al. 2019; Miller and Brown 2018). It provides analysis capabilities and a learning process by processing large datasets (Wang et al. 2019). Currently, many AI applications such as Alexa and Siri are actively used to make daily life easier (Koch 2018). In addition, AI is a promising candidate to pioneer radical changes in various fields such as health, engineering, and science (Holzinger et al. 2019; Jordan and Mitchell 2015).

A rapid digitalization process has begun in all sub-branches of medicine with the emergence of AI-supported systems, making it a hot topic in the medical field (Wilhelm et al. 2020). AI is believed to have an innovative and revolutionary capacity to bring about a "paradigm shift" in healthcare. In other words, it is thought that this technology can have an effect similar to the significant changes in daily life

R. Jagtap (✉)
Division of Oral and Maxillofacial Radiology, Department of Care Planning and Restorative Sciences, University of Mississippi Medical Center, Jackson, MS, USA

Department of Radiology, School of Medicine, University of Mississippi Medical Center, Jackson, MS, USA

S. K. Bayrakdar
Division of Oral and Maxillofacial Radiology, Department of Care Planning and Restorative Sciences, University of Mississippi Medical Center, Jackson, MS, USA

Department of Periodontology, School of Dentistry Eskisehir Osmangazi University, ESOGÜ Meşelik Yerleşkesi, Eskisehir, Turkey

K. Orhan
Faculty of Dentistry, Department of Dentomaxillofacial Radiology, Ankara University, Ankara, Turkey

K. Orhan, R. Jagtap (eds.), *Artificial Intelligence in Dentistry*,
https://doi.org/10.1007/978-3-031-43827-1_14

caused by the invention of smartphones or motor vehicles in the field of health (Koschmann 1996; Gore 2020).

AI can be utilized in various specialized tasks in dentistry, including diagnosis, treatment planning, robotic treatment, patient information recording systems, teledentistry, and dentistry education (Joda and Zitzmann 2022; Katne et al. 2019). Overall, AI and augmented intelligence are preferred in the dental field to enable more accurate, faster, and more efficient work, as well as to simplify and enhance all dental-related processes (Roy et al. 2021; ADA 2022). However, along with their rapid development, these systems have raised ethical concerns, risks, and legal problems that are often associated with technological advancements (D'Antonoli 2020; Keskinbora 2019; Guan 2019). This book chapter aims to systematically present the advantages and disadvantages of these systems in the dental field. Thus, it will enable dentists, academicians, and technology developers to better understand these technologies, guide their development within the framework of general ethical and social expectations, and engage in more comprehensive integrated planning while considering potential risks.

Advantages of AI in Dental Health

All technological advances arise from the search for solutions to needs or problems and offer advantages such as improving existing functionality, accessibility, accuracy, or working speed (Rip and Kemp 1998). AI is an innovative technology in dentistry and undoubtedly offers numerous advantages and benefits in the field, both directly and indirectly (Ossowska et al. 2022; Kurup et al. 2020; Rizk 2023; Tandon and Rajawat 2020). The following sections aim to discuss these advantages with relevant examples.

Automatic operation: AI technologies enable the automation of various processes in business operations, reducing the reliance on human operators (Abdalla-Aslan et al. 2020; Kalappanavar et al. 2018; Grischke et al. 2020; Rong et al. 2020; Verghese et al. 2018). In the field of health and dentistry, AI is used to create automatic diagnosis/treatment planning systems, appointment reminder systems, patient satisfaction evaluation systems, and treatment billing systems (AlMuhaideb et al. 2019; Miller 2012; Wang 2022; Alugubelli 2016). For instance, Lahoud et al. (2021) reported that AI-supported systems can accurately perform tooth segmentation automatically and at a speed 6–12 times faster than manual methods. Moreover, these systems can be utilized to provide automated pre-reminders to healthcare providers regarding conditions such as systemic diseases and allergies, which have been previously recorded in the patient registration system (Bhat et al. 2020). This advantage can also be extended to dentistry education. For example, AI can automatically score multiple-choice or short-answer questions and compare students' responses in dental education (Yang et al. 2021).

Providing uninterrupted service: AI-supported machines and computer systems have the potential to enhance accessibility and continuity in the dental field (Shuborna et al. 2021). Unlike humans, machines and computer systems do not require sleep or breaks, making them well suited for tasks that demand uninterrupted operation in dentistry (Bhbosale et al. 2020). AI-based personal assistant support can be utilized at various stages, such as patient appointment requests through phone or email, enabling patients to schedule appointments at any time of the day (Srinivasan and Madheswari 2018). Additionally, patients can engage with chatbots to receive advice for basic situations (FDI n.d.). In emergencies and other critical situations, AI-based integrated systems facilitate easier access to patients' medical records, medical history, or discharge summaries at any time of the day (Mazzanti et al. 2018).

Increasing communication: AI technology facilitates diagnosis and treatment planning by improving communication between healthcare professionals through the development of intelligent patient information and consultation systems in the medical and dental fields (Bindushree et al. 2020; Amisha et al. 2019; Mao and Zhang 2021). AI systems offer advantages in communication with individuals with disabilities through features such as speech recognition, natural language processing, and computer vision (Gevarter 1984; Wah et al. 1993). These applications can enhance the dental health service quality for disabled individuals. Additionally, AI systems have the potential to address communication issues arising from language incompatibility. Interlingual translation capabilities can be easily incorporated into these systems, suggesting that they may serve as a solution for language barriers between patients and healthcare providers in the future (Basu et al. 2020).

Increasing employee comfort: AI technology has the potential to eliminate repetitive, tedious, and monotonous tasks, allowing human efforts to be utilized more effectively (Ivanov and Webster 2017; Monterubbianesi et al. 2022). As a result, it enhances the comfort and productivity of dentists, dental assistants, academics, and other dental professionals (Alauddin et al. 2021; Banerjee 2021).

Increasing reliability, efficiency, accuracy, and precision: It enables more reliable, effective, and accurate decision-making (Ossowska et al. 2022; Bindushree et al. 2020). It minimizes errors caused by human factors such as fatigue, intensity, distraction, and lack of experience (Park et al. 2020; Schwalbe and Wahl 2020; Kurt Bayrakdar et al. 2021). Additionally, it helps find more effective solutions to complex problems in dental diagnosis (Kalappanavar et al. 2018). Numerous AI-based studies in the field of dentistry demonstrate that these systems diagnose with higher accuracy compared to decision-makers such as assistant physicians and dentistry students (Ossowska et al. 2022; Khanagar et al. 2021a). For instance, Mertens et al. (2021) reported that these systems improve dentists' diagnostic accuracy and provide a more precise approach when deciding on invasive treatment for enamel-level lesions. Similarly, in their study, Murata et al. (2019) demonstrated that AI exhibits greater success in detecting maxillary sinus from panoramic radiographs compared to dental residents. When the literature is examined, many studies support these examples, further reinforcing the benefits of AI in dental diagnosis.

Standardization: AI algorithms developed with appropriate protocols, methods, and guidelines offer standardized results and solutions (Tandon and Rajawat 2020; Chen et al. 2020; Bansod and Pisulkar 2021). They provide access to more calibrated information in the acquisition of patient records. For instance, Carrillo-Perez et al. (2022) reported that AI models enabling full characterization of tooth color can be developed for use in aesthetic dentistry applications, leading to more successful tooth restorations with standardized color. These systems also enhance the comparability and interpretability of patient records taken at different time intervals. By enabling the utilization of data in academic studies within an objective and consistent framework (Chen et al. 2020), AI facilitates the evaluation of large datasets in a fast and standardized manner, enabling comprehensive epidemiological studies (Kalappanavar et al. 2018; Listl and Chiavegatto Filho 2021).

Monitoring and regular data recording: AI systems offer the advantage of processing, interpreting, monitoring, and archiving raw data to provide more comprehensive information (Tandon and Rajawat 2020; Carrillo-Perez et al. 2022). For instance, AI algorithms can analyze various diagnostic images used in dental practice, including oral pathology preparations, radiology images, and intraoral photographs (Schwalbe and Wahl 2020; Askar et al. 2021; Duong et al. 2021). These systems enable the automatic detection of anatomical variations, dental diseases, and pathologies within these images (Patil et al. 2022; Zhang et al. 2022). The monitored and regularly recorded data of this nature can be easily utilized in various areas such as clinical operations, academic processes, and educational stages within dentistry.

Time planning and time-saving: AI allows for increased productivity within a shorter timeframe (Ossowska et al. 2022; Tandon and Rajawat 2020; Khanna 2010). It provides additional time-savings by assisting dentists in making faster decisions, developing more ergonomic work plans, and addressing tasks that would otherwise require significant human effort (Khanna 2010). This technology enables professionals to focus on essential and critical processes. Furthermore, by facilitating early diagnosis, AI supports the prompt resolution of certain dental conditions that may require complex and long-term treatment (Kalappanavar et al. 2018). Additionally, it is widely recognized that AI systems are significantly faster than humans when it comes to consolidating diagnostic data such as dental/medical history, intraoral photographs, and radiographic images (Khanna and Dhaimade 2017).

Analytical forecasting: AI systems possess comprehensive forecasting capabilities (Awotunde et al. 2021; Agrawal and Nikhade 2022). They can easily analyze situations that may be challenging for physicians to predict, such as identifying the most suitable treatment method and determining the appropriate follow-up interval (AlMuhaideb et al. 2019). Moreover, these systems can provide prognostic estimations by considering various factors such as genetic characteristics, individual habits, environmental effects, age, and gender, based on historical data (Khanna 2010; Khanagar et al. 2021b). Certain studies in the literature demonstrate that AI systems can accurately estimate patient gender and age solely by interpreting radiographs (Balan et al. 2022; Batool and Gilanie 2023). This finding supports their reliable use in fields like forensic dentistry, ultimately enabling personalized treatment plans (Chen et al. 2020). This advantage enhances patient motivation and facilitates the implementation of the most suitable treatment plan (Chen et al. 2020). Additionally, AI systems can be easily utilized for simple analytical computational measurements, such as determining the caries risk group for each patient and assessing the severity of periodontal disease, thereby improving routine diagnostic decision-making (Alotaibi et al. 2022; Schwendicke et al. 2022; Fontana et al. 2020).

A more economical business plan: While the software development and updating phases can be costly (Tandon and Rajawat 2020; Bhat et al. 2020), AI systems offer a more cost-effective long-term working plan (Abubaker Bagabir et al. 2022; Taheri et al. 2022; Peng et al. 2020). They enable certain tasks to be performed in less time and with fewer employees, resulting in reduced expenses (Morrison et al. 2022). Furthermore, with their advantages such as early diagnosis, accurate diagnosis, and prognostic estimation, AI systems facilitate informed decision-making regarding the most suitable treatment, thus preventing unnecessary waste of time and money. A study conducted on telemedicine screenings in the healthcare field in China reported that AI-based result interpretation and grading can be achieved at a significantly lower cost compared to manual techniques (Lin et al. 2023). Based on this information, it can be inferred that these systems can be preferred in dental research as well, as they are likely to be more cost-effective.

Risk reduction/elimination: AI systems offer the advantage of predictive capability, enabling the identification and mitigation of certain risks (Kurup et al. 2020; Grischke et al. 2020). For instance, they reduce or eliminate the risk of misdiagnosis when making treatment decisions (Tandon and Rajawat 2020; FDI n.d.; Chang et al. 2022). Moreover, AI systems provide an additional benefit in various calculations, including financial calculations, as they operate with minimal errors. This makes them suitable for tasks such as patient billing and financial calculations in clinical and hospital management, delivering more reliable and accurate results compared to manual methods (Wagner 2019; Bhatia et al. 2020).

The advantages of AI algorithms extend beyond clinical functionality. They also elevate dental administrative work, technical services, and dental laboratory

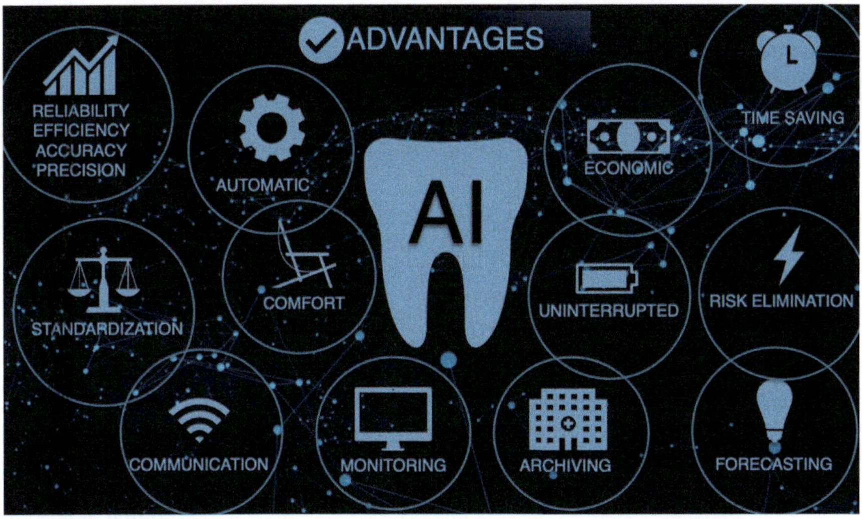

Fig. 14.1 What kind of advantages do AI systems provide in the field of dentistry?

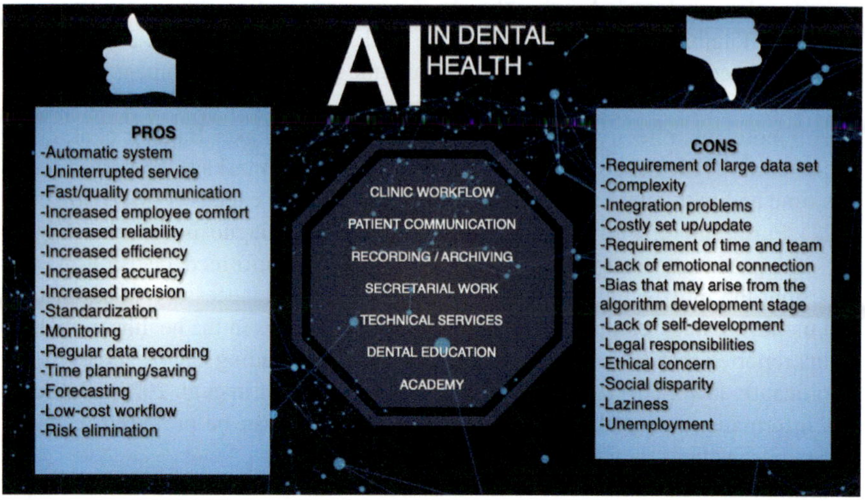

Fig. 14.2 Summary: application of AI systems in dental health and their advantages/disadvantages

processes to higher standards. Additionally, AI enhances the quality of academic studies and improves the efficiency of educational processes (Figs. 14.1 and 14.2). Undoubtedly, AI brings forth the advantages of emerging applications like teledentistry and robotic technologies, which have gained popularity through its integration. As the routine use of AI systems in dentistry continues to expand, the benefits they provide will become increasingly apparent, and innovations related to these technologies will offer even more comprehensive advantages.

Disadvantages and Limitations of AI in Dental Health

In addition to the advantages and benefits of using AI in the dental and medical fields, there are also certain disadvantages and limitations (Fig. 14.2). These can be summarized as follows:

Need for big data access: AI systems rely on accessing and processing vast amounts of data (Miller and Brown 2018; Bindushree et al. 2020). To make accurate decisions, AI systems need to be developed considering all possibilities. For instance, an AI system used as a decision support system in diagnosis should be capable of detecting specialized and rare cases. This requires access to comprehensive information and data archives for each scenario. Without sufficient data access, the system may produce incorrect results in unexpected cases or situations it does not recognize (Kurup et al. 2020). The need for big data presents challenges such as data quality issues, standardization deficiencies, and the need to improve electronic health records (Lee and Yoon 2017).

System complexity and integration issues: Shifting from manual to digitalized AI-powered systems can be complex initially (Tandon and Rajawat 2020; Bindushree et al. 2020). Users of the technology require specific knowledge and skills, potentially necessitating additional training (Grischke et al. 2020; Santos et al. 2021). Integration problems may arise when incorporating AI systems with existing dental devices and software, requiring the development of a modern technical infrastructure for seamless integration.

High cost and workload in algorithm development and updates: Developing and implementing AI algorithms can be costly (Kurup et al. 2020; Tandon and Rajawat 2020; Grischke et al. 2020; Bhat et al. 2020). The process requires trained experts in technical infrastructure creation, hardware and software, data collection, and data processing, thereby increasing costs (Bynagari 2015; Lemley et al. 2017). AI systems are complex machines with high energy consumption, necessitating compliance with the latest requirements and continuous updates, leading to additional financial expenses (Ben Ayed and Hanana 2021).

Need for a team and time: Algorithms yield successful results within their specific domains. Achieving near-perfect results requires extensive datasets, a large team working in harmony, and time for algorithm development. It should be noted that achieving full success may take many years (Kurup et al. 2020).

Lack of emotional communication: Effective communication and behavior management skills, along with knowledge of patient psychology, are crucial for healthcare professionals, including dental practitioners (Moore 2022; Yamalik 2005; Skaret and Soevdsnes 2005; Armfield and Heaton 2013). AI systems still lack the ability to empathize, convey emotions, and engage in fluent communication to address issues like patient anxiety and fear (Bhat et al. 2020). Similarly, in dental education, these systems cannot replace trainers with excellent communication skills.

Subjective results and lack of causality: Biased or incomplete preparation of datasets used in AI algorithms can result in subjective or biased outcomes (Tandon and Rajawat 2020; Bhat et al. 2020; FDI n.d.; Sunarti et al. 2021). Users should be aware of these potential disadvantages.

Inability to fully emulate the human brain and lack of self-development: AI systems, despite attempting to imitate the human brain, are incapable of self-development. They lack common sense, emotional skills, and empathy, limiting their ability to handle complex real-life information (Bhat et al. 2020; Bindushree et al. 2020).

Legal responsibility and ethical concerns: The use of AI systems raises concerns regarding personal data protection, patient privacy, and data privacy, leading to legal responsibility and ethical considerations (Eschert et al. 2022; Mintz and Brodie 2019; Hamet and Tremblay 2017). Inaccurate or biased results, bias creation, or overriding the physician's judgment can arise if AI diagnostic tools are not developed responsibly. Determining primary responsibility in misleading situations remains a topic of debate, even with the physician as the ultimate decision-maker (Elmore and Lee 2022).

Social disparity: Access to advanced technologies may be limited for certain socioeconomic groups, resulting in social inequality and differences in access to treatment and employee standards (Korda et al. 2011; Currie and Rohren 2022).

Laziness: There is a concern that intelligent systems and AI technologies may make individuals intellectually lazy, as they become increasingly reliant on technology in various domains (Bhat et al. 2020; Aiken and Epstein 2000). This may apply to dentists, dental students, and personnel in the field, as continuous technology use fosters dependence (Khanzode and Sarode 2020).

Unemployment: Since AI automates many tasks, there are concerns about potential job displacement and an increase in unemployment rates in the future (Wah et al. 1993; Mutascu and Hegerty 2023; Doğaner 2021; Priyadarshini and Sahoo 2020). This trend may also affect certain job roles in dentistry, resulting in a reduced need for employees or the elimination of certain positions. For instance, various stages of procedures in dental laboratories can be facilitated by AI and digitalized systems, reducing the reliance on manual labor. Additionally, tasks like patient appointment tracking can be efficiently managed using smart computer systems alone.

Efforts are underway to address these disadvantages and limitations, aiming to develop more advanced technologies and overcome these challenges. Minimizing limitations will contribute to the rapid development of AI in dentistry. As the use of AI becomes more prevalent, its benefits and advantages will become better understood by dental professionals, patients, and individuals within the field of influence.

References

Abdalla-Aslan R, Yeshua T, Kabla D, Leichter I, Nadler C. An artificial intelligence system using machine-learning for automatic detection and classification of dental restorations in panoramic radiography. Oral Surg Oral Med Oral Pathol Oral Radiol. 2020;130(5):593–602.

Abubaker Bagabir S, Ibrahim NK, Abubaker Bagabir H, Hashem AR. Covid-19 and Artificial intelligence: genome sequencing, drug development and vaccine discovery. J Infect Public Health. 2022;15(2):289–96.

ADA. SCDI white paper. 2022 (White paper no. 1106 Approved by SCDI).

Agrawal P, Nikhade P. Artificial intelligence in dentistry: past, present, and future. Cureus. 2022;14(7):e27405.

Aiken RM, Epstein RG. Ethical guidelines for AI in education: starting a conversation. Int J Artif Intell Educ. 2000;11(2):163–76.

Alauddin MS, Baharuddin AS, Mohd Ghazali MI. The modern and digital transformation of oral health care: a mini review. Healthcare (Basel). 2021;9(2):118.

AlMuhaideb S, Alswailem O, Alsubaie N, Ferwana I, Alnajem A. Prediction of hospital no-show appointments through artificial intelligence algorithms. Ann Saudi Med. 2019;39(6):373–81.

Alotaibi G, Awawdeh M, Farook FF, Aljohani M, Aldhafiri RM, Aldhoayan M. Artificial intelligence (AI) diagnostic tools: utilizing a convolutional neural network (CNN) to assess periodontal bone level radiographically—a retrospective study. BMC Oral Health. 2022;22(1):399.

Alugubelli R. Exploratory study of artificial intelligence in healthcare. Int J Innov Eng Res Technol. 2016;3(1):1–10.

Amisha MP, Pathania M, Rathaur VK. Overview of artificial intelligence in medicine. J Family Med Prim Care. 2019;8(7):2328–31.

Armfield JM, Heaton LJ. Management of fear and anxiety in the dental clinic: a review. Aust Dent J. 2013;58(4):390–407; quiz 531.

Askar H, Krois J, Rohrer C, Mertens S, Elhennawy K, Ottolenghi L, et al. Detecting white spot lesions on dental photography using deep learning: a pilot study. J Dent. 2021;107:103615.

Awotunde JB, Folorunso SO, Jimoh RG, Adeniyi EA, Abiodun KM, Ajamu GJ. Application of artificial intelligence for COVID-19 epidemic: an exploratory study, opportunities, challenges, and future prospects. In: Artificial intelligence for COVID-19. 2021. pp. 47–61.

Balan H, Alrasheedi AF, Askar S, Abouhawwash M. An intelligent human age and gender forecasting framework using deep learning algorithms. Appl Artif Intell. 2022;36(1):2073724.

Banerjee M. Artificial intelligence in dentistry: a ray of hope. Artif Intell. 2021;13(2):58.

Bansod AV, Pisulkar SK. Artificial intelligence & its contemporary applications in dentistry. Turk J Comput Math Educ. 2021;12(6):4192–6.

Basu K, Sinha R, Ong A, Basu T. Artificial intelligence: how is it changing medical sciences and its future? Indian J Dermatol. 2020;65(5):365.

Batool SN, Gilanie G. CVIP-net: a convolutional neural network-based model for forensic radiology image classification. Comput Mater Con. 2023;74(1):1319–32.

Ben Ayed R, Hanana M. Artificial intelligence to improve the food and agriculture sector. J Food Qual. 2021;2021:1–7.

Bhat PR, Trasad VA, Naik B. Artificial intelligence—an emerging intelligence. Guident. 2020;13(12):34–6.

Bhatia N, Trivedi H, Safdar N, Heilbrun ME. Artificial intelligence in quality improvement: reviewing uses of artificial intelligence in noninterpretative processes from clinical decision support to education and feedback. J Am Coll Radiol. 2020;17(11):1382–7.

Bhbosale S, Pujari V, Multani Z. Advantages and disadvantages of artificial intelligence. Aayushi Int Interdiscip Res J. 2020;77:227–30.

Bindushree V, Sameen R, Vasudevan V, Shrihari T, Devaraju D, Mathew NS. Artificial intelligence: in modern dentistry. J Dent Res Rev. 2020;7(1):27.

Bynagari NB. Machine learning and artificial intelligence in online fake transaction alerting. Eng Int. 2015;3(2):115–26.

Carrillo-Perez F, Pecho OE, Morales JC, Paravina RD, Della Bona A, Ghinea R, et al. Applications of artificial intelligence in dentistry: a comprehensive review. J Esthet Restor Dent. 2022;34(1):259–80.

Chang L, Wu J, Moustafa N, Bashir AK, Yu K. AI-driven synthetic biology for non-small cell lung cancer drug effectiveness-cost analysis in intelligent assisted medical systems. IEEE J Biomed Health Inform. 2022;26(10):5055–66.

Chen YW, Stanley K, Att W. Artificial intelligence in dentistry: current applications and future perspectives. Quintessence Int. 2020;51(3):248–57.

Currie G, Rohren E. Social asymmetry, artificial intelligence and the medical imaging landscape. Semin Nucl Med. 2022;52(4):498–503.

D'Antonoli TA. Ethical considerations for artificial intelligence: an overview of the current radiology landscape. Diagn Interv Radiol. 2020;26(5):504–11.

Doğaner A. The approaches and expectations of the health sciences students towards artificial intelligence. Karya J Health Sci. 2021;2(1):5–11.

Duong DL, Kabir MH, Kuo RF. Automated caries detection with smartphone color photography using machine learning. Health Informatics J. 2021;27(2):14604582211007530.

Elmore JG, Lee CI. Artificial intelligence in medical imaging-learning from past mistakes in mammography. JAMA Health Forum. 2022;3(2):e215207.

Eschert T, Schwendicke F, Krois J, Bohner L, Vinayahalingam S, Hanisch M. A survey on the use of artificial intelligence by clinicians in dentistry and oral and maxillofacial surgery. Medicina (Kaunas). 2022;58(8):1059.

FDI. White paper, artificial intelligence for dentistry. FDI Artificial Intelligence Working Group. n.d.

Fontana M, Carrasco-Labra A, Spallek H, Eckert G, Katz B. Improving caries risk prediction modeling: a call for action. J Dent Res. 2020;99(11):1215–20.

Gevarter WB. Artificial intelligence, expert systems, computer vision, and natural language processing. 1984.

Gore JC. Artificial intelligence in medical imaging. Elsevier; 2020. p. A1–A4.

Grischke J, Johannsmeier L, Eich L, Griga L, Haddadin S. Dentronics: towards robotics and artificial intelligence in dentistry. Dent Mater. 2020;36(6):765–78.

Guan J. Artificial intelligence in healthcare and medicine: promises, ethical challenges and governance. Chin Med Sci J. 2019;34(2):76–83.

Hamet P, Tremblay J. Artificial intelligence in medicine. Metabolism. 2017;69s:S36–40.

Holzinger A, Langs G, Denk H, Zatloukal K, Müller H. Causability and explainability of artificial intelligence in medicine. Wiley Interdiscip Rev Data Min Knowl Discov. 2019;9(4):e1312.

Ivanov SH, Webster C. Adoption of robots, artificial intelligence and service automation by travel, tourism and hospitality companies—a cost-benefit analysis. 2017.

Joda T, Zitzmann NU. Personalized workflows in reconstructive dentistry-current possibilities and future opportunities. Clin Oral Investig. 2022;26(6):4283–90.

Jordan MI, Mitchell TM. Machine learning: trends, perspectives, and prospects. Science. 2015;349(6245):255–60.

Kalappanavar A, Sneha S, Annigeri RG. Artificial intelligence: a dentist's perspective. J Med Radiol Pathol Surg. 2018;5(2):2–4.

Katne T, Kanaparthi A, Gotoor S, Muppirala S, Devaraju R, Gantala R. Artificial intelligence: demystifying dentistry—the future and beyond. Int J Contemp Med Surg Radiol. 2019;4(4):D6–9.

Keskinbora KH. Medical ethics considerations on artificial intelligence. J Clin Neurosci. 2019;64:277–82.

Khanagar SB, Al-Ehaideb A, Maganur PC, Vishwanathaiah S, Patil S, Baeshen HA, et al. Developments, application, and performance of artificial intelligence in dentistry—a systematic review. J Dent Sci. 2021a;16(1):508–22.

Khanagar SB, Naik S, Al Kheraif AA, Vishwanathaiah S, Maganur PC, Alhazmi Y, et al. Application and performance of artificial intelligence technology in oral cancer diagnosis and prediction of prognosis: a systematic review. Diagnostics (Basel). 2021b;11(6):1004.

Khanam S, Tanweer S, Khalid S, Rosaci D. Artificial intelligence surpassing human intelligence: factual or hoax. Comput J. 2019;64(12):1832–9.

Khanna S. Artificial intelligence: contemporary applications and future compass. Int Dent J. 2010;60(4):269–72.

Khanna SS, Dhaimade PA. Artificial intelligence: transforming dentistry today. Indian J Basic Appl Med Res. 2017;6(3):161–7.

Khanzode KCA, Sarode RD. Advantages and disadvantages of artificial intelligence and machine learning: a literature review. Int J Lib Inf Sci. 2020;9(1):3.

Koch M. Artificial intelligence is becoming natural. Cell. 2018;173(3):531–3.

Korda RJ, Clements MS, Dixon J. Socioeconomic inequalities in the diffusion of health technology: uptake of coronary procedures as an example. Soc Sci Med. 2011;72(2):224–9.

Koschmann T. Paradigm shifts and instructional technology: An introduction. In: CSCL: theory and practice of an emerging paradigm, vol 116. 1996. pp. 1–23.

Krittanawong C, Zhang H, Wang Z, Aydar M, Kitai T. Artificial intelligence in precision cardiovascular medicine. J Am Coll Cardiol. 2017;69(21):2657–64.

Kurt Bayrakdar S, Orhan K, Bayrakdar IS, Bilgir E, Ezhov M, Gusarev M, et al. A deep learning approach for dental implant planning in cone-beam computed tomography images. BMC Med Imaging. 2021;21(1):86.

Kurup RJ, Sodhi A, Sangeetha R. Dentistry and artificial intelligence. Acta Sci Dent Sci. 2020;4(10):26–32.

Lahoud P, EzEldeen M, Beznik T, Willems H, Leite A, Van Gerven A, et al. Artificial intelligence for fast and accurate 3-dimensional tooth segmentation on cone-beam computed tomography. J Endod. 2021;47(5):827–35.

Lee CH, Yoon HJ. Medical big data: promise and challenges. Kidney Res Clin Pract. 2017;36(1):3–11.

Lemley J, Bazrafkan S, Corcoran P. Deep learning for consumer devices and services: pushing the limits for machine learning, artificial intelligence, and computer vision. IEEE Consum Electron Mag. 2017;6(2):48–56.

Lin S, Ma Y, Xu Y, Lu L, He J, Zhu J, et al. Artificial intelligence in community-based diabetic retinopathy telemedicine screening in urban China: cost-effectiveness and cost-utility analyses with real-world data. JMIR Public Health Surveill. 2023;9:e41624.

Listl S, Chiavegatto Filho AD. Big data and machine learning. In: Oral epidemiology: a textbook on oral health conditions, research topics and methods. 2021. pp. 357–365.

Mao Y, Zhang L. Optimization of the medical service consultation system based on the artificial intelligence of the internet of things. IEEE Access. 2021;9:98261–74.

Mazzanti M, Shirka E, Gjergo H, Hasimi E. Imaging, health record, and artificial intelligence: hype or hope? Curr Cardiol Rep. 2018;20(6):48.

Mertens S, Krois J, Cantu AG, Arsiwala LT, Schwendicke F. Artificial intelligence for caries detection: randomized trial. J Dent. 2021;115:103849.

Miller PL. Selected topics in medical artificial intelligence. Springer Science & Business Media; 2012.

Miller DD, Brown EW. Artificial intelligence in medical practice: the question to the answer? Am J Med. 2018;131(2):129–33.

Mintz Y, Brodie R. Introduction to artificial intelligence in medicine. Minim Invasive Ther Allied Technol. 2019;28(2):73–81.

Monterubbianesi R, Tosco V, Vitiello F, Orilisi G, Fraccastoro F, Putignano A, et al. Augmented, virtual and mixed reality in dentistry: a narrative review on the existing platforms and future challenges. Appl Sci. 2022;12(2):877.

Moore R. Maximizing student clinical communication skills in dental education—a narrative review. Dent J (Basel). 2022;10(4):57.

Morrison SL, Dukhovny D, Chan RVP, Chiang MF, Campbell JP. Cost-effectiveness of artificial intelligence-based retinopathy of prematurity screening. JAMA Ophthalmol. 2022;140(4):401–9.

Murata M, Ariji Y, Ohashi Y, Kawai T, Fukuda M, Funakoshi T, et al. Deep-learning classification using convolutional neural network for evaluation of maxillary sinusitis on panoramic radiography. Oral Radiol. 2019;35(3):301–7.

Mutascu M, Hegerty SW. Predicting the contribution of artificial intelligence to unemployment rates: an artificial neural network approach. J Econ Financ. 2023;47:400.

Ossowska A, Kusiak A, Świetlik D. Artificial intelligence in dentistry—narrative review. Int J Environ Res Public Health. 2022;19(6):3449.

Park CW, Seo SW, Kang N, Ko B, Choi BW, Park CM, et al. Artificial intelligence in health care: current applications and issues. J Korean Med Sci. 2020;35(42):e379.

Patil S, Albogami S, Hosmani J, Mujoo S, Kamil MA, Mansour MA, et al. Artificial intelligence in the diagnosis of oral diseases: applications and pitfalls. Diagnostics (Basel). 2022;12(5):1029.

Peng J, Zeng X, Townsend J, Liu G, Huang Y, Lin S. A machine learning approach to uncovering hidden utilization patterns of early childhood dental care among Medicaid-insured children. Front Public Health. 2020;8:599187.

Priyadarshini SR, Sahoo PK. Artificial intelligence: the future in dentistry. Indian J Forensic Med Toxicol. 2020;14(4):8168–71.

Rip A, Kemp R. Technological change. In: Human choice and climate change, vol 2. 1998. pp. 327–399.

Rizk S. Artificial intelligence in dentistry. Biomed J. 2023;2(2):29–45.

Rong G, Mendez A, Assi EB, Zhao B, Sawan M. Artificial intelligence in healthcare: review and prediction case studies. Engineering. 2020;6(3):291–301.

Roy P, Vivekananda L, Singh GP. Artificial intelligence in dentistry and its future. GSC Adv Res Rev. 2021;7(1):82–6.

Santos JC, Wong JHD, Pallath V, Ng KH. The perceptions of medical physicists towards relevance and impact of artificial intelligence. Phys Eng Sci Med. 2021;44(3):833–41.

Schwalbe N, Wahl B. Artificial intelligence and the future of global health. Lancet. 2020;395(10236):1579–86.

Schwendicke F, Grano C, de Oro J, Garcia Cantu A, Meyer-Lueckel H, Chaurasia A, Krois J. Artificial intelligence for caries detection: value of data and information. J Dent Res. 2022;101(11):1350–6.

Shuborna NS, Islam SS, Jahan SS, Apu EH, Noor OB, Chowdhury MTHCH. Teledentistry: limitation and challenges. Update Dent Coll J. 2021;11(2):1–3.

Skaret E, Soevdsnes EK. Behavioural science in dentistry. The role of the dental hygienist in prevention and treatment of the fearful dental patient. Int J Dent Hyg. 2005;3(1):2–6.

Srinivasan A, Madheswari AN. The role of smart personal assistant for improving personal healthcare. Int J Adv Eng Manag Sci. 2018;4(11):268274.

Sunarti S, Fadzlul Rahman F, Naufal M, Risky M, Febriyanto K, Masnina R. Artificial intelligence in healthcare: opportunities and risk for future. Gac Sanit. 2021;35(Suppl 1):S67–70.

Taheri H, Gonzalez Bocanegra M, Taheri M. Artificial intelligence, machine learning and smart technologies for nondestructive evaluation. Sensors (Basel). 2022;22(11):4055.

Tandon D, Rajawat J. Present and future of artificial intelligence in dentistry. J Oral Biol Craniofac Res. 2020;10(4):391–6.

Verghese A, Shah NH, Harrington RA. What this computer needs is a physician: humanism and artificial intelligence. JAMA. 2018;319(1):19–20.

Wagner JB. Artificial intelligence in medical imaging. Radiol Technol. 2019;90(5):489–501.

Wah BW, Huang TS, Joshi AK, Moldovan D, Aloimonos J, Bajcsy RK, et al. Report on workshop on high performance computing and communications for grand challenge applications: computer vision, speech and natural language processing, and artificial intelligence. IEEE Trans Knowl Data Eng. 1993;5(1):138–54.

Wang Y. Research on the influence of service quality of hotel intelligent system on customer satisfaction based on artificial intelligence evaluation. Math Probl Eng. 2022;2022:1.

Wang R, Pan W, Jin L, Li Y, Geng Y, Gao C, et al. Artificial intelligence in reproductive medicine. Reproduction. 2019;158(4):R139–54.

Wilhelm D, Bouarfa L, Navab N, Meining A, Müller-Stich B, Jarc A, et al. Artificial intelligence in visceral medicine. Visc Med. 2020;36(6):471.

Yamalik N. Dentist-patient relationship and quality care 3. Communication. Int Dent J. 2005;55(4):254–6.

Yang SJ, Ogata H, Matsui T, Chen N-S. Human-centered artificial intelligence in education: seeing the invisible through the visible. Comput Educ Artif Intell. 2021;2:100008.

Zhang X, Liang Y, Li W, Liu C, Gu D, Sun W, et al. Development and evaluation of deep learning for screening dental caries from oral photographs. Oral Dis. 2022;28(1):173–81.

Applications of Machine Learning and Artificial Intelligence in the COVID-19 Pandemic

15

Ingrid Różyło-Kalinowska and Kaan Orhan

Introduction

The COVID-19 pandemic has caused a global health crisis, with millions of cases and hundreds of thousands of deaths worldwide. It has posed significant challenges to healthcare systems all around the world. With the rapid spread of the virus, healthcare systems had to adapt and find new ways to manage the spread of the virus, diagnose and treat infected individuals, as well as develop effective treatments and vaccines (Vamathevan et al. 2020). To address these challenges, machine learning (ML) and artificial intelligence (AI) have been employed to aid in the fight against the virus and played a significant role in these efforts, providing new tools and approaches to address the dangers posed by the pandemic. Machine learning (ML) and artificial intelligence (AI) have been applied in predictive modeling for disease spread and resource allocation, identification of high-risk individuals and populations for targeted testing and interventions, real-time monitoring and tracking of COVID-19 cases, monitoring social media and identifying potential outbreaks, providing chatbots and virtual assistants, image diagnosis, drug discovery and repurposing, as well as telehealth. This chapter aims to summarize various applications of these technologies in response to the pandemic (Fig. 15.1) and provide an overview of the current state of these applications.

I. Różyło-Kalinowska
Department of Dental and Maxillofacial Radiodiagnostics, Medical University of Lublin, Lublin, Poland
e-mail: rozylo.kalinowska@umlub.pl

K. Orhan (✉)
Faculty of Dentistry, Ankara University, Ankara, Turkey
e-mail: kaan.orhan@dentistry.ankara.edu.tr

K. Orhan, R. Jagtap (eds.), *Artificial Intelligence in Dentistry*,
https://doi.org/10.1007/978-3-031-43827-1_15

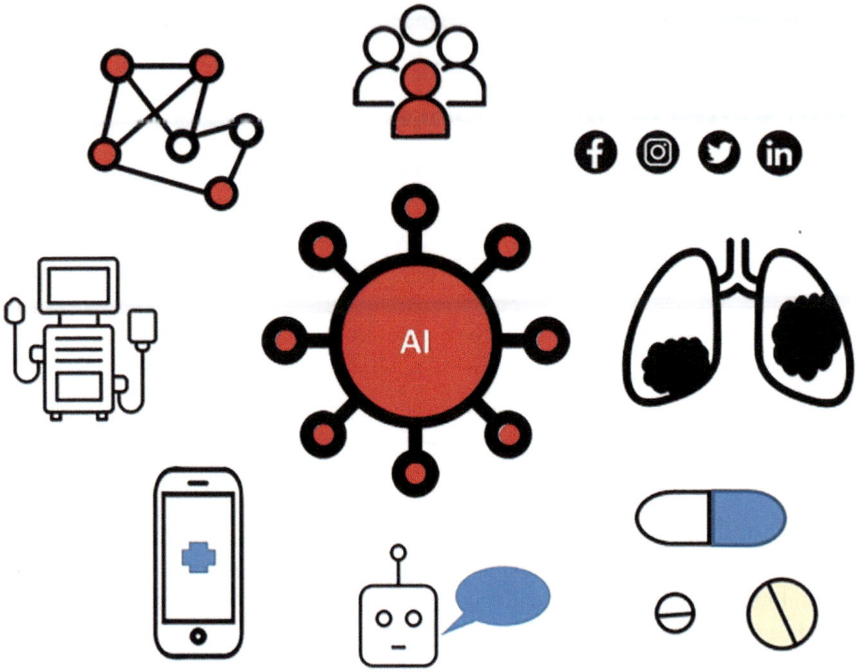

Fig. 15.1 Schematic representation of applications of artificial intelligence (AI) in the COVID-19 pandemic

Application of Artificial Intelligence in COVID-19 Diagnosis and Management

Predictive Modeling for Disease Spread and Resource Allocation

Predictive modeling is a crucial aspect of the response to the COVID-19 pandemic, as it enables healthcare systems to anticipate the spread of the virus and prepare accordingly. Prediction of such factors as epidemic peak, transmission, and developmental trends is fundamental. Implementation of AI-based prediction of the epidemic trend of COVID-19 also leads to the limitation of outbreaks. In general, the faster a country can predict an outbreak and spread, the faster it implements protective measures and targeted interventions, the more lives can be saved (Williams et al. 2021). Accurate prediction of the evolution of cases of infection facilitates the timely implementation of isolation and quarantine procedures as well as allows for early interventions in patients requiring treatment (Bouchareb et al. 2021). Various factors, such as incidence, the number of confirmed cases, deaths and recoveries, the rate of transmission, and the population density of affected areas, have been analyzed by machine learning algorithms in order to create models that predict the spread of the virus. AI-based prediction of the unreported number of infections is important in the assessment of the pandemic's evolution, including daily incidence, infection and death rates, transmission laws, and developmental trends (Wang et al. 2021). Some models also take into account the impact of climate-associated factors in infection rate. Machine learning models have been developed to predict the number of hospital beds and intensive care units needed for the treatment of COVID-19 patients. These models provide valuable information for healthcare systems, allowing them to allocate resources such as hospital beds, ventilators, and other medical equipment, in a timely and efficient manner. By predicting the potential number of cases in a given area, healthcare systems can prepare and allocate necessary resources, reducing costs and increasing the effectiveness of therapies and interventions.

Several AI models have been implemented for the prediction of COVID-19 spread, and they include adaptive neuro-fuzzy interference system (ANFIS), autoregressive integrated moving average (ARIMA), multilayer perception (MLP), long short-term memory (LSTM), the latter in combination with natural language processing (NLP). AI methods offer high-quality predictive models and exceed traditional statistical modeling methods. The above-mentioned algorithms proved effective in short-term forecasting; however, further studies are required to validate long-term efficacy. However, direct comparison of the models is challenging as they were trained and applied to different datasets (Ghafouri et al. 2021).

AI and ML can aid mass vaccination planners in the effective distribution of vaccines while at the same time monitoring already vaccinated people (Asgary et al. 2020).

Real-Time Monitoring and Tracking of COVID-19 Cases

Real-time monitoring and tracking of COVID-19 cases is critical for the effective response to the pandemic. Machine learning and artificial intelligence have been used to quickly and accurately track cases of the virus, helping to identify hotspots and potential outbreaks, thus providing valuable information for healthcare systems and public health organizations. For example, machine learning algorithms have been used to analyze data from various sources, such as news reports, social media, and official health reports. These algorithms can quickly analyze large amounts of data from multiple sources, providing a more comprehensive and up-to-date picture of the spread of the virus. Based on the prediction of epidemic trends of COVID-19, policymakers and health managers can efficiently allocate healthcare resources.

Additionally, machine learning and artificial intelligence have been used to develop early warning systems, which can quickly identify potential outbreaks and alert public health organizations, allowing them to respond quickly and effectively. For example, these systems can analyze data from sources such as Google search trends and social media to identify spikes in searches for COVID-19-related symptoms, indicating a potential increase in cases.

Artificial intelligence and machine learning have been applied in contact tracing, which is based on the reverse revision of an individual's activities and movements in order to identify the chain of transmission following exposure to infectious contagion (Bragazzi et al. 2020). Smart bracelets and smartphones can be used for

AI-driven, real-time monitoring of isolated infections (Adly et al. 2020). Internet of Things (IoT) is used to track patient zero and transmission chain, as well as to recognize and track those who do not follow social distancing rules (Javaid et al. 2020). Surveying of populations was also carried out by means of infrared thermal cameras paired with AI-based face recognition systems. They were used to observe whether social distancing rules were applied and facial masks worn (Wang et al. 2021).

Helping to Identify High-Risk Individuals and Populations for Targeted Testing and Interventions

One of the key challenges in the response to the COVID-19 pandemic has been the need to prioritize limited resources, including testing and interventions, to those who are at greatest risk of contracting the virus. Machine learning algorithms have been used to identify individuals and populations at high risk of contracting the virus, allowing for targeted testing and interventions. For example, algorithms have been developed to analyze demographic and health data to identify populations at high risk based on factors such as age, underlying health conditions, and occupation. These algorithms can also consider other aspects, such as social and economic determinants of health, to identify high-risk populations that may not be immediately evident. By targeting testing and interventions to those who are at greatest risk, healthcare systems can more effectively control the spread of the virus and minimize its impact on the population. In addition, by focusing on high-risk populations, healthcare systems can reduce the number of false negatives and improve the accuracy of test results. In low-income countries, where financing for healthcare services is limited, machine learning–based, accurate patient triage may lead to a decrease in costs and lower the burden on human resources as well as medical facilities (Hamid et al. 2020).

Natural Language Processing for Monitoring Social Media and Identifying Potential Outbreaks

Natural language processing (NLP) is a field of machine learning that focuses on the interaction between computers and humans through language. Machine learning algorithms have been developed to analyze social media posts, online forums, and other sources of information to identify individuals who have tested positive for the virus or are exhibiting symptoms. These algorithms can quickly analyze large amounts of data, allowing for real-time monitoring of the spread of the virus. For example, NLP algorithms can analyze social media posts for keywords related to COVID-19, such as "fever" or "cough", to identify individuals who may have the virus. This way machine learning and natural language processing have been used to monitor social media and other online sources to identify potential outbreaks and track the spread of the virus. Additionally, NLP algorithms can also analyze other sources of information, such as news reports, to identify outbreaks and monitor the spread of the virus. NLP methods can be used for automated processing of literature, which results in unlocking information from unstructured text which otherwise would have been inaccessible. More effective data mining leads to the identification of relevant papers.

Providing Chatbot and Virtual Assistants

Another major challenge in the response to the COVID-19 pandemic has been the need to provide accurate and up-to-date information to the public. Currently humans are subjected to an enormous amount of data derived from different sources, some of which are accurate and some are not. Therefore the term "infodemia" was created. Machine learning and artificial intelligence tools have been applied to distinguish between true and false information, and to prevent the spread of the latter. AI in "infodemiology" was applied in order to raise awareness about hygiene and sanitation by combining validated sources of information with daily news (Pandey et al. 2020; Patel et al. 2022). Machine learning and natural language processing have been used to develop chatbots and virtual assistants that can answer common questions about the virus and provide guidance on self-care. Chatbots and virtual assistants provide a convenient and accessible means of obtaining information about COVID-19. For example, chatbots have been developed to provide information on the symptoms, transmission, and treatment of COVID-19 and to provide guidance on self-isolation and quarantine procedures. These regularly updated chatbots can handle large volumes of inquiries and provide consistent and accurate information, reducing the burden on healthcare systems and allowing individuals to access information quickly and easily. In addition, natural language processing algorithms have been used to enhance the capabilities of these chatbots and virtual assistants, allowing them to understand and respond to complex questions, providing a more natural and conversational interaction with users. AI-based dialogue chatbots can also be used in screening patients for symptoms of COVID-19.

Image and Signal Processing for Rapid and Accurate Diagnosis and Prognosis

Machine learning algorithms have been used to analyze medical data such as radiographic images, computed tomography (CT) scans, and other signals for screening, diagnosis, and prognosis of COVID-19. These algorithms can quickly analyze large amounts of imaging data and provide a diagnosis in a matter of minutes, reducing the time and resources required for manual analysis. Application of AI models to quickly screen patients allows for fast identification of cases that must be prioritized. Differentiation between COVID-19-induced pneumonia and infections caused by other viruses is crucial in patient management. Also the classification of the severity of pneumonia is of utmost importance as it allows for early interventions. Machine learning and deep learning (DL) models have demonstrated their ability to enhance the efficiency of radiology reporting, achieving performance levels that are at least comparable to radiologists and, in some cases, even surpassing them.

Application of AI in the analysis of medical images is based on advanced automated image analysis, including radiomics, which aims at the extraction of quantitative features from segmented regions of interest (ROI) or on the application of neural networks in deep learning (DL). The advantage of the latter is no need of image segmentation into ROIs, as well as focusing on important areas in large datasets. On the other hand, radiomics performs better in small and medium datasets. Moreover the integration of the two methods in the form of "deep radiomics" is available (Bouchareb et al. 2021).

Machine learning has been employed to analyze digital radiographs, CT, and ultrasound images for patterns characteristic of lesions related to the COVID-19 infection. The following models of ML have been studied in the diagnosis and/or prognosis of COVID-19: Decision Tree (DT), Multinomial Naïve Bayes (MNB), Logistic Regression (LR), Random Forrest (RF), Rebadging (BAG), Recursive Feature Elimination (RFE), Support Vector Machine (SMV), and others. The accuracy of radiomics in the detection of COVID-19 features in diagnostic imaging studies is reported in a wide range from 33% to 99%, depending on applied algorithms.

Machine learning algorithms have also been developed to detect characteristic patterns in CT scans that are indicative of the COVID-19 infection. As far as chest CT is concerned, deep learning algorithms have been employed not only for the identification of features of lesions in CT images but also for dose reduction in CT scans by means of the generation of high-quality images from ultra-low-dose CT images. Sensitivity of differentiation between COVID-19 pneumonia and pneumonia induced by other pathogens, both viral and bacterial, is reported in the range from 87 to 97%, while the specificity reaches 92%.

As far as deep learning is concerned, convolutional neural networks (CNNs) and recurrent neural networks (RNNs) are most frequently used. However, a drawback of the CNN model is the necessity of applying a large amount of training data as well as considerable technical skills in order to determine the best model architecture. Moreover the preparation of annotations of training data by radiologists is time consuming and, taking into account the common paucity of radiology specialists in many regions of the world, challenging.

Sensitivity of the image-based COVID-19 detection (chest X-rays and/or chest CT) falls within the range of 42–100% for human observers, 60–95% for AI models, and is the highest in the case of AI-supported human reading, reaching 81–98%. Also when specificity is taken into account, it is the highest when human observers are supported by AI algorithms, and the values are from 78 to 99%. Studies on human observers provided specificity values from 26 to 100%, while AI-only models performed at the specificity levels of 61–96% (Kriza et al. 2021).

Comparison of the area under curve (AUC) for a neural network and radiologists resulted in confirmation of a higher score for the network, i.e., 0.90 vs. 0.85 (Zhang et al. 2021).

Apart from radiography and CT, also ultrasound is used in the assessment of the condition of the lungs in COVID-19-induced pneumonia. AI-driven methods allow for ultrasound image analysis and prediction of disease severity scores (Roy et al. 2020).

Machine learning algorithms have been used to analyze signals from other sources, such as chest X-rays and pulse oximetry, to provide a more comprehensive picture of a patient's condition and support the diagnosis of COVID-19. Moreover, combining clinical variables, such as patient demographics (e.g., gender, age, weight, height, BMI), clinical signs, and symptoms of infection (e.g., fever, cough, sore throat, headache, dyspnea, musculoskeletal pain, ageusia, and anosmia), concomitant diseases, as well as blood test results with the scoring of chest radiographs performed by radiologists, allowed for quick, accurate, cost-effective, and relatively simple differentiation between COVID-19 and viral pneumonia induced by other pathogens (Shiri et al. 2021; Xia et al. 2021). Such hybrid approaches are reported to outperform clinical-only or radiomics-only models (Shiri et al. 2021).

The ability to identify the risk of developing critical illness based on patient's characteristics at hospital admission results in appropriate, targeted patient management as well as effective medical resource allocation. Early determination of the patient's prognosis influences the prompt onset of treatment, resulting in reduced mortality from COVID-19. Many studies reported that machine and deep learning algorithms could aid in decision-making in an intensive care unit environment, regarding risk stratification and the deterioration of patient conditions.

Nevertheless, not all reports on the application of AI in COVID-19 imaging are enthusiastic. Potential difficulties, obstacles, and sources of error or bias include limited access to training datasets owing to their privacy or low number of cases with certain diseases (e.g., mycoplasma infections or CT in pediatric patients), problems in the validation of research studies as well as standardization of imaging protocols for application in clinical practice. It is also highlighted that radiographic and CT patterns of COVID-19-related pneumonia vary depending on the host factor. Last but not least, the method of segmentation of features matters. Manual or semi-automated methods may result in missing some ill-limited or small lesions; thus it is recommended to replace these with fully automated segmentation methods.

Drug Discovery and Repurposing Using AI-Assisted Techniques

Drug discovery is based on developing therapies, such as cell therapy, as well as drugs such as antibodies, peptides, and small molecules, that are designed to modulate the activity of a molecular target, thus changing the disease state. There are numerous applications of deep neural networks in drug discovery (Spitzer et al. 2019). They include molecular design as well as the prediction of synthesis and bioactivity.

Target identification and prioritization on the basis of existing evidence is the first step in the validation of the target in ex vivo and in vivo models. Taking into account that medicine is extremely rich in data, including clinical and genetic materials, machine learning can contribute to target identification and validation by being able to analyze large datasets. ML algorithms may focus on specific diseases or therapeutic areas such SARS-Co-19, so that they can predict specific drug effects. Early identification of predictors of the success of target-based drug discovery programs is one of the most desired outcomes of the application of machine learning in this field. Prediction of future clinical trial success may result in the reduction of failed drug discovery programs and aid in avoiding costly, long-term late-stage clinical trials. Deep neural networks are also employed in planning the chemical synthesis of drugs in order to identify the most efficient routes of synthesis.

Rapid discovery of effective treatments for COVID-19 is critical for the active response to the pandemic. Machine learning and artificial intelligence have been used to identify potential drugs and repurpose existing drugs for the treatment of COVID-19. For example, algorithms have been developed to analyze large datasets of chemical compounds to identify those with potential antiviral properties. These algorithms can quickly search through thousands of compounds and predict which may be effective against the virus, thus reducing the time and resources required for manual analysis and experimentation. By analyzing data on the molecular structure and behavior of the virus, the algorithms can identify existing drugs that may have potential as treatments for COVID-19, allowing for faster and more efficient drug repurposing. Shortening of the time from drug discovery to its validated application in clinical practice is of utmost importance during the COVID-19 pandemic, as effective therapies for this new virus infection are essential, and there is no time to wait for the long-term results of clinical studies. AI has been used, for instance, to identify 13 drugs active against feline coronavirus infection (feline infectious peritonitis—FIP), which later were tested in clinical settings and proved effective against SARS-CoV-2 (Ke et al. 2020). Another example is the identification of baricitinib used in the treatment of rheumatoid arthritis as having antiviral effects in the course of scouring of medical literature performed by an AI start-up company (Bragazzi et al. 2020).

Elaboration of safe and effective vaccines is one of the strategies to combat the pandemic. The development of vaccines is related to many obstacles, such as virus mutation, variability between populations as well as individual variability, and the complexity of the human immune system. Therefore, the process of developing a new vaccine is also time consuming and costly, just like in case of drug development. AI algorithms can aid in modeling mutations of SARS-Co-2 for the development of new vaccines, as well as in screening compounds that can be potential adjuvants for vaccines. Machine learning was used, for instance, in the prediction of the adhesion of tested proteins to virus particles thus the most promising candidate for the vaccine component (Wong et al. 2019).

Telemedicine in the Era of COVID-19

The use of telemedicine, otherwise called telehealth, has increased tremendously since the onset of the COVID-19 pandemic. Recurring lockdowns, prolonged periods of isolation and quarantine, Covid morbidity among healthcare staff, relocation of staff from general practice, and specialist wards to units dedicated to the treatment of patients with COVID-19 resulted in limited access to some healthcare services. It is worth underlining that during the pandemic some patients, especially from groups of risk, deliberately refrained from face-to-face medical consultations due to fear of contracting the disease in healthcare facilities, especially when social distancing rules were not obeyed and protective facial masks not worn. One of the factors facilitating the implementation of telemedicine is the enormous popularity of smartphones and other mobile devices, also in low-income countries with limited access to healthcare services. Teleconsultation turned into an accepted medical service, allowing the detection of signs and symptoms of infection without direct contact with a sick person. In the pandemic new reality a doctor under quarantine still can work remotely, and assistance to patients is not jeopardized. Application of AI tools in telemedicine is associated with cost-effectiveness and availability; it can also compensate for limitations of humans, e.g., in the case of analysis of large datasets. The role of artificial intelligence in telehealth is attributed to providing a framework for telemedicine services, taking into account the distribution of diagnosis and treatment needs, geographical patterns, time constraints, healthcare facilities, and human resources. This way subjective person-to-person communication in providing emergency patient management will be eliminated. Medical wearables as a part of the Internet of Things are thought to be able to supply AI-based smart healthcare and individualized treatment.

In the era of the pandemic AI-based telemedicine solutions using, e.g., virtual reality can also be implemented in the education of healthcare practitioners. AI-assisted education, also known as the educational intelligence, is based on making informed decisions that positively influence learning outcomes (Rodriguez-Rodriguez et al. 2021).

The remote use of robotic technologies during pandemics results in decreased exposure of medical staff to infection. Care-providing robots may replace humans in such tasks as disinfection, distribution of food and drugs, or measuring vital signs. The possibility of two-way communication via robots may be beneficial for patients under isolation or quarantine regimens.

The possible danger of telemedicine applying AI approach lies in the potential loss of skills of human doctors. In opposition to human healthcare workers, who are trained to be prepared for contingencies, AI methods follow rigid algorithms including decision-making trees thus may not readily respond to unexpected changes or experience difficulties in differentiation between relevant and non-relevant information (Bhaskar et al. 2020).

AI in Supervision of Medical Devices

Apart from prognosis and diagnosis, artificial intelligence can also play a role in the management of medical devices. During the COVID-19 pandemic machine learning was applied to determine pressure volume curve in a group of ventilated patients, enabling more effective treatment regimen (Ghanzaert et al. 2002). Other machine learning algorithms were developed in order to detect machine faults (Lei et al. 2020).

Conclusion

In conclusion, the use of machine learning algorithms for identifying high-risk individuals and populations has proven to be a valuable tool in the response to the COVID-19 pandemic, allowing for targeted testing and interventions and helping to control the spread of the virus, providing accurate and up-to-date information on the spread of the virus, and enabling healthcare systems and public health organizations to respond quickly and effectively. The use of image and signal processing with machine learning algorithms has proven to be a valuable tool in the rapid and accurate diagnosis of COVID-19, reducing the time and resources required for manual analysis and providing a more comprehensive picture of a patient's condition. However, AI should not be used as an independent tool but to assist diagnosis, as there is little evidence for a direct comparison of the performance of humans and AI in actual clinical practice. AI-driven solutions in telemedicine and robotics also play an important role in the era of the pandemic.

Bibliography

Adly AS, Adly AS, Adly MS. Approaches based on artificial intelligence and the internet of things to prevent the spread of COVID-19: a scooping review. J Med Internet Res. 2020;2(8):e19104.

Arif M, Zaidi AK. COVID-19 pandemic and the role of machine learning in predicting its spread. J King Saud Univ Comput Inform Sci. 2021;33(2):109–18.

Asgary A, Valtchev SZ, Chen M, Najafabadi MM, Wu J. Artificial intelligence model of drive-through vaccination simulation. Int J Environ Res Public Health. 2020;18:268.

Bhaskar S, Bradley S, Sakhamuri S, Moguilner S, Chattu VK, Pandaya S, Schoeder S, Ray D, Banach M. Designing futuristic telemedicine using artificial intelligence and robotics in the COVID-19 era. Front Public Health. 2020;8:556789.

Bouchareb Y, Khaniabadi PM, Al Kindi F, Al Dhuhli H, Shirir I, Zaidi H, Rahmin A. Artificial intelligence-driven assessment of radiological images for COVID-19. Comput Biol Med. 2021;136:104665.

Bragazzi NL, Dai H, Damiani G, Behzadifar M, Martini M, Wu J. How big data and artificial intelligence can help better manage the COVID-19 pandemic. Int J Environ Res Public Health. 2020;17:3176.

Chen Z, Wu Z, Wei Y, Lai X, Jia Y. Machine learning in diagnosis of COVID-19 based on CT images. J Med Syst. 2020;45(12):865–71.

Ghanzaert S, Guttmann J, Kersting K, Kuhlen R, Putensen C, Sydow M, Kramer S. Analysis of respiratory pressure-volume curves in intensive care medicine using inductive machine learning. Artif Intell Med. 2002;26:69–86.

Ghafouri-Fard S, Mohammad-Rahimi H, Motie P, Minabi MAS, Taheri M, Nateghinia S. Application of machine learning in the prediction of COVID-19 daily new cases: a scoping review. Heliyon. 2021;7:e08143.

Guo X, Yin H. A machine learning approach for COVID-19 spread prediction based on different types of data sources. Chaos, Solitons Fractals. 2021;142:110766.

Hamid H, Abid Z, Amir A, Rehman TU, Akram W, Mehboob T. Current burden on healthcare systems in low- and middle-income countries: recommendations for emergency care of COVID-19. Drugs Ther Perspect. 2020;36:466–8.

Javaid M, Haleem A, Vaishya R, Bahl S, Suman R, Vaish A. Industry 4.0 technologies and their applications in fighting COVID-19 pandemic. Diabetes Metab Syndr. 2020;14:419–22.

Karimzadeh A, Forouzan F, Roohi NH, Moosavi RZ. The role of machine learning in predicting COVID-19: a comprehensive review. J Med Syst. 2020;45(12):818–28.

Ke YY, Peng TT, Yeh TK, Huang WZ, Chang SE, Wu SH, et al. Artificial intelligence approach fighting COVID-19 with repurposing drugs. Biomed J. 2020;43:355–62.

Kriza C, Amenta V, Zeni A, Panidis D, Chasaigne H, Urban P, Hozwarth U, Sauer AV, Reina V, Griesinger CB. Artificial intelligence for imaging-based COVID-19 detection: systematic review comparing added value of AI versus human readers. Eur J Radiol. 2021;145:110028.

Lei Y, Yang B, Jiang X, Jia F, Li N, Nandi AK. Applications of machine learning to machine fault diagnosis: a review and roadmap. Mech Syst Signal Process. 2020;138:106587.

Li X, Li Z, Li H, Li J, Li H, Li H, Li Y. Predicting the spread of COVID-19 by deep learning. Math Biosci Eng. 2021;18(2):855–71.

Mistry AK, Anderson ER, Zhang H, Brown JA, Grau-Moya J, De Oliveira D. Machine learning for COVID-19 triage, screening and risk stratification: a systematic review. J Med Syst. 2021;45(5):348.

Nie Y, Wei J, Sun J. Machine learning models for predicting the number of confirmed COVID-19 cases in different regions. Chaos Solitons Fractals. 2020;140:110610.

Pandey R, Gautam V, Pal R, Bandhey H, Dhingra LS, Misra V, Sharma H, Jain C, Bhagat K, Arushi Sawyer J. Artificial intelligence-driven smart healthcare services and personalized clinical care in COVID-19 telemedicine. Am J Med Res. 2020;7:71–7.

Patel L, Agarwal M, Agrawal S, Jalan R, Wadhwa A, Garg A, Agrawal Y, Rana B, Kumaraguru P, Sethi T. A machine learning application for raising WASH awareness in the times of covid-19 pandemic. Sci Rep. 2022;12(1):810.

Rodriguez-Rodriguez I, Rodriguez J-V, Shirvanizadeh N, Ortiz A, Pardo-Qules D-J. Applications of artificial intelligence, machine learning, big data and the internet of things to the COVID-19 Pandemic: A scientometeric review using text mining. Int J Environ Res Public Health. 2021;18(16):8578.

Roy S, Menapace W, Oei S, Luijten B, Fini E, Saltori C, Huijben I, Chennakeshava N, Mento F, Sentelli A, et al. Deep learning for classification and localization of the COVID-19 markers in point-of-care lung ultrasound. IEEE Trans Med Imaging. 2020;39:2676–87.

Shiri I, Sorouri M, Geramifar P, Nazari M, Abdollahi M, Salimi Y, et al. Machine learning-based prognostic modeling using clinical data and quantitative radiomic features from chest CT images in COVID-19 patients. Comput Biol Med. 2021;132:104304.

Spitzer M, Zhao S. Applications of machine learning in drug discovery and development. Nat Rev Drug Discov. 2019;18(6):463–77.

Vamathevan J, Clark D, Czodrowski P, Dunham I, Ferran E, Lee G, Li B, Madabhusi A, Shah P, Ong E, Wong MU, Huffman A, He Y. COVID-19 coronavirus vaccine design using reverse vaccinology and machine learning. Front Immunol. 2020;11:1581.

Vu KT, Nguyen SV, Lee B. Machine learning in drug discovery and development for COVID-19. J Med Syst. 2020;46(10):833–44.

Wang L, Zhang Y, Wang D, Tong X, Liu T, Zhang S, Huang J, Zhang L, Chen L, Fan H, Clarke M. Artificial intelligence for COVID-19: a systematic review. Front Med. 2021;8:704256.

Williams CM, Chaturvedi R, Urman RD, Waterman RS, Gabriel RA. Artificial intelligence and a pandemic: an analysis of the potential uses and drawbacks. J Med Syst. 2021;45:26.

Wong ZSY, Zhou J, Zhang Q. Artificial intelligence for infectious disease big data analytics. Dis Health. 2019;24(1):44–8.

Xia Y, Chen W, Ren H, Zhao J, Wang L, Jin R, Zhou J, Wang Q, Yan F, Zhang B, Lou J, Wang S, Li X, Zhou J, Xia L, Jin C, Feng J, Li W, Shen H. A rapid screening classifier for diagnosing COVID-19. Int J Biol Sci. 2021;17(2):539–48. https://doi.org/10.7150/ijbs.53982. eCollection 2021.

Xu JJ, Chen YC, Wu YJ. Artificial intelligence in COVID-19 pandemic: a review. J Med Syst. 2020;45(12):829–38.

Yang XL, Deng MT, Huang ZL, Liu YH, Liu XF. Artificial intelligence and deep learning for COVID-19: a review. J Med Syst. 2020;45(12):801–17.

Zhang R, Tie X, Qi Z, Bevins NB, Zhang C, Griner D, et al. Diagnosis of coronavirus disease 2019 by chest radiographs: value of artificial intelligence. Radiology. 2021;298(2):E88–97.

Medico-Legal Problems of Artificial Intelligence

16

Kaan Orhan, Melis Mısırlı Gülbeş, Aniket Jadhav, and Rohan Jagtap

An Overview of Human Rights, Democracy, and the Rule of Law

> **Each and every human right is global, indivisible, interdependent, and interconnected.**
> **—Vienna Declaration of the United Nations, 1993**

Since Classical Antiquity, privacy and secrecy have been two of the primary foundations of medical ethics, although they may not have always been defined in those terms. The concept and scope of privacy have been a persistent source of debate among scholars and philosophers, and this debate continues today. In the 1948 United Nations General Assembly's Universal Declaration of Human Rights (UDHR), privacy was identified as a basic human right. However, there was no agreement on what constitutes privacy, its breadth, or its boundaries.

There is a strong relationship between human rights, democracy, and the rule of law. The ability of legitimate governments to effectively protect human rights

K. Orhan (✉)
Faculty of Dentistry, Department of Dentomaxillofacial Radiology, Ankara University, Ankara, Turkey

M. M. Gülbeş
Faculty of Dentistry, Department of Dentomaxillofacial Radiology, Final University, Lefkoşa, Cyprus
e-mail: melis.gulbes@final.edu.tr

A. Jadhav
American Board of Oral and Maxillofacial Radiology, Oral Diagnostics Sciences, VCU School of Dentistry, Richmond, VA, USA
e-mail: abjadhav@vcu.edu

R. Jagtap
Division of Oral and Maxillofacial Radiology, Department of Care Planning and Restorative Sciences, Department of Radiology, School of Medicine, University of Mississippi Medical Center, Jackson, MS, USA

K. Orhan, R. Jagtap (eds.), *Artificial Intelligence in Dentistry*,
https://doi.org/10.1007/978-3-031-43827-1_16

depends on the interdependence of strong and accountable democratic institutions, inclusive and transparent decision-making systems, and an independent and impartial judiciary that upholds the rule of law. Human rights are the fundamental rights and freedoms possessed by every person in the world from birth to death, preserving and protecting the inviolable dignity of every individual regardless of race, ethnicity, gender, age, sexual orientation, class, religion, disability status, language, nationality, or any other ascribed characteristic.

These basic rights and liberties impose on governments the duty to respect, preserve, and fulfill human rights. Individuals are entitled to legal remedies that permit the remedy of any human rights abuses if these obligations are not met (Leslie et al. 2021).

The Development of Human Rights over the Years

In the aftermath of the horrors and suffering of World War II, the collection of fundamental rights and ideas known today as human rights arose for the first time in the middle of the twentieth century.

1948

The United Nations adopts the Universal Declaration of Human Rights (UDHR), the first worldwide baseline for basic rights and liberties. While not legally binding, this declaration would serve as the foundation for the numerous treaties, conventions, and charters on human rights that have been enacted globally to date.

1953

The European Convention on Human Rights (ECHR) was incorporated. This international treaty, initially established by the Council of Europe in 1950, enshrines the civil and political rights to which the 47 Member States of the Council are legally obliged. In addition to creating fundamental rights designed to defend the inviolable dignity of every individual, the ECHR obligated governments to protect ordinary people from human rights infringements.

1961

The European Social Charter (ESC) is released by the Council of Europe for signatures. This convention enlarges the scope of fundamental rights to encompass social and economic rights pertaining to health, working conditions, housing, migrant labor, gender equality, and social security. In 1988, further procedures were implemented to promote employment opportunity equality, worker involvement, and protection for the poor and elderly. In 1996, a new ESC was adopted.

1966

The International Covenant on Civil and Political Rights (ICCPR) and the International Covenant on Economic, Social, and Cultural Rights (ICESCR) are adopted by the United Nations. Included in the ICCPR are freedom from torture, the right to a fair trial, nondiscrimination, and the right to privacy. The ICESCR enhances fundamental rights to include rights to fair working conditions, health, quality of living, education, and social security. The UN's UDHR, ICCPR, and ICESCR are now collectively referred to as the International Bill of Human Rights.

2009

The Treaty of Lisbon gives the Charter of Fundamental Rights of the European Union (CFR) full legal effect. This entrenches in EU law a fundamental set of civil, political, social, economic, and cultural rights for EU people. The categories of human rights addressed by the CFR include human dignity, basic freedoms, equality, solidarity, economic rights, and the right to participate in the community's life (Leslie et al. 2021).

The Privacy of Patients in the Age of Big Data

The Privacy Rule of the Health Insurance Portability and Accountability Act (HIPAA) establishes the regulatory framework and strikes a balance between access to health information (HI) for secondary (scientific) use and protective measures. The rule specifies the circumstances under which health information is legally protected and how such information may be de-identified for secondary use.

Human subjects research is defined as any biological study that incorporates personal identifiers of the subject of the information in the United States. Health information (HI) is described as information pertaining to an individual's past, present, and future Healthcare or health condition, as well as payment-related health information. Personally, identifiable health information is a subset of health information (HI) and consists of identifiers or other information that may be used to identify the health information's subject. The majority of personally identifiable health data are protected health information (PHI). In 1996, the US Congress established the Health Insurance Portability and Accountability Act (HIPAA) and mandated that the Secretary of Health and Human Services (HHS) issue guidelines to fulfill its provisions: "(1) The rights that a subject of personally identifiable information should have. (2) Procedures for the exercise of such rights. (3) The disclosures and uses of such information that should be approved or mandated". In 1999, HHS proposed the original iteration of the Privacy Rule as a set of privacy protection guidelines for the management and transmission of individuals' protected health information (PHI). The current version of the rule incorporates revisions to the 2008 Genetic Information Nondiscrimination Act (GINA) and the Health Information Technology for Economic and Clinical Health (HITECH) Act. The

Privacy Rule forbids selling protected health information or using it for marketing purposes without the individual's explicit consent. If the selling/marketing party receives compensation, it must be disclosed openly.

PHI may be used by the provider for the purpose of the individual's treatment (i.e., for main use) and disclosed to other providers for the same reason or to health insurance services for notice of payment. Individuals may also authorize another person (such as a family member) to receive their PHI. The individual has the right to be notified before making these disclosures and to prohibit them. At the individual's death, the provider may disclose PHI to a family member or other individual selected by the individual, unless the individual has requested against such disclosures. In certain cases, PHI may also be used or disclosed for secondary (non-care-related) purposes. If required by law, the provider may disclose PHI without the individual's agreement to a public health or government body, to approved workers' compensation programs, or to organizations participating in tissue/organ banks or transplants. Disclosures must always be restricted to the smallest amount of PHI "required to achieve the stated purpose of the use, disclosure, or request". Companies can restrict employee access to protected health information (PHI) to only those components that are essential for them to fulfill their tasks. A hospital registrar may view the names and addresses of patients, but not their diagnostic codes or clinical reports.

Privacy regulation for scientific research: Researchers are permitted to utilize protected health information (PHI) if they get consent from the subjects of the PHI. Without such authorization, commonly known as informed consent, researchers must request a waiver of authorization from the institutional review board (IRB). Typically, informed consent entails general agreement to treat, consent for a specific technique, or participation in a research project; however, big data frequently necessitates pooling and analyzing data in the future for reasons that were not envisaged at the time of consent (Kayaalp 2018; Balthazar et al. 2018).

Effect of AI and Machine Learning on Human Rights, Democracy, and the Rule of Law: Opportunities and Threats

Artificial intelligence (AI) technologies provide a variety of avenues for enhancing the quality of human life. The strength, scalability, and speed of AI systems may increase efficiency and effectiveness in several fields, such as Healthcare, transportation, education, and government. Humans can be relieved of boring, risky, unpleasant, and difficult duties. AI technologies have the potential to have harmful effects on human rights, democracy, and the rule of law. These benefits and threats should be seen in light of AI's "socio-technical" nature; AI is a broad spectrum of sophisticated technologies designed to work in human contexts and achieve human-defined goals. Thus, AI systems mirror the attitudes and preferences of their creators and users.

AI may be used to generate predictions about human behavior, discover illness indications, and evaluate threats to the interests or well-being of others. All of these responsibilities have the potential to influence the rights, opportunities, and well-being of individuals who are subject to them. Hence, accountability is a crucial part of developing and utilizing these systems. While AI can take over tedious or complicated tasks from humans, the choices involved in the construction and use of AI systems can result in the reproduction of harmful biases and other fallibilities of human judgment that negatively impact affected individuals and society in ways that are more difficult to identify than when performed by humans.

The desired output from the AI algorithm is completely dependent on the quality, quantity, and type of the data fed into the system creating AI technology. Hence it is crucial that when an AI model is being curated, the QA of the data must be governed and done under the supervision of experts to minimize the risk, should it be caused by the AI outcome. The aviation industry has been utilizing AI for decades and has also been known for disastrous and tragic failures such as Boeing 737 Max airplanes (Mongan and Kohli 2020). Kohli et al. further jotted down the five lesions for the implementation of AI and stated that malfunctioning AI can create safety hazards in patient care, and hence the accuracy of inputs in the AI algorithm is as important as the accuracy of the algorithm itself. It is important to recognize that human interaction and the ability to retrospectively assess AI performance would be crucial in the future in cases of biased data output. Training new-generation physicians, radiologists, and Healthcare providers on AI is a crucial need in Healthcare so that this workforce is ready to tackle any adverse outcome due to the failure of AI systems.

European and North American multisocieties further elaborated on the ethics of AI in radiology and broadly classified it according to data, algorithms, and practice (Geis et al. 2019). As the quality and privacy of data are important, so is the assessment of its outcome, which may pose a significant risk of causing harm to a subset of patients based on their gender, sexual orientation, ethnicity, and socioeconomic background. Supreme Court Justice Cardozo in 1914 set forth the ethical principle of autonomy, which states, "Every human being of adult years and sound mind has a right to determine what shall be done with his own body" (Schloendorff 1914).

Given that AI is a technological tool and hence cannot process this ethical decision, it becomes the moral duty of Healthcare professionals to respect and prioritize this ethical principle. The three other principles of ethics, such as beneficence, nonmaleficence, and justice, are equally important. Many prime organizations worldwide took initiative to incorporate the four principles into AI. According to the Harvard Data Science Review, these four principles may not perfectly blend into AI, and hence they proposed the fifth principle of Explicability. This fifth principle incorporates intelligibility (How it works) and accountability (Who is responsible for the way it works) (Schloendorff 1914).

In addition to examining the technical characteristics of a given system or technology, AI responsibility necessitates that we examine the possible risks and benefits to persons and communities. Among the possible drawbacks is explicit prejudice, such as when AI algorithms make discriminatory predictions or otherwise treat a certain demographic group or identify unjustifiably differently from others. Due to the opaque nature of some AI systems, it is more difficult to evaluate their potential for causing damage. In addition to being developed utilizing specialized knowledge, it can be difficult to comprehend or explain the operation of AI systems due to their technological complexity and intellectual property protections. The European Convention on Human Rights (ECHR) and the European Social Charter (ESC), including its specific guarantees regarding liberty and justice, privacy, freedom of expression, equality and nondiscrimination, and social and economic rights, provide insight into the specific human rights implications of AI systems. There are further consequences of artificial intelligence on democracy and the rule of law that do not explicitly fit under the rules of the ECHR and the ESC but are still as significant. A comprehensive analysis of the risks and opportunities posed by AI systems will help us determine where existing rights and freedoms provide needed protections, where existing rights and freedoms require further clarification, and where new rights and freedoms must be tailored to the novel challenges and opportunities posed by AI and machine learning.

Privacy: AI can access and analyze vast quantities of data about persons with amazing speed. AI may anticipate a person's behavior, mental state, and identity by detecting data that is not necessarily deemed personal or private, such as facial expressions, heart rate, physical location, and other seemingly banal or publicly accessible information. This can have the impact of invading a person's feeling of privacy, as well as the so-called panoptic consequences of altering a person's behavior out of fear of being viewed or analyzed.

The Committee of Ministers of the Council of Europe agreed the terms of reference for the Ad Hoc Committee on Artificial Intelligence in September 2019 (CAHAI). The CAHAI is tasked with assessing the viability and potential components of a legal framework for the creation, design, and deployment of AI systems based on Council of Europe norms in the interconnected areas of human rights, democracy, and the rule of law. As a vital first step in carrying out this task, the CAHAI's Feasibility Study, accepted by its plenary in December 2020, proposes nine principles and goals designed to underlie a framework of binding and non-binding legislative instruments.

Human Dignity

All persons are intrinsically and inviolably deserving of respect by virtue of their human position alone. People should be considered as moral subjects, not as things to be evaluated or manipulated algorithmically.

Human Freedom and Independence

Humans should be able to independently and judiciously decide if, when, and how to deploy AI technologies. These technologies should not be used to condition or control human beings but rather to enhance their capacities.

Protection from Hurt

The physical and mental integrity of individuals and the biosphere's sustainability must be safeguarded, and further protections must be implemented to protect the vulnerable. AI systems should not be authorized to negatively harm human or global health.

Nondiscrimination, Gender Equality, Fairness, and Diversity

All individuals have the right to nondiscrimination, equality, and equal treatment under the law. The good effects and distribution of hazards of AI systems must be intended to be fair, equal, and inclusive.

AI System Transparency and Explainability

When a product or service employs an AI system, affected individuals must be informed. Similarly, meaningful information must be supplied on the logic driving its results.

Accountability and Responsibility

All parties participating in the design and deployment of AI systems must be held accountable for any violations of relevant legal standards or unfair harm to end-users or others. Individuals who are harmed must have access to appropriate remedies for restitution.

Democracy

Transparent and inclusive monitoring methods are required to defend democratic decision-making processes, pluralism, access to information, autonomy, and economic and social rights in the context of the design and implementation of AI systems.

The Rule of Law

AI technologies must not compromise judicial impartiality, independence, or due process. To guarantee this, the data's openness, integrity, and fairness, as well as the data processing techniques, must be safeguarded.

Information Security and the Right to Privacy

The design and implementation of AI systems that rely on the processing of personal data must respect an individual's right to private and family life, including the right to govern one's own data. Consent that is informed, freely provided, and unequivocal must play a role here (Leslie et al. 2021).

De-identification of Various Forms of Data

Four sorts of data exist: tabular, image/video, signal, and text. If field standards are established, de-identification of tabularly organized data is trivial. The Privacy Rule mandates the removal of full-face photographs and photos that may be used to identify an individual; however it is feasible to delete certain facial elements from photographs. For instance, the faces of all people seen in Google Street View photographs are obscured, as are the letters and numbers on car license plates. Face and text recognition software are required for doing this task with photos.

With the development of artificial intelligence and computational linguistics, computational text de-identification algorithms offer findings that are de-identified almost as good as those produced by human specialists, but considerably more quickly, reliably, and for free. Current clinical text de-identification solutions open the way for big data and provide scientists with access to de-identified health information while ensuring patient confidentiality.

Disclosure of patient information for patient care is permissible, but publication of the same information for study, experimentation, or development requires informed permission. Although the distinction between patient care and research is well acknowledged, its application to novel approaches can evade even the most competent companies. Imaging is a reliable source of phenotypic data suited for the use of big data, artificial intelligence, and customized medicine techniques. Long ago, we adopted ethical and regulatory frameworks to govern our use of patient and research subject data. In many instances, it is unclear how to apply these standards in the age of big data and artificial intelligence, with their seemingly insatiable thirst for more data. The terms "big data", "artificial intelligence", "personalized medicine", "population health", and "predictive analytics" belong to a family of similar but distinct ideas (Kayaalp 2018).

Big Data

The phrase "big data" is frequently used informally in Healthcare to refer to any dataset containing more than a few thousand data points. However, the definition of big data is not based on sample size thresholds; rather, the scale and challenge of "big data" in the modern era are that datasets are now so large that storage or processing of the data strains the computational capacity of a single computer and necessitates the use of more specialized computing solutions. In Healthcare, large datasets may contain numerous rows containing the patient records of millions of patients and/or several columns matching the multiple patient characteristics recorded.

High-variety, high-volume, and/or high-velocity information assets comprise the "3V's" of big data classification. They are particularly suited for radiology data, which consists of massive quantities of pictures and reports in a range of imaging modalities, body parts, and formats (unstructured text and structured DICOM), which are rapidly created and possibly evaluated in real time or near real time. The most used standard for representing and transmitting clinical picture data is DICOM. Each DICOM image dataset is made up of a header comprising structured (tabular) data and image pixels (Balthazar et al. 2018; Wang et al. 2020).

The volume, velocity, and variety of big data in Healthcare, coupled with recent advancements in data storage and processing technologies, have created a fertile environment for the development of artificial intelligence (AI) models that can perform a wide range of classification and prediction tasks.

The increasing adoption of electronic health records (EHRs) since 2008, driven by the Meaningful Use program of the HITECH Act, and the concurrent development and widespread adoption of standards for health data exchange have enabled the aggregation of health data from multiple sources, thereby creating a new, rich environment for big data and artificial intelligence.

Standards for health data interchange establish formats and fields for the storing of health data from diverse health systems and sources, hence providing the syntactic interoperability necessary for machines to read data from diverse sources employing standard standards. Digital Imaging and Communications in Medicine (DICOM), which was created in 1993, is the gold standard for imaging in radiology and ophthalmology. Through different versions of the Health Level-7 guidance and the development of the new Fast Healthcare Interoperability Resources (FHIR), standards for EHR data have undergone significant evolution. FHIR is the next-generation standards framework for EHR data that supports the most recent web service technologies. FHIR holds data in modular components called resources that are meant to be flexible, interoperable, and simple to deploy concurrently. These standard data exchange formats enable the aggregation of data from various sources into ever-larger datasets, which in turn enables the development of powerful AI predictive algorithms that can be validated across different settings, such as predicting hospitalization mortality, length-of-stay, and readmissions across various Healthcare systems using a common deep learning approach (Wang et al. 2020).

Developing an AI model on such a massive amount of data necessitates substantial computational resources. Cloud-based computing and storage infrastructures, many of which contain HIPAA-compliant security mechanisms for the storage and processing of protected health information, have supplanted the need of local supercomputing gear.

These cloud-based systems have the capacity to store and analyze massive amounts of data, enabling the training of sophisticated AI models. Once a model has been trained, the process of utilizing it to create predictions is referred to as inference. Inference technology is very affordable and growing more widespread:

voice-activated assistants on smartphones, picture search, spam filtering, and product recommendation apps all employ inference to understand instructions. In hospitals and Healthcare settings, however, this sort of infrastructure must be improved to maximize the future benefits of deploying AI models to support and improve clinical treatment decisions.

Artificial Intelligence

Artificial intelligence is a subfield of computer science concerned with automating intelligent behavior. In contrast to the first generation of artificial intelligence (AI) systems, which relied on the curation of medical knowledge by experts and the formulation of robust decision rules, recent AI research has utilized machine learning methods, which can account for complex interactions, to identify patterns in the data.

The definition of artificial intelligence (AI) is "A system's capacity to accurately understand external inputs and use those learnings to achieve specified goals and tasks through flexible adaptation". AI employs complicated computer algorithms to simulate human intellect, with the added ability to analyze vast datasets. The area of artificial intelligence is advancing quickly and has made substantial inroads into nearly every element of human existence, including Healthcare. It is anticipated that the adoption of AI-based tools and approaches would enhance Healthcare delivery by making treatment more accessible and inexpensive and by enhancing its quality. CT images, for instance, may be automatically interpreted by AI as well as radiologists. Using AI with chest x-rays, it is possible to screen for tuberculosis with equivalent accuracy to molecular testing, and mammography images may be used to forecast the beginning of breast cancer before visible symptoms appear. As a result, AI for health has been identified as a core topic by both researchers and governments. A morally competent policy framework is required to govern the development and implementation of AI technology in Healthcare. Moreover, when AI technologies are further researched and implemented in clinical decision-making, it is crucial to establish safeguarding and protection procedures that address responsibility in the event of mistakes. Like with any other diagnostic instrument, AI-based solutions cannot be held accountable for their own conclusions and assessments. At all phases of the development and implementation of AI for health, it is consequently essential to assign accountability and duty.

In spite of all the potential benefits, adopting AI for Health raises a number of ethical, legal, and societal issues, particularly in relation to its development and implementation. The topic can be widely led by well-established principles of health research, but the development and implementation of AI-based solutions in Healthcare must address a number of concerns, such as those pertaining to data safety, data sharing, data privacy, etc. For instance, AI-based solutions can empower the masses by enabling easy and early diagnosis and access to health facilities, but the unsupervised use of such tools and approaches might be dangerous. Hence, an ethical and regulatory framework is required before AI for Health is integrated into health research and Healthcare delivery. While the broad principles of biomedical research and Healthcare delivery are applicable to AI for health, the subject also includes a number of distinct ethical challenges.

In building AI technology for use in Healthcare, same ethical criteria can be adhered to. Due to the particular methodological and interpretive issues posed by AI technology and the fast-developing Healthcare environment, the recommendations were developed in conjunction with professionals from both domains. The purpose of these guidelines is not to restrict innovation or recommend any disease-specific diagnostic or therapeutic approach, but rather to guide the development, deployment, and adoption of AI-based technologies in biomedical research and Healthcare delivery in a manner that is both effective and safe (Cohen and Gordon 2022; Chan et al. 2020; Yu et al. 2018).

General Ethical Considerations for Health Research

To ensure protection of the safety, dignity, rights, and welfare of the community and the participants, all health and biomedical research, whether AI-based or using conventional methods, should adhere to the fundamental ethical principles of doing good (beneficence), respect for persons (autonomy), doing no harm (non-malfeasance), and distributive justice.

These four basic principles have been expanded into ten general principles in the 2017 ICMR National Ethics Guidelines. These broad ethical principles cover the majority of the ethical considerations involved in biomedical and health research. Despite this, AI for health relies heavily on data collected from human participants, which raises additional problems including possible biases, data management, interpretation, autonomy, risk reduction, professional competence, data sharing, and confidentiality. Thus, it is essential to create an ethical framework that tackles AI for Health-specific challenges.

Ethical Standards for AI Health Technology

All key parties must adhere to and apply ethical norms and principles in the development and deployment of artificial intelligence technology in Healthcare. Machine learning (ML), a branch of artificial intelligence, consists of data-driven approaches, such as deep learning, that are used to discover patterns and anticipate behavior with minimal human interaction. The system "learns" by studying training data and makes predictions based on a fresh dataset.

Variations of Machine Learning

Basic machine-learning algorithms broadly fall into two groups, supervised and unsupervised, based on the sorts of problems they are intended to answer.

Supervised Education

Models of supervised learning are taught using datasets including labeled data. In these models, "learning" happens when several instances are used to train an algorithm to translate input variables (commonly referred to as features) to desired outputs (also called target variables or labels). On the basis of these instances, ML models are able to find patterns between inputs and outcomes. These ML models may then repeat these patterns by utilizing the rules refined during training to classify or predict fresh inputs. Using factors such as the existence of the words "lottery" and "you won" to predict whether an email should be categorized as spam or not is a classic example of supervised learning. Supervised learning can take the form of classification, such as predicting if an email is spam or not, or regression, which determines the connection between input factors and a target variable. While linear regression and classification are the basic kinds of supervised learning, support vector machines and random forests are also often used. Classification, regression, and the characterization of the similarity between examples with identical result labels are among the most common applications of supervised machine-learning models.

Unsupervised Instruction

Unsupervised learning infers the underlying patterns in unlabeled data in order to discover sub-clusters of the original data, identify outliers in the data, or generate low-dimensional representations of the data. It should be noted that the identification of low-dimensional representations for labeled cases can be accomplished more successfully through supervision. Methods of machine learning enable the construction of artificial intelligence applications that simplify the identification of previously undiscovered patterns in the data without the need to set decision rules for each unique job or account for complicated connections between input elements. Hence, machine learning is now the chosen foundation for developing AI utilities (Leslie et al. 2021; Yu et al. 2018).

Repetition Learning

Reinforcement learning models acquire knowledge via their interactions with a virtual or actual environment, as opposed to existing data. Reinforcement learning "agents" seek the ideal approach to finish a task by performing a set of actions that maximize the chance of success. Based on the success or failure of their actions, individuals are awarded or punished. These "agents" are trained to maximize their reward by choosing their actions. They "learn" from prior successes and mistakes, improve via numerous cycles of trial and error, and may be engineered to build long-term plans to maximize their total return, as opposed to focusing just on the next step.

Reproducibility is crucially dependent on the following when training AI models on huge data:

(1) The labeling of the data used to train the AI model, (2) the underlying structure and properties of the data, and (3) the model architecture's specifics. When creating and assessing AI models based on big data, each of these elements is crucial to consider.

This approach shows promise in radiology for preliminary lesion identification and differential diagnosis generation, with the potential to increase radiologists' sensitivity and precision. Natural language processing, a branch of artificial intelligence, focuses on comprehending the complete meaning of written or spoken material by combining concepts and methods from a variety of areas.

Although promising, the complexity of such "machine-driven" analytical methods has caused health practitioners and academics to exercise caution. Unlike other domains of AI, AI for Health has the potential to have significant consequences for all aspects of patients' lives. Before these algorithms can be included into the ordinary Healthcare sector, a careful, nonintrusive, and ethical approach is required. At all phases of the development and implementation of AI for Healthcare, the safety and confidentiality of patients' health data must be treated with concern.

The ten ethical principles presented in Fig. 16.1 address concerns unique to AI for health. These patient-centric principles are intended to guide all stakeholders in the development and deployment of accountable and trustworthy AI for health. These principles include the following:

Autonomy

The implementation of AI technology in Healthcare may raise concerns about decision-making authority being placed in the hands of computers. It is essential that AI-based Healthcare systems and medical decision-making remain under human control. Artificial intelligence technologies should never interfere with patient autonomy.

To ensure human oversight, the "Human in the Loop" (HITL) approach for AI technology allows for continuous human monitoring of the system's operation and performance. In cases where clinical choices made by AI technology and physicians differ, it can create uncertainty for the user/patient about whom to trust. In such situations, the patient should be presented with both alternatives.

Before adopting any AI technology in Healthcare, a permission process should be in place for all research studies and assessment programs. Patients must be fully informed about the medical, psychological, and social risks associated with the use of AI technology. Patients should have complete discretion over whether to accept or decline the use of AI technology. Throughout all stages of AI research and deployment, it is crucial to effectively and transparently monitor human values and moral considerations. Participants or patients should have the right to decline consent (Johnson 2020).

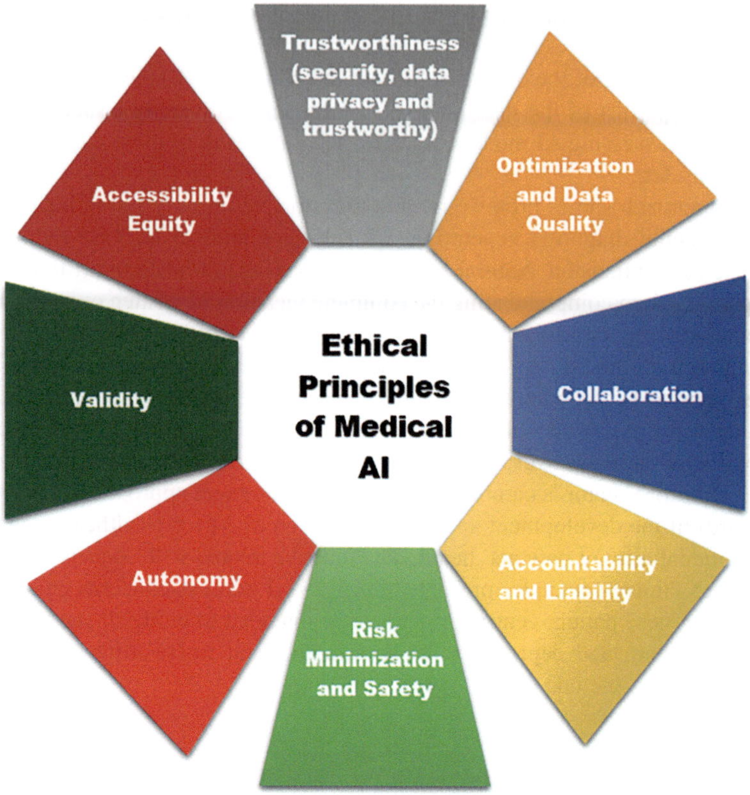

Fig. 16.1 Ethical principles in AI for Healthcare

Safety and Risk Reduction

Before widely implementing an AI technology-based system, it is crucial to ensure its secure and reliable operation. All parties involved in the development and deployment of AI-based technologies bear the responsibility of safeguarding the participants' safety. The risk of using AI-enabled technologies in areas with a high potential for patient harm must be carefully assessed. Listed below are some key risk reduction and safety considerations:

1. A comprehensive set of control mechanisms is necessary to prevent accidental or intentional misuse.
2. Due to the sensitive nature of Healthcare data, having secure systems and software is of utmost importance and an absolute necessity.
3. AI technologies should be developed with a preventative approach to risks, ensuring consistent functionality while minimizing unexpected repercussions and outcomes.

4. AI technologies are vulnerable to cyber-attacks, which can compromise the security and confidentiality of patients' data and information. Therefore, it is essential to verify that the data is entirely anonymized and disconnected from the global technology landscape to ensure its utmost safety.
5. The Ethics Committee (EC) and other relevant stakeholders should conduct a thorough benefit-risk analysis. The potential benefits must outweigh the associated risks. Considering the societal and scientific significance of AI technology, the risks must be reasonable and well managed.
6. The researcher shall take all feasible precautions for the protection of participants/patients. The measures should be evaluated by the European Commission and other regulatory organizations.
7. AI technologies should be developed in accordance with the country's legal and data protection requirements while carefully respecting ethical values.
8. A robust, expressly stated method for regularly monitoring the performance, vulnerabilities, and safety criteria of the AI technology should be in place.
9. Regarding patient data, AI technology must adhere to the strictest security standards. The manufacturer and all other stakeholders must ensure that security requirements are promptly upgraded. Publicizing patient data protection procedures allows for rigorous scrutiny, building public trust.
10. Precautions must be taken to protect and shield patients/participants from prejudice or stigmatization based on their health status, which may be disclosed by the usage of AI technology. Before adopting AI technology in Healthcare, the EU and competent authorities must carefully examine these steps.
11. Similar to clinical trials for new pharmaceuticals and devices, if new evidence of unintended harm linked with the use of AI technology emerges, the researcher/manufacturer and all other relevant stakeholders are required to notify the applicable ethics committee and data safety monitoring board. Uncommon and novel technology-related unintended harm must be tracked and recorded after introduction, akin to Phase 4 studies. The patient/participant must be made aware of the elevated risk of injury. Individuals must have the option to withdraw from the study/treatment or to continue participation.
12. AI systems with the potential to inflict physical or mental harm should be equipped with extra safety precautions. Further security measures will be evaluated by the appropriate regulatory organizations and discussed with ethical committees.
13. If vulnerable populations are engaged in the creation of AI technology at any point, additional security safeguards must be taken to protect their rights and safety. The researcher must provide justification for their inclusion.
14. All AI technologies and algorithms must undergo validation with scientific rigor in their intended environments. The algorithm's performance must be assessed across various races, ethnic groups, age groups, socioeconomic classes, and other pertinent human traits.
15. Ensuring the safety and security of vulnerable individuals requires special attention. The mix and quality of training datasets may not adequately represent the target population for the AI system. Minority populations and vulnerable

groups might be underrepresented, leading to skewed or inadequate AI performance. The European Commission, sponsors, and all other stakeholders must guarantee that the data used sufficiently represent the population. Exposing patients to unwarranted risks is unethical.
16. AI technology used to forecast the likelihood of contracting a disease may predispose the patient/participant to emotional and psychological stress, potentially leading to stigmatization of individuals or groups. The researcher and Ethics Committee (EC) must explore means of reducing this harm. Patients/participants must be thoroughly informed about the potential effects of using AI technology, including the risks of stigmatization and injury.
17. The evaluation of AI technologies and methodologies must consider the risks arising from the use of information generated by the technology, which may cause discomfort or unintended physical, psychological, social, economic, or legal harm.
18. Depending on the risk assessment of the circumstance, relevant oversight bodies/committees may be incorporated to ensure the fairness of AI technology and method development and deployment.
19. Risk reduction is an ongoing activity, and all stakeholders must ensure that the aim and impact of the technology align with its intended performance.
20. Before deploying AI technology on a large scale, it is necessary to evaluate the likelihood and severity of any harm caused by the technology. Artificial intelligence systems must not inflict significant bodily harm or mental discomfort.
21. AI developers, the EC, and relevant regulatory organizations shall examine the risk mitigation measures applied. The European Commission and other regulatory agencies can offer advice on risk mitigation techniques.

Trustworthiness

In AI for Healthcare, the most desirable attribute of any diagnostic or prognostic tool is reliability. Doctors must develop trust in the tools they employ, and AI technologies are no exception. Clinicians and Healthcare professionals require a straightforward, systematic, and reliable method for testing the validity and dependability of AI technologies to employ them successfully. A reliable AI-based solution should also possess the following characteristics:

1. Legal compliance, adhering to all applicable rules and regulations.
2. Ethical conformity, aligning with the community's treasured ethical ideals and values.
3. Dependable and valid, both from technical and social standpoints, ensuring the predictability of the outputs and consequences of AI-based solutions when implemented in various clinical situations.

4. Explainable, i.e., the outcomes and interpretations generated by AI-based algorithms must be explicable in terms of scientific plausibility. To ensure that AI technology is legitimate, trustworthy, and accountable, it must be feasible to comprehend the reasoning behind the outcomes. The absence of transparency on the decision-making processes of AI algorithms has led some to refer to it as a "black box", which can hinder its widespread adoption. It is anticipated that a well-explained AI-based solution would boost the confidence of both patients and medical practitioners.
5. In cases where a diagnostic AI technology generates results that conflict with physicians' perspectives or decisions on sickness, the credibility of both the system and the physician may be questioned. In such situations, the physician may seek advice from peers or AI developers. The patient should be informed about both the doctor(s) and AI technology's recommendations and should have the exclusive discretion to accept or reject the AI-generated conclusion.
6. Transparent, i.e., all stakeholders must have easy access to information on the development and deployment to make an educated choice. Developers of AI should offer openness at every stage so that customers can make informed decisions on data sharing and AI use. To ensure that the end-user is not exploited by AI technology, they must be presented with sufficient information in a language they can comprehend. The end-user must be made aware of the purpose, outcome, and limitations of AI technology. Without adequate information on the procedures involved, widespread adoption of AI for Health is unlikely. This is particularly significant for legal and regulatory considerations, especially when AI technologies may lead to poor Healthcare consequences due to erroneous interpretation or suggestion. Therefore, transparency, explainability, and functional comprehension are required for the regulation, adoption, and implementation of AI technology. Limitations in system transparency hinder validation, clinical advice, and the identification of mistakes and biases.
7. Before employing AI technology in the Healthcare industry, it is crucial to provide sufficient information widely. A suitable forum for public engagement and debate should be established to address design, usage, safety, and other relevant factors. Regular publication and documentation of this information are essential.
8. All AI technology must adhere to legal standards. Developers must demonstrate and ensure AI compliance with data and privacy regulations. Upgrades to the software or privacy policies for established AI systems must comply with applicable regulatory requirements.
9. Ethical obligations apply equally to artificial intelligence technologies produced outside of India. They must be openly transparent and compliant with the law, just like domestically developed AI technologies. The assessment process should be the same for any AI technology, regardless of its origin.
10. Conflicts of interest that arise at any stage of the development process must be declared and made accessible on public platforms.

Data Privacy

At all phases of development and implementation, AI-based technologies should preserve privacy and personal information. Retaining the confidence of all stakeholders, including the recipients of Healthcare, regarding the safe and secure use of personal data is crucial to the widespread use and success of AI. Personal data must be protected against unauthorized access, alteration, and/or loss. The use of AI on personal data must not unduly restrict the actual or perceived liberty of individuals. In the Healthcare industry, where medical information constitutes sensitive data that, if mishandled, might harm patients or lead to inadvertent discrimination, these standards are vital. Individual patient data should be anonymized unless preserving it in a format that allows for identification is necessary for therapeutic or research purposes (Australia's Artificial Intelligence Ethics Framework n.d. https://www.industry.gov.au/data-and-publications/australias-artificial-intelligence-ethics-frame). Prior to any data exchange, any algorithms handling patient-related data must anonymize the data appropriately. Importantly, patient identification might exist as both "Metadata" and "on-image" data, and both must be anonymized successfully. The challenges surrounding data ownership are complicated and vary depending on national or regional laws and regulations. Moreover, it relies on the level of data anonymization. Since data for constructing AI applications is frequently gathered from multiple diverse sources (e.g., medical and insurance records, pharmaceutical data, genetic data, social media data, and GPS data), it may become easier to trace that data to a patient and (intentionally or unintentionally) undermine privacy goals (https://www.industry.gov.au/data-and-publications/australias-artificial-intelligence-ethics-frame).

Responsibility and Accountability

Accountability is defined as the requirement for a person or organization to account for their activities, accept responsibility for their actions, and report the outcomes in a transparent manner. The artificial intelligence (AI) technology planned for use in the health sector must be prepared to undergo review by relevant authorities at any time. Regular internal and external audits must be conducted on AI technology to ensure their optimal functioning. These audit reports must be made available to the public.

Enhancement of Data Quality

AI is a data-driven technology whose outputs depend heavily on the data utilized for training and testing. This is of particular relevance in the field of AI for Health, since a dataset that is both skewed and insufficiently large can lead to data bias, mistakes, discrimination, etc. Data bias is seen as the greatest challenge to data-driven technologies such as AI for Healthcare. Due diligence is required to guarantee that the "training data" is devoid of known biases and accurately reflects substantial portions of the target population.

1. Before adopting AI technology, the possibility of biases must be acknowledged, detected, and evaluated rigorously.
2. Datasets utilized by AI systems should sufficiently represent the population for whom they are designed. The data of ethnic minorities, marginalized people, and populations situated in distant areas should be sufficiently represented; otherwise, oversampling may be necessary to provide the same quality of results as found with populations with higher representation.
3. The presence of bias in the dataset may impact the performance of AI technology. If there are any allegations of prejudice or indications of bias in an AI system, its functioning must be immediately suspended. The maker is responsible for removing the prejudice.
4. The process of data collecting and development of AI algorithms presents a number of obstacles and compromises, and developers and researchers must guarantee that the best data is used for their particular use case.
5. Before any AI-based technology is employed in Healthcare, these inherent data-related issues may be addressed by rigorous clinical validation.
6. All developing technologies, including AI, must undergo a rigorous evaluation procedure relevant to all fields of biological research and clinical treatment. In reality, it is advisable to develop a "pre-deployment testing" procedure to ensure that data gathering techniques are fair and comprehensive and that any deficiencies or misrepresentations are identified.
7. Low data quality and improper or inadequate data representations can result in biases, discrimination, mistakes, and inferior AI performance.

Accessibility, Fairness, Inclusion, and Equality

The use of computers for the development and implementation of AI technologies in Healthcare requires greater infrastructure availability. It is well known that the digital gap exists in virtually all nations and is more pronounced in low- and middle-income nations (LMICs).

Furthermore, the high dependence on technology may impede the widespread implementation of promising solutions in regions where it is anticipated to have a bigger impact.

1. AI developers and relevant agencies must guarantee equitable sharing of AI technologies. Different user groups should be provided with equal opportunities and access to AI technology by organizations. Particular care must be given to those that are disadvantaged or lack the necessary infrastructure to utilize this technology.
2. Artificial intelligence technology may lead to discrimination in ways that are not obvious or that violate the fundamental rights of persons.

3. AI developers and other stakeholders should prioritize making these technologies accessible to socially and economically disadvantaged groups.
4. The patient's opinion on AI technology is influenced by socioeconomic and cultural factors. AI technology must be built to accommodate a broad variety of user attributes, including gender, race, ethnicity, financial level, and others.
5. AI developers should pay extra attention to hiring individuals from varied social strata and cultural backgrounds.
6. AI systems may include local languages into its user interface to eliminate the language barrier associated with technology accessibility. It enhances AI technology acceptability and user compliance in general.
7. Certain AI systems may require internet access, technical knowledge, energy, and other infrastructure. Relevant stakeholders of AI technology should guarantee that enough infrastructure is available for the optimal and seamless operation of AI technologies designed for usage in low-resource environments.
8. The phrase "digital divide" refers to the unequal distribution of access to and utilization of information and communication technologies among a variety of various groups. The government and other key stakeholders must erase the existing digital gap in order for new technologies to be universally accepted and utilized. The deployment of advanced AI technology should not result in or exacerbate the digital gap between populations/groups.
9. Everyone participating in the creation of AI technologies, including individuals who have provided data for AI research, is morally permitted to use the technology.
10. Interoperability of artificial intelligence software must be addressed wherever feasible so that various applications may operate easily on different platforms. It expands the accessibility options available to user groups.
11. The user interface of AI technology may support many language options in order to overcome the language barrier and close the digital gap (https://main.icmr.nic.in/sites/default/files/whats_new/AI_Ethical_Guidlines.pdf).

Collaboration

The field of health-related AI is data driven. A substantial collection of meticulously managed datasets is required for any significant use of AI in Healthcare. This can only be accomplished by encouraging collaboration on all levels. Due to the quickly evolving nature of AI technology, it is essential that AI professionals collaborate throughout research and development in order to apply the most applicable approaches and algorithms to any Healthcare challenge. During the development and deployment of AI-based solutions, collaboration between AI researchers and health professionals is anticipated to increase the output of this promising technology.

1. While inter-disciplinary collaboration should be encouraged, it is essential that prospective trials of AI technologies have no negative impact on patients whose data may be utilized to develop or test algorithms.
2. Motivations for cooperation and possible conflicts of interest should be expressed publicly and, if necessary, thoroughly reviewed to prevent harm to any stakeholders.
3. Prior to beginning, any overseas partnerships or support relating to biomedical and health research must be presented to the Health Ministry's Screening Committee (HMSC) for permission (Draft Ethical Guidelines for Application of Artificial Intelligence in Biomedical Research and Healthcare. Indian Council of Medical Research. https://main.icmr.nic.in/sites/default/files/whats_new/AI_Ethical_Guidlines).

Data Collecting

The bulk of research to date on the use of deep learning in medical imaging has produced extremely promising results that frequently outperformed the performance of physicians, elevating hopes for AI tools. Unfortunately, the majority of research utilized tiny training sets, and the trained models have not been subjected to rigorous validation using huge test data from the actual world. Unknown at this time is the generalizability of these deep learning models to new patients or to various therapeutic contexts. A sufficiently enough training sample set with validated reference truth that is representative of the features of the population of interest is one of the fundamental prerequisites for developing a robust machine-learning algorithm. The unusually high number of weights in the structure of deep convolutional neural networks (DCNN) makes training deep learning even more difficult. Even with good regularization approaches to prevent overfitting, the generality of the learnt feature representations depends on how much of the training set they cover.

1. It is expensive to collect medical imaging data that are typical of the patient population and include trustworthy annotation or reference truth. While it is relatively simple to gather a high number of normal instances for a screening modality, it is challenging to collect enough abnormal cases, especially considering that the different classes in the dataset should ideally be balanced. Among the screening population, there are just a few instances per thousand for diseases like breast cancer, which is the most frequent malignancy in women. Due to factors such as patient age, breast density and size, habitus, race, ethnicity, imaging procedures, and processing methods, it is difficult to gather enough breast cancer mammograms or tomosynthesis to cover the variations in picture characteristics. Even more difficult is the collection of normal and abnormal cases with special imaging modalities, such as MR or PET, because a relatively small number of patients will undergo these examinations, and their availability may depend on the protocols for various types of diseases in various health systems.

2. Research has proved the viability of gathering a significant number of annotated cases through data mining and natural language processing of the electronic medical record (EMR) and clinical annotations in the picture archiving and communication system (PACS). It would be advisable for suppliers and users to establish uniform reporting techniques and structures across the many data archiving systems to ease the future collection of large amounts of data for the advancement of AI toward precision medicine.
3. Moreover, establishing standardized protocols for secure electronic transmission of patient files among hospitals for referral patients will not only improve the Healthcare of referral patients by transferring patient data accurately and efficiently but also increase the accuracy of data mining in these cases. Ultimately, multi-institutional collaboration may be the best way to build a large database that can encompass a wide range of heterogeneous imaging protocols and equipment, clinical settings, and patient characteristics in order to expedite the development of robust deep learning models for each type of disease that may be more applicable to a variety of clinical environments.
4. Data sharing for any national or international cooperation while protecting privacy and security is crucial in the case of employing Healthcare data in the research and development of an AI system, since it may contain very sensitive participant information. The observance of Indian laws and guidelines (DISHA and PDP norms) is required. Suitable MOUs and/or MTAs must be in place to protect the interests of participants and assure compliance (addressing concerns of confidentiality, data sharing, and joint publishing). For efficient data use, it is crucial to involve individuals whom the data are intended to benefit. Engagement of stakeholders and participation of varied interest groups improve technological communication, guaranteeing that the AI technology satisfies user requirements. (Chan et al. 2018).

Principles of Nondiscrimination and Fairness

1. The data collection used to train the algorithm must be accurate and representative of the target population. The researcher is accountable for ensuring data quality.
2. Inaccuracies and biases might result in poor or dysfunctional AI technology. External, independent algorithmic audits and ongoing end-user feedback analysis should be conducted to prevent inaccuracies and biases. The creators and researchers of AI must recognize any inherent biases and make appropriate efforts to eliminate them.
3. AI should never be used to exclude individuals. Underrepresented and vulnerable populations, such as children, ethnic minorities, and people with impairments, require special consideration. Developers of artificial intelligence should actively promote the participation of women and minority groups.

4. Developers should pay special attention to promoting and maintaining individual equality. Freedom, rights, and dignity should be handled fairly and with respect.
5. AI technology should be created for widespread use. It is immoral to discriminate against individuals or groups based on race, age, caste, religion, or social standing.
6. The reversibility of judgments made by AI technology should be evaluated if any patient or participant has been harmed. Before adopting the technology, the option for decision reversibility must be incorporated into the architecture of the AI.
7. In the event that any bad occurrences result from the malfunction of AI technology, the victim should have access to an adequate recourse mechanism. The maker must guarantee that there is adequate recourse for customer complaints.
8. There must be a secure way to communicate concerns about AI technology; these problems may be technical, functional, ethical, or related to the misuse of technology. There should be a suitable protection framework for whistleblowers.

Validity

Before being applied to patients/participants, AI technology in Healthcare must undergo extensive clinical and field validation. These validations are required to guarantee safety and efficacy. Due to discrepancies in the datasets used for training AI systems, algorithmic divergence may be exacerbated. Therefore, there must be an internal method to monitor such issues and provide developers with pertinent input while keeping the clinical context in mind (Draft Ethical Guidelines for Application of Artificial Intelligence in Biomedical Research and Healthcare. Indian Council of Medical Research. https://main.icmr.nic.in/sites/default/files/whats_new/AI_Ethical_Guidlines).

References

Australia's Artificial Intelligence Ethics Framework | Department of Industry, Science, Energy and Resources. n.d.. https://www.industry.gov.au/data-and-publications/australias-artificial-intelligence-ethics-frame.

Balthazar P, Harri P, Prater A, Safdar NM. Protecting your patients' interests in the era of big data, artificial intelligence, and predictive analytics. J Am Coll Radiol. 2018;15(3):580–6. https://doi.org/10.1016/j.jacr.2017.11.035.

Chan HP, Samala RK, Hadjiiski LM, Zhou C. Deep learning in medical image analysis. Adv Exp Med Biol. 2020;1213:3–21. https://doi.org/10.1007/978-3-030-33128-3_1.

Cohen EB, Gordon IK. First, do no harm. Ethical and legal issues of artificial intelligence and machine learning in veterinary radiology and radiation oncology. Vet Radiol Ultrasound. 2022;63(1):840–50. https://doi.org/10.1111/vru.13171.

Draft Ethical Guidelines for Application of Artificial Intelligence in Biomedical Research and Healthcare. Indian Council of Medical Research 2018. https://main.icmr.nic.in/sites/default/files/whats_new/AI_Ethical_Guidlines.

Geis JR, Brady AP, Wu CC, Spencer J, Ranschaert E, Jaremko JL, Langer SG, Kitts AB, Birch J, Shields WF, van den Hoven van Genderen R. Ethics of artificial intelligence in radiology: summary of the joint European and north American multisociety statement. Can Assoc Radiol J. 2019;70(4):329–34.

Johnson J. What is human in the loop (HITL) machine learning? (2020); BMC Software | Blogs. https://www.bmc.com/blogs/hitl-human-in-the-loop/. Accessed 5 July 2022.

Kayaalp M. Patient privacy in the era of big data. Balkan Med J. 2018;2018(35):8–17.

Leslie D, Burr C, Aitken M, Cowls J, Katell M, Briggs M.. Artificial intelligence, human rights, democracy, and the rule of law: a primer. The Council of Europe. 2021.

Mongan J, Kohli M. Artificial intelligence and human life: five lessons for radiology from the 737 MAX disasters. Radiol Artif Intell. 2020;2(2):e190111.

Schloendorff V. Society of New York Hospital. New York: Court of Appeals; 1914. p. 92.

Wang SY, Pershing S, Lee AY. Big data requirements for artificial intelligence. Curr Opin Ophthalmol. 2020;31(5):318–23. https://doi.org/10.1097/ICU.0000000000000676.

Yu KH, Beam AL, Kohane IS. Artificial intelligence in Healthcare. Nat Biomed Eng. 2018;2(10):719–31. https://doi.org/10.1038/s41551-018-0305-z.

Deep Learning in Image Processing: Part 1—Types of Neural Networks, Image Segmentation

17

Ruben Pauwels and Alexandros Iosifidis

Introduction

Image processing gained traction in the 1970s and 1980s, owing to the increased digitization in radiography as well as the introduction of advanced imaging modalities, such as computed tomography (CT) and magnetic resonance imaging (MRI). Throughout the following decades, a variety of advanced image processing algorithms have been developed. Strictly speaking, several of these algorithms can be considered as 'artificial intelligence' (AI), as they often involve the replacement of a human task. For example, automatic segmentation techniques offer an alternative to manual recognition and delineation of objects in an image. However, the introduction of deep learning, and particularly that of convolutional neural networks (CNN) trained on graphics processing units (GPU), has revolutionized the image processing field in recent years.

In this chapter and the subsequent one, an overview of AI applications in image processing will be provided. The focus will be on *deep learning* (DL); with the exception of unsupervised clustering methods used in segmentation, all applications shown or mentioned in this chapter involve the use of a type of deep *neural network* (NN). In this chapter, a brief description of NN types and architectures that are commonly used in image processing is provided, followed by an overview of DL applications in image segmentation. The next chapter will focus on applications in image

R. Pauwels (✉)
Department of Dentistry and Oral Health, Aarhus University, Aarhus, Denmark

Department of Radiology, Faculty of Dentistry, Chulalongkorn University, Bangkok, Thailand
e-mail: ruben.pauwels@dent.au.dk

A. Iosifidis
DIGIT, Department of Electrical and Computer Engineering, Aarhus University, Aarhus, Denmark
e-mail: ai@ece.au.dk

K. Orhan, R. Jagtap (eds.), *Artificial Intelligence in Dentistry*,
https://doi.org/10.1007/978-3-031-43827-1_17

enhancement, reconstruction, and registration. An exhaustive literature review is beyond the scope of this chapter; in-depth reviews on particular applications will be cited accordingly.

Types of Neural Networks Used in Image-to-Image Processing

Convolutional Neural Networks

Encoder-Decoder

An encoder-decoder network is typically formed by two connected neural networks, an encoder and a decoder. The encoder receives an input (e.g., a vector, an image, a video, or text) and produces a new representation of it in a new space, usually called a latent space. The decoder receives a representation of the input in the latent space and produces an output which has the same dimensions as the input to the encoder (Fig. 17.1). By training these two connected neural networks jointly, i.e., by optimizing their parameters with the output of the decoder corresponding to the desired output (or target) for the input to the encoder, this type of neural network is suitable for performing various types of input-to-output mappings (e.g., image-to-image mapping). When the target for the decoder corresponding to an input to the encoder is that same input, the neural network takes the form of an autoencoder. When the input to the encoder is a noisy version of the target of the decoder, the neural network takes the form of a *denoising autoencoder* (Vincent et al. 2010). When the latent space representation of the entire training set is forced to follow a predefined distribution (commonly a multidimensional Gaussian distribution) and

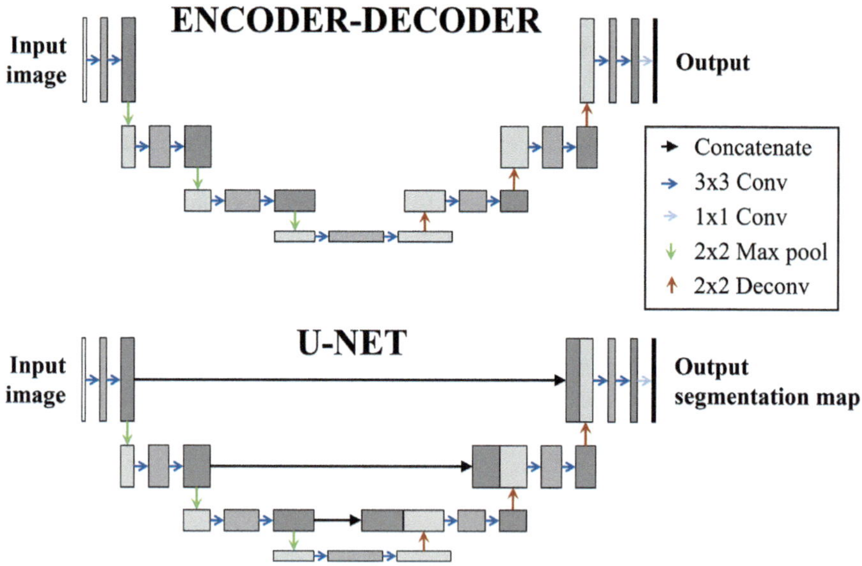

Fig. 17.1 Examples of a typical encoder-decoder (*top*) and U-Net (*bottom*) architecture

the input to the decoder is randomly sampled from that distribution, the neural network takes the form of a *variational autoencoder* (Kingma and Welling 2014). Here we need to mention that encoder-decoder networks do not necessarily need to be autoencoders, i.e., the target for the decoder does not necessarily need to be the input to the encoder (or a denoised version of it) but rather a target which has the same dimensions as the input to the encoder. An example of such a case is that of color image segmentation, where an input image corresponding to a tensor of *WxHx3* elements (where the last dimension corresponds to the three color channels of the image) is introduced to the encoder and the target for the decoder is a map with *WxH* elements, each corresponding to the segment label of a pixel in the input image.

U-Net

A U-Net CNN is a commonly used network architecture for (semantic) image segmentation, introduced in 2015 (Ronneberger et al. 2015). It is similar to an image encoder-decoder in the sense that it consists of two mirrored paths, i.e., a contracting and an expansive path (Fig. 17.1). The contracting path comprises successive convolutional layers, pooling and downsampling. In the original version of the network, the 2D input image has a size of 572 × 572 pixels, and the contracting path results in a tensor with 32 × 32 × 512 elements. In the expansive path of the network, upsampling (i.e., deconvolution) and concatenation of feature maps of the outputs of layers in the contracting path are used to combine features from each resolution step into a segmentation map. This concatenation of feature maps produced by the contracting and expansive paths is expressed in the form of *skip connections* (see also section "Residual Neural Network"). This allows for the extraction of both low-resolution and high-resolution features in the image to produce the final output segmentation map.

The main difference between an encoder-decoder-type and a U-Net-type NN is the connections between the two mirrored paths for the latter. An encoder-decoder network can be split up and used as separate parts; in fact, the encoder would be similar to an image compression-type network, and the decoder would be similar to a generative network producing its output based on the latent representation of the input image. For a U-Net-type NN, the skip connections make the output mapping at a given level of the network depend on the lower-resolution level of the expansive path as well as the same-resolution level of the contracting path.

Residual Neural Network

The residual neural network (ResNet) was introduced in 2015 to address the vanishing/exploding gradient issue for networks with a large number of layers (He et al. 2016). ResNet makes use of *skip connections*, which, as their name implies, allow for layers that negatively affect the model's performance to be bypassed. More importantly, these skip connections allow the gradients of the error (i.e., loss) to follow a shorter path for reaching the earlier layers of the network, which leads to more effective training of all layers in deep neural networks. ResNet architectures and pretrained models, such as ResNet50 and ResNet152, are widely used for a variety of applications, most notably for image classification. The general principle of having multiple pathways in an NN, effectively skipping certain layers, is also applied in other NN architectures. A commonly used NN with a large degree of skip connections is DenseNet (Huang et al. 2017).

Generative Adversarial Network

A generative adversarial network (GAN) is a particular type of machine learning framework, in which two neural networks are in competition with each other. The first one, the *generator*, attempts to generate synthetic data in accordance with a set of 'real' training data. The second, the *discriminator*, attempts to distinguish real data from synthetic data (Fig. 17.2). The result is a zero-sum game in which the generator attempts to generate more realistic data throughout the training process (or, more correctly, data that fools the discriminator), and the discriminator attempts to improve its recognition ability of characteristics that distinguish real from synthetic data.

GANs used to generate images by using convolutional layers are typically referred to as deep convolutional generative adversarial networks (DCGAN). Variations of GANs with use for image-to-image translation include conditional adversarial networks (cGAN; Isola et al. 2016) and cycle-consistent adversarial networks (cycleGAN; Zhu et al. 2017); the latter can be used when paired data is not available.

One of the main challenges in GAN training is the rate at which the two components learn. If the generator learns too fast, this can lead to mode collapse (i.e., an inability to generalize). On the other hand, if the discriminator learns too fast, the vanishing gradient problem may occur, in which the generator is unable to improve using gradient-based optimization. A popular variant of GAN that addresses these,

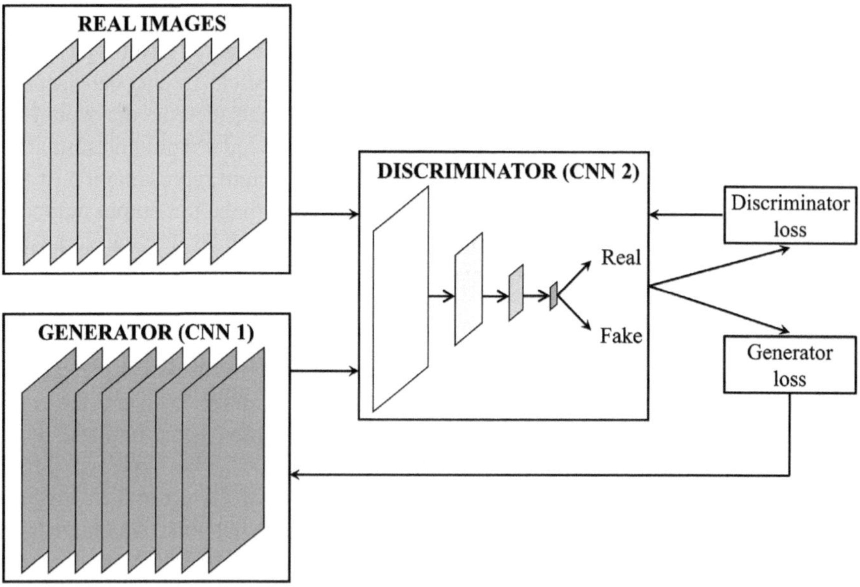

Fig. 17.2 General principle of a generative adversarial network (GAN)

and other, issues is the Wasserstein GAN (WGAN; Arjovsky et al. 2017). A WGAN uses a different metric for the discriminator, leading to improved overall learning stability and an increased ability to fine-tune hyperparameters. Alternative approaches for a more stable learning outcome for GANs include progressive growing (Karras et al. 2018) and spectral normalization (Miyato et al. 2018).

Region-Based Convolutional Neural Network (R-CNN)

R-CNNs (Girshick et al. 2013) are a family of NNs, initially aimed at object detection but covering various other tasks nowadays. The general principle involves a sequence of regions of interest (ROIs) detection, feature extraction, and classification (Fig. 17.3). This could be considered a more efficient and flexible approach compared to patch-based or sliding-window techniques, as it allows for irrelevant parts of the image to be ignored and for ROIs to be adapted to the size of the object(s) of interest.

Several versions of R-CNN have been developed over the years. The initial version used selective search (Uijlings et al. 2013) to identify ROIs, followed by introducing each of these ROIs to the CNN for classifying them to object classes. Subsequent variations/improvements included:

- *Fast R-CNN,* a commonly used variation, in which an NN operates on the whole image, and ROI-specific features are extracted at the end (Girshick 2015)
- *Faster R-CNN*, which incorporates the ROI generation into the NN rather than using selective search, allowing for real-time data throughput (Ren et al. 2017)
- *Mask R-CNN*, which allows, for instance, segmentation rather than object detection, as well as the use of subpixels (He et al. 2020)
- *Mesh R-CNN,* which builds on Mask R-CNN to predict 3D meshes from 2D images (Gkioxari et al. 2019)

Vision Transformers

A Transformer neural network is based on the *attention* principle (Luong et al. 2015). Attention learning, in a very general sense, allows an NN to focus on certain parts or aspects of the input data. In the case of Transformers, attention helps in

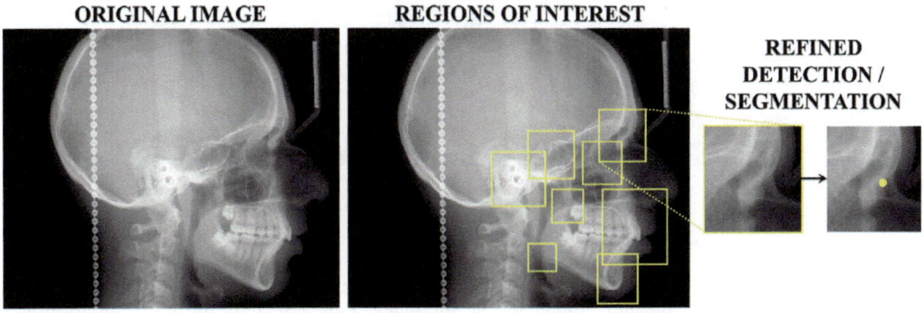

Fig. 17.3 General principle of region-based convolutional neural networks

making associations between the different parts of the input in a data-driven manner. This is achieved by determining relationships between sets of input tokens using the scaled dot-product attention mechanism.

While Transformers were initially applied in natural language processing, they have also been adapted for image processing tasks in the form of Vision Transformers (ViT; Cordonnier et al. 2019). The overall principle is to assess relationships between pixels (or voxels) within small subsections of an image. While this can be considered as a type of encoding, which would make it suitable for image classification tasks, the addition of a Transformer Decoder allows for image-to-image processing. One of the drawbacks of Transformers is that they need to receive as input the entire sequence of tokens used for providing their output, leading to much slower operation compared with recurrent neural networks (RNNs), which receive as input the tokens as a sequence. The Continual Transformer (Co-Trans) reformulates the scaled dot-product attention, allowing the Transformer Encoder layer to operate in a token-by-token manner (Hedegaard et al. 2023).

Graph Neural Networks

In graph theory, a graph can be defined as a structure composed of *nodes* (also called vertices or points) and *edges* (also called lines or links). The simplicity of the graph data structure makes it highly flexible, with endless applications in mathematics, physics, biology, social sciences, etc.

An image can be considered as a special type of graph, in which the nodes are equally spaced on a Euclidean grid as pixels or voxels (Fig. 17.4). Thus, convolutional neural networks can be considered as a type of GNN that involves convolutional filters and pooling operators for processing structured data. However, when data is not structured on a grid, CNNs cannot be applied. Thus, geometric deep learning has emerged as an area that explores graphs in non-Euclidean spaces in particular (Bronstein et al. 2017).

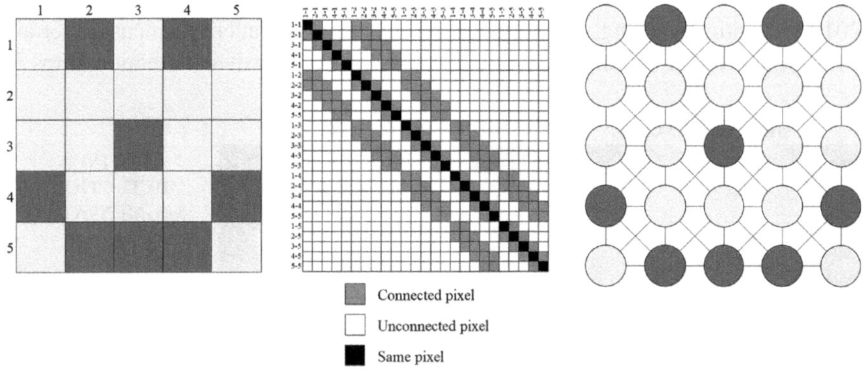

Fig. 17.4 An image can be represented in various ways. *Left*: conventional representation as a grid of pixels. *Middle*: adjacency matrix, indicating pixels that are connected. *Right*: graph representation of an image

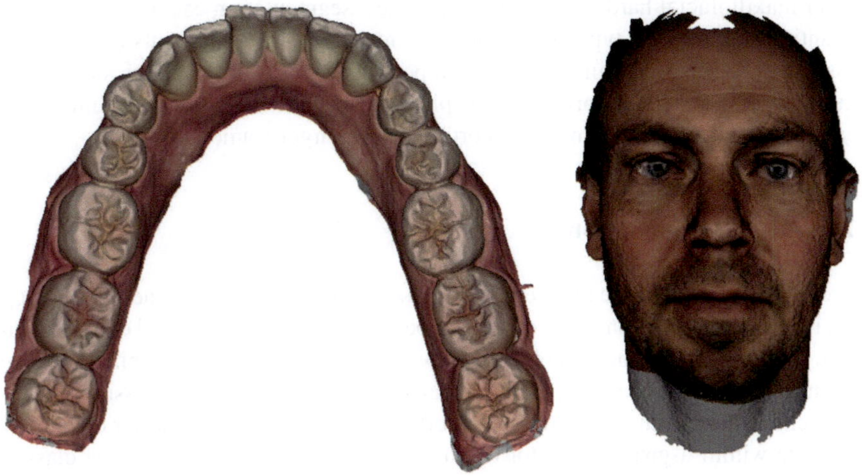

Fig. 17.5 Examples of mesh-type data used in dentistry. *Left*: intra-oral scan. *Right*: facial scan. (Courtesy of Mohammedreza Sefidroodi and Peter Bangsgaard Stoustrup, Section of Orthodontics, Department of Dentistry, Aarhus University, Denmark)

A typical type of data that does not follow the grid-like structure of images is a *polygon mesh*. While CNNs cannot be readily used on mesh data, GNNs can easily be adapted for this purpose, as a mesh can be considered as a set of vertices and edges. In medical imaging, several examples can be found of mesh-type data that could benefit from the use of GNNs. Intra-oral scanning is often used within digital dentistry and facial scanning/photogrammetry is used in orthodontics and orthognathic surgery, among others (Fig. 17.5). Furthermore, surface renderings (e.g., from CT or CBCT data) are used for visualization and for the creation of surgical guides. For this type of data in particular, GNNs can be of interest. However, they can also be of benefit in image processing, e.g., through the use of superpixels that do not follow the Euclidean grid-like structure of the original image.

Several variations of GNNs have been explored in recent years, including the *graph convolutional network* (GCN; Kipf and Welling 2016) and *graph attention network* (GAT; Veličković et al. 2017), which are able to learn transformations of the input representations of the graph nodes by exploiting information of node connectivity expressed in the graph structure and, in the case of GAT, by learning new connections between graph nodes in a data-driven manner based on graph attention.

AI in Image Segmentation

Image segmentation involves the partitioning of images into specific regions. Several uses of segmentation can be found in medical imaging. In many cases, anatomical structures of interest require segmentation for advanced visualization; a typical example is the creation of volume/surface renderings of the jaws, teeth, and other maxillofacial hard tissues. In many cases, segmentation can also be used for quantitative purposes, typically involving dimensional measurements (e.g., airway assessment). Finally, segmentation of important anatomical structures such as the mandibular canal can be pivotal in the planning and risk assessment of third molar extractions, implant placement, and orthognathic surgery, among others.

Types of Segmentation

In computer vision, three different types of segmentation can be defined (Fig. 17.6). An important distinction between these types of segmentation is based on the countable nature of the segmented objects. In *instance segmentation*, each pixel/voxel of an image is assigned to a (typically predefined) class. Examples of possible classes on a clinical image are 'hard tissues', 'soft tissues', 'air', etc. No further distinction is made within a given class; for example, if 'hard tissues' is one of the classes, semantic segmentation will make no distinction between the individual bones or teeth. In other words, semantic segmentation does not assume that the segmented objects are countable; this is typically referred to as the segmentation of *stuff*. In contrast, *instance segmentation* makes a distinction between individual objects within a given class. For example, whereas semantic segmentation may distinguish 'teeth' voxels from 'non-teeth' voxels on an image, instance segmentation will result in separate individual teeth; such individual instances are referred to as *things*.

While both types of segmentation can be applicable for image processing tasks in medicine, it can often be beneficial to consider an image as a combination of *stuff* and *things*. To this end, *panoptic segmentation* was introduced in 2018 (Kirillov et al. 2018). This approach combines semantic and instance segmentation; it aims to provide both a semantic label and a unique instance identifier to each pixel in an image.

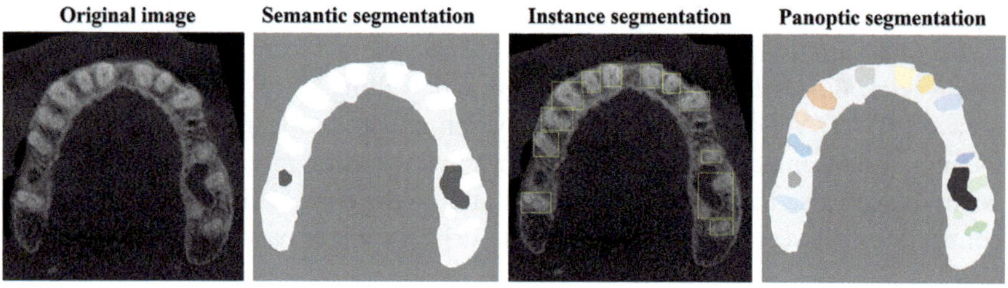

Fig. 17.6 Examples of semantic segmentation (pixel-based classification of bone, teeth, and sinus), instance segmentation (bounding box detection of individual teeth), and panoptic segmentation (combining semantic and instance segmentation)

Supervised Segmentation: Clinical Applications

The following subsections describe the most common clinical applications of DL-based segmentation of anatomical structures in dentistry: hard tissues (bones and teeth), mandibular canal, air-filled structures (sinus and upper airways), and cephalometric landmarks. A number of research studies are briefly summarized; an exhaustive review of all literature on the topic is beyond the scope of this chapter.

Bone/Tooth Segmentation

Segmentation of the mandible, maxilla, and other bones in the maxillofacial region can be useful for several purposes, such as 3D visualization (surface/volume rendering) and computer-assisted surgery. Tooth segmentation can be split up into (1) segmenting the crowns as part of a 3D *hard tissue* model of the mandible and/or maxilla, (2) segmenting the *entire tooth* (incl. root) for applications such as autotransplantation and 3D orthodontic planning, and (3) tooth identification and *numbering* for the purpose of charting. The use of deep learning for segmenting dentomaxillofacial bones and teeth has been explored for several imaging modalities.

(Cone-Beam) Computed Tomography

Accurate segmentation of bones and teeth on CT or CBCT scans can be complicated using conventional intensity- or edge-based segmentation methods. Individual tooth segmentation can be difficult due to the close contact between neighboring teeth and the narrow (and sometimes interrupted) periodontal ligament space. Furthermore, metal artifacts can affect tooth segmentation quality considerably. Another challenge, particularly for CBCT segmentation, is the high variability in image quality (sharpness, contrast, noise, geometric accuracy) between scanners from different manufacturers (Pauwels et al. 2012; Liang et al. 2010; Kosalagood et al. 2015). Furthermore, the unreliability of Hounsfield Unit (HU) calibration in CBCT complicates any threshold-based approach toward segmentation due to differences in gray value distribution between patients, scan protocols, and region of interest (ROI) positions relative to the field of view (Pauwels et al. 2015).

In a study by Minnema et al. (2019), the mandible and tooth crowns were segmented on CBCT scans in the presence of metal artifacts. They reported mean Dice similarity coefficients (DSCs) between 0.86 and 0.87 for DL-based segmentation models (mixed-scale dense CNN, U-Net, and ResNet), which outperformed a semi-automatic clinical benchmark algorithm based on thresholding and seed points. Another study by Minnema et al. (2018), involving CNN-based segmentation of skulls on CT data, showed a DSC of 0.92 and mean absolute deviations of 0.44 mm. Dot et al. (2022a) used a self-configuring U-Net-type network for the segmentation of various craniomaxillofacial structures on head CT scans; they found a DSC for segmented volumes of 0.962 for the upper skull, 0.942 for the mandible, and 0.948/0.944 for upper/lower teeth. Average surface distances were within 0.2 mm for all structures.

It can be seen that the majority of studies involve the use of a U-Net-type network as the main backbone of their segmentation process. However, due to the small voxel sizes that are generally used in CBCT, it can be challenging to use U-Nets on the entire dataset due to GPU memory limitations. Instead, a two-phase approach has been proposed for mandibular segmentation of CBCT scans, in which the first 3D U-Net performs a rough segmentation of downsampled scans and a second one performs a fine segmentation on smaller patches (Verhelst et al. 2021). This method showed DSCs of 0.972 and 0.971 and root mean square (RMS) distances of 0.263 mm and 0.269 mm for fully automated and manually refined DL-based segmentations, respectively, compared with a conventional semi-automatic segmentation method. The same approach was used for segmenting the maxillofacial complex (Preda et al. 2022), showing a DSC of 0.926 and RMS distance of 0.5 mm for DL segmentations vs. fully manual segmentations, which significantly outperformed a semi-automated segmentation method (DSC: 0.687; RMS: 1.76 mm). Alternatively, modified versions of U-Net can be used that do not require as many high- and low-resolution representations of the input image. For example, Yan et al. (2018) compared various networks for mandible segmentation on CT, including a traditional 2D U-Net architecture and different end-to-end symmetric CNNs (SCNNs) without pooling or upsampling. The best-performing SCNN network architecture resulted in a DSC of 0.922. Another study proposed the use of a DenseNet for mandibular segmentation, which resulted in a DSC of 0.938 and slightly outperformed original and modified U-Net architectures (DSC: 0.919 and 0.931, respectively; Torosdagli et al. 2019). Further study is needed to determine optimal network architectures for a given segmentation task, considering accuracy, training/inference speed, and memory consumption.

Several studies focused specifically on the segmentation of individual teeth, in which deep learning was combined with other image processing methods. Chen et al. (2020) proposed a DL method using a dual-branch fully convolutional network, which yields separate probability maps for the tooth bodies and tooth surfaces, and a post-processing step to combine these two segmentation maps into a final result (Fig. 17.7). The new method resulted in a DSC of 0.936 and an error (i.e., average symmetric surface distance, ASSD) of 0.363 mm. A 3D U-Net and 3D DenseNet showed similar segmentation performance, with the latter showing a slightly larger error of 0.450 mm. All deep learning-based methods greatly outperformed alternative segmentation approaches using connected region extraction (mean error: 3.6 mm) or a level-set method (mean error: > 4 mm). Rao et al. (2020) used a residual network to yield a segmentation probability map of teeth on CBCT scans, along with a dense conditional random field method for obtaining the final semantic segmentation result, showing an ASSD of 0.25. The combination of a U-Net with a dense block also resulted in improved segmentation performance for teeth on CBCT scans (DSC: 0.918) compared with an original U-Net or a level-set method (Lee et al. 2020). Another study combined a modified U-Net and level-set method for tooth segmentation on CT scans; they found that the combined use of the two methods outperformed both individual methods (Gou et al. 2019).

In some cases, bone segmentation serves as an intermediary step for determining certain landmarks of interest (Torosdagli et al. 2019; Zhang et al. 2020). See section "Cephalometry" for more on DL-based cephalometric landmark detection.

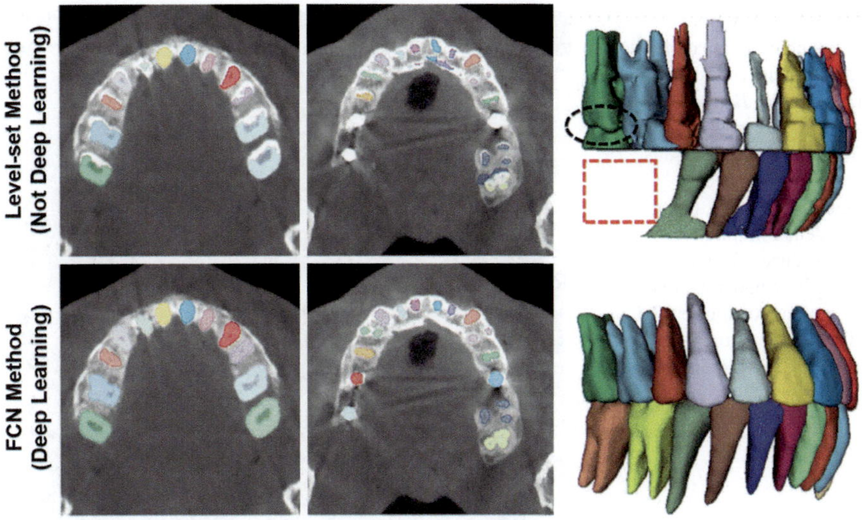

Fig. 17.7 Deep learning for tooth segmentation on cone-beam computed tomography scans. *Top row*: Conventional segmentation using level-set method. *Bottom row*: multi-task 3D fully conventional network (FCN) with marker-controlled watershed transform. The *black circle* and *red rectangle* indicate specific regions in which the level-set method failed. (Reproduced from Chen et al. 2020 under a Creative Commons Attribution 4.0 International License; relabeled version of original figure)

Panoramic Radiography

Segmentation of anatomical structures on panoramic radiographs can serve many purposes, from charting to initial diagnosis and treatment planning. Due to the unique geometry of panoramic radiography, resulting in anatomical overlap (incl. double and ghost images), accurate detection and segmentation can be non-trivial. Therefore, most research studies involved a combination of multiple neural networks for this purpose.

As mentioned in section "Types of Segmentation", depending on the structure that is segmented, either semantic or instance segmentation can be used. Thus, a comprehensive segmentation of various anatomical structures on panoramic radiographs may require a combination of both types of segmentation. Cha et al. (2021) developed a panoptic segmentation model for different structures on panoramic radiographs using the Panoptic-DeepLab network architecture by Cheng et al. (2020), which contains a semantic segmentation branch and instance segmentation branch. For the maxillary sinus, maxilla, mandible, and mandibular canal, they used semantic segmentation, whereas for normal teeth, treated teeth, and dental implants, instance segmentation was used (Fig. 17.8). For bone and teeth, intersection-over-union (IoU) values of 0.886 and 0.895 were reached, respectively. The average precision was 0.772 for normal teeth, 0.490 for treated teeth, and 0.714 for dental implants.

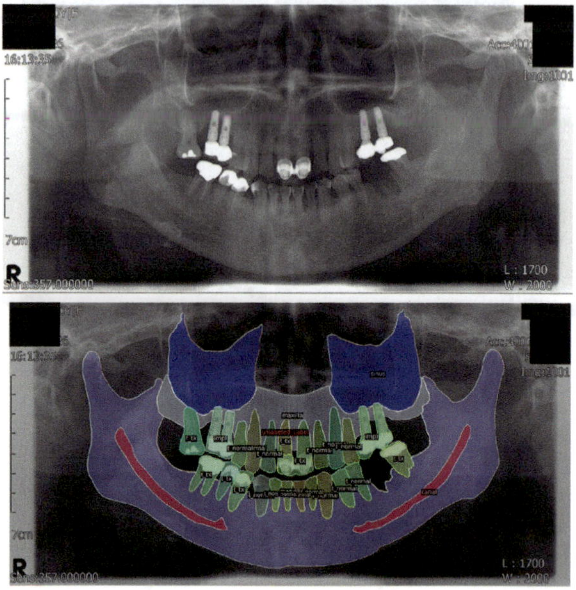

Fig. 17.8 Panoptic segmentation on panoramic radiographs. *Top*: original radiographs. *Bottom*: color-coded segmentation maps for maxillary sinus, maxilla, mandible, mandibular canal, teeth, and dental implants. (Reproduced from Cha et al. 2021 under a Creative Commons Attribution (CC BY) license; cropped version of original figure)

Several studies focused specifically on tooth numbering on panoramic radiographs, which could involve either a bounding box (using an object detection model) or an exact outline of each tooth (using a semantic segmentation model). The most commonly found network architectures for this task are U-Nets and (Mask or Faster) R-CNNs. Adnan et al. (2023) combined a U-Net with a Faster R-CNN, with the former yielding semantic segmentation maps and the latter resulting in bounding boxes; this combined approach is comparable to panoptic segmentation. A similar approach was proposed by Chandrashekar et al. (2022), using a Mask R-CNN and Faster R-CNN for tooth segmentation and identification. Their collaborative model resulted in an accuracy of 0.988 for segmentation, which outperformed a singular Mask R-CNN and U-Net. For identification, the accuracy was 0.984, which was only outperformed by a YOLO-v5 network (0.995); the latter is based on a Cross Stage Partial Network (CSPN) architecture (Wang et al. 2019a). Prados-Privado et al. (2021) also applied a Mask R-CNN for an initial segmentation map, followed by a ResNet-101 network for tooth classification. They found an accuracy of 0.992 for tooth detection and 0.938 for tooth numbering. Another study using a Mask R-CNN with ResNet-101 resulted in a precision, recall, and F1 score of 1.000, 0.972, and 0.947 for segmentation, and 0.944, 0.952, and 0.933 for tooth numbering, which outperformed 'classical' neural network classifier architectures, such as AlexNet, GoogLeNet, and MobileNet, by a significant margin (Yaren Tekin et al. 2022). Bilgir et al. (2021) used a Faster R-CNN Inception v2 model for tooth detection and numbering, showing a precision of 0.965, sensitivity of 0.956, and F1 score of 0.961. Estai et al. (2022) proposed a three-step procedure for tooth detection and numbering, comprising a U-Net for initial segmentation, a Faster R-CNN for tooth identification, and a VGG-16 network (i.e., a contractive CNN with 13 convolutional layers and 3 dense layers) for numbering. Tooth detection was performed with a precision and sensitivity of 0.99, whereas tooth numbering showed a precision, sensitivity, and F1 score of 0.98. Tuzoff et al. (2019) opted for an approach in which semantic segmentation is not performed as a first step; instead, they used a Faster R-CNN for tooth detection and a VGG-16 architecture for tooth numbering.

A few studies explored detection and numbering of primary and permanent teeth on *pediatric* panoramic radiographs, which is a more challenging task due to the crowding of teeth and the incomplete development of permanent teeth. Kaya et al. (2022) used a YOLO-v4 model for this purpose; they reported a precision of 0.922, sensitivity of 0.944, and F1 score of 0.91. Kılıc et al. (2021) used the same Faster R-CNN Inception v2 network as Bilgir et al. (2021) for deciduous tooth detection and numbering on pediatric panoramic radiographs, showing similar performance to the adult tooth numbering model in the aforementioned study, with a precision of 0.957, sensitivity of 0.980, and F1 score of 0.969.

Intra-oral Radiography

Similar to studies involving panoramic radiography, DL has been explored in intra-oral radiography for *tooth numbering* and/or *delineation*. Kabir et al. (2022) used a U-Net/ResNet-34 network for segmentation of bone and teeth on periapical radiographs, followed by a tooth detection/numbering algorithm. In addition, they applied DL models for periodontal diagnosis and caries detection. For tooth segmentation and numbering, a DSC of 0.93, and a precision and sensitivity of 0.96 was reported, respectively. Several other studies used region-based CNNs (R-CNN). Chen et al. (2019a) used a residual R-CNN for teeth detection along with a separate NN for predicting missing teeth on periapical radiographs. They found a precision of 0.988, sensitivity of 0.985 and a mean IoU of 0.91, which is on par with human observers (Fig. 17.9). A pretrained R-CNN (Inception v3) with transfer learning for tooth detection/numbering on periapical radiographs showed a precision of 0.781, sensitivity of 0.987, and F1 score of 0.872 (Görürgöz et al. 2022). Another study using an R-CNN for tooth detection and numbering on bitewing radiographs showed a precision of 0.929, a sensitivity of 0.975 and an F1 score of 0.952 (Yasa et al. 2021).

Intra-oral Scans

With the increasing use of intra-oral scans (IOS) in the digital dental workflow, several studies have explored the segmentation and numbering of tooth crowns on IOS. Due to the different nature of this data (see 2.3), conventional convolution-based neural networks such as U-Nets cannot be readily used. To this end, Xu et al. (2019) proposed a segmentation approach in which features are extracted from the IOS mesh data and organized in 20x30 patches, after which CNNs are used to label the teeth, followed by several refinements. Their method resulted in a mean segmentation error of 0.085 mm.

Hao et al. (2022) proposed a two-step segmentation process in which (1) the IOS is resampled as a point cloud, followed by segmentation using a Dynamic Graph CNN (DGCNN; Wang et al. 2019b) and further optimization using a graph cut algorithm, and (2) a confidence evaluation, which indicates a need for manual

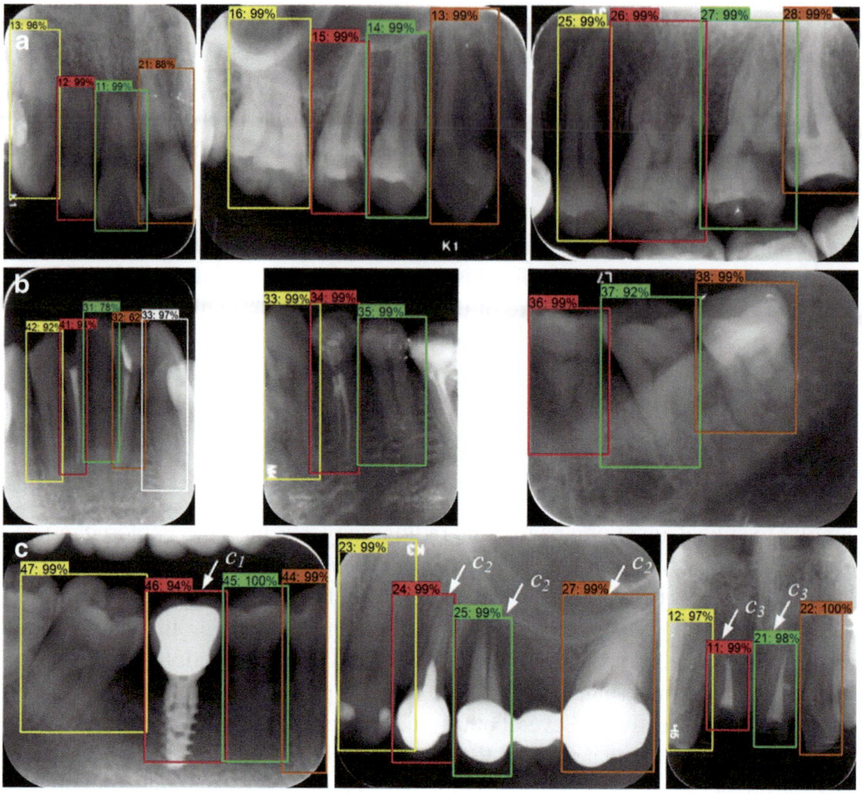

Fig. 17.9 Tooth detection and numbering on intra-oral radiographs. Each *bounding box* denotes the estimated tooth number and corresponding probability for (**a**) upper teeth, (**b**) lower teeth, (**c**) complicated cases (Reproduced from Chen et al. 2019a under a Creative Commons Attribution 4.0 International License)

correction. A clinical evaluation of their method showed that 2.9% of the segmentations were flagged for correction, and 0.2% actually needed to be redone manually. The model requires approx. 24 s to generate segmentations vs. 15 min by human experts. Liu et al. (2023) proposed a contrastive self-supervised framework consisting of (1) resampling to a point cloud and preprocessing to 'region-level' and 'point-level' input pairs, (2) parallel learning modules for the region- and point-level data, and (3) supervised fine-tuning using the aforementioned DGCNN-type layers and dense layers. The proposed method resulted in a DSC of 0.949, outperforming other supervised and unsupervised methods.

Wu et al. (2022) adapted and modified networks developed for mesh data (MeshSegNet) and point-cloud data (PointNet) for tooth segmentation and landmark identification, respectively, in a two-stage framework. Similar to the study by Hao et al. (2022), they used a graph cut approach to refine the initial segmentation, resulting in a DSC of 0.964. The mean absolute error for landmark detection, comprising contact points, gingival points, cusps, and mesial/distal line angles, was

0.597 mm. Notably, the segmentation only required 0.6 s of computational time per IOS.

Intra-oral Photographs/Videos

Apart from the aforementioned applications of DL on radiographic, tomographic, and IOS data, there is an interest in automated processing of photographic data as well, owing to the increasing use of intra-oral cameras. In this case, segmentation of the tooth surface can be performed as an intermediary step for caries detection or other tasks (Fig. 17.10; Park et al. 2022).

Mandibular Canal (MC) Segmentation

The MC—containing the inferior alveolar nerve, artery, and vein—is an important anatomical structure due to its proximity to the lower teeth and the risk of injury during treatment, especially implant placement, third molar extraction, and orthognathic surgery. Therefore, several studies explored DL for MC segmentation, mostly within the context of implant planning or third molar assessment.

Cone-Beam Computed Tomography

Similar to bone/teeth segmentation (see above), MC segmentation on CBCT using DL can be challenging due to the relatively high resolution of the scans, causing excessive GPU memory consumption. However, as the MC is a continuous structure with a relatively consistent shape, it makes sense to retain the 3D information

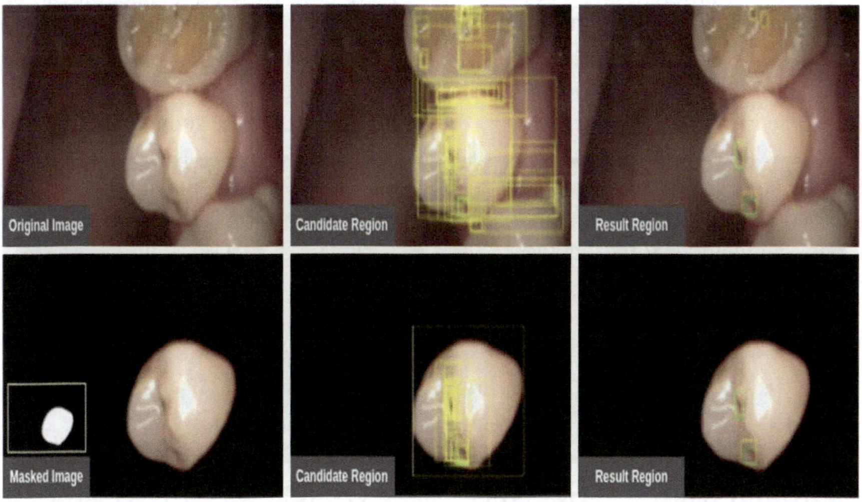

Fig. 17.10 Segmentation of tooth area on intra-oral photographs/videos. *Top row*: A Faster R-CNN for caries detection applied directly to the original image. *Bottom row:* the same model applied to a tooth segmented using a U-Net. The latter approach can improve the detection accuracy considerably by masking irrelevant parts of the image. (Reproduced from Park et al. 2022 under a Creative Commons Attribution 4.0 International License; cropped version of original figure)

provided by the entire CBCT scan throughout the segmentation process. When using a 2D segmentation approach, e.g., on a series of coronal slices, the overall accuracy may be affected and discrepancies between consecutive images may be present, leading to a jagged segmentation result. Kwak et al. (2020) evaluated different 2D and 3D U-Net-like network architectures for MC segmentation on CBCT scans (Fig. 17.11). A 3D U-Net resulted in the highest overall performance, with a class accuracy of 0.96 and mean IoU of 0.577, although it required splitting up the scans into smaller 3D patches due to GPU memory limitations. Jaskari et al. (2020) also used a 3D U-Net-like architecture and patch-based approach, resulting in a mean DSC of 0.575 and mean curve distance (MCD) of 0.56 mm (Fig. 17.12). Kurt Bayrakdar et al. (2021) used 3D U-Net architectures as well to segment various structures for the purpose of implant planning; for the MC, they reported a 72.2% correct detection frequency, with the detection accuracy being highest in the molar region (97.5%). A study by the same group used segmentation to ultimately assess impacted third molars, with a correct MC detection frequency of 92.9% (Orhan et al. 2021). Liu et al. (2022) performed 2D U-Net-based segmentation as an intermediary step for evaluating the relation between the mandibular third molar and MC; for the MC, the mean DSC was 0.925 and the mean IoU was 0.900.

Panoramic Radiography

MC segmentation on panoramic radiographs is somewhat more complicated due to anatomical overlap with the mandibular bone and, in some cases, the roots. The aforementioned panoptic segmentation study by Cha et al. (2021) showed an IoU of 0.639 for the mandibular canal (Fig. 17.8). Vinayahalingam used a U-Net for MC segmentation on panoramic radiographs, reporting a mean DSC of 0.847 (Fig. 17.13).

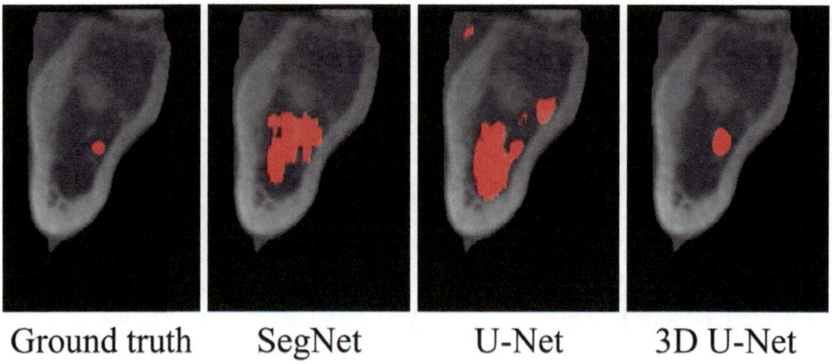

Fig. 17.11 Segmentation of the mandibular canal using 2D U-Net-type networks (SegNet/U-Net) vs. a 3D U-Net. Whereas the 2D U-Nets' segmentation maps encompassed the canal, they grossly overestimated its dimensions. A 3D U-Net yielded a much more accurate result (albeit still a slight overestimation). (Reproduced from Kwak et al. 2020 under a Creative Commons Attribution 4.0 International License; cropped version of original figure)

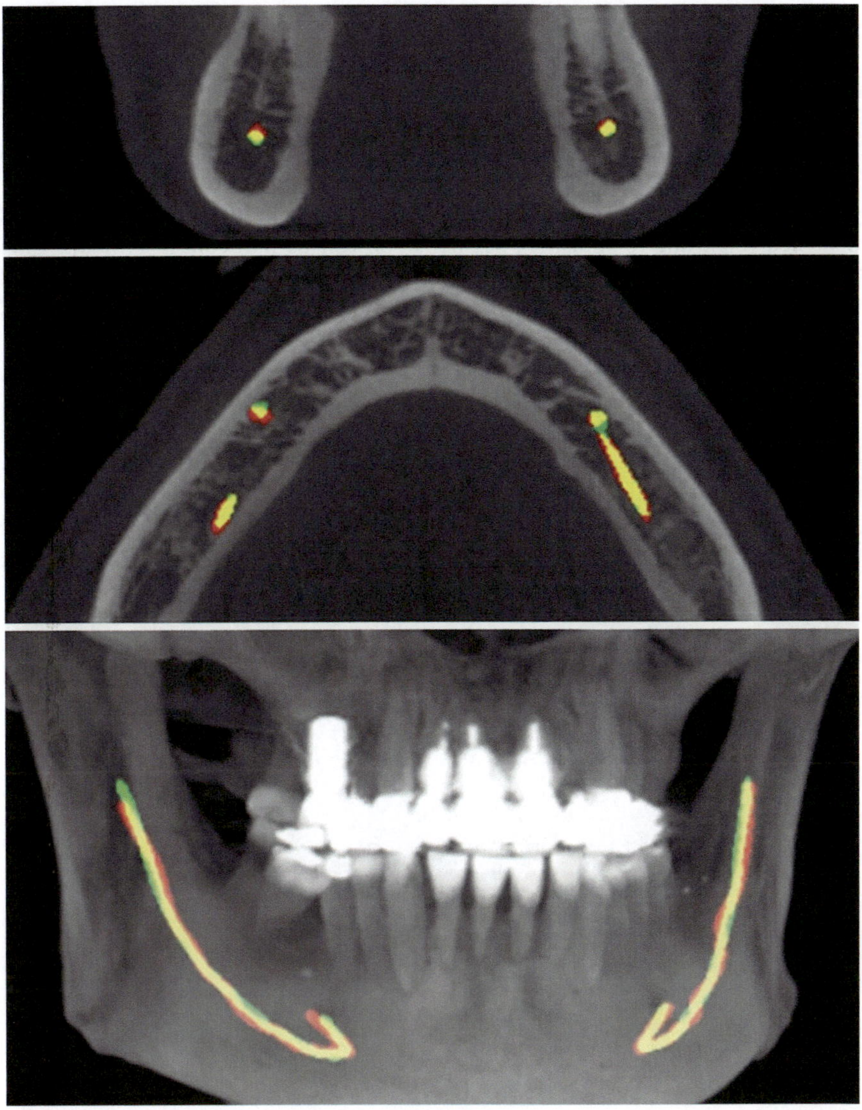

Fig. 17.12 Segmentation of the mandibular canal using a 3D U-Net. The *yellow line* indicates the overlap between the model's output and the annotation (*red line*). (Reproduced from Jaskari et al. 2020 under a Creative Commons Attribution 4.0 International License; cropped version of original figure)

Maxillary Sinus/Airway Segmentation

Segmentation of various parts of the respiratory system can serve several purposes. Within the dental field, the main regions of interest are (1) the maxillary sinus, due to its close contact with the upper teeth, resulting in potential odontogenic sinus pathosis, especially after implant placement and endodontic treatment; and (2) the upper airways, due to their relation with craniofacial development and issues such as obstructive sleep apnea (OSA).

Steybe et al. (2022) developed a patch-based 3D U-Net-based segmentation model for several structures on head CT scans; for the maxillary sinus, their approach resulted in a DSC of 0.94. and an ASSD of 0.16 mm (Fig. 17.14). On CBCT data, due to the limited contrast and relatively high degree of noise, the maxillary sinus may appear somewhat cloudy, even when healthy. When the sinus is opacified (e.g., due to sinusitis), segmentation can be particularly difficult. Choi et al. (2022) trained a 2D U-Net on CBCT scans comprising a mixture of clear and opacified maxillary sinuses. After post-processing using a connected components

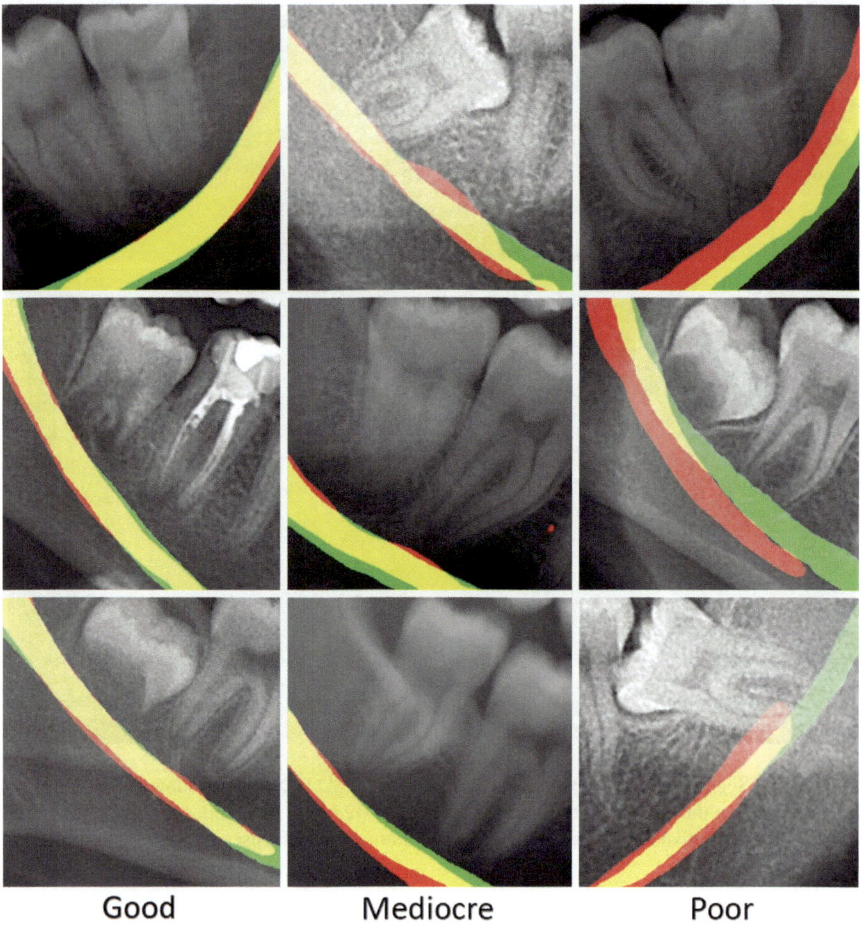

Fig. 17.13 Examples of mandibular canal segmentation on panoramic radiographs using U-Net. Images with *good, mediocre*, and *poor* segmentation accuracy are shown. *Green*: manual segmentation. *Red*: U-Net-based segmentation. Yellow: overlap between manual and U-Net-based segmentations. (Reproduced from Vinayahalingam et al. 2019 under a Creative Commons Attribution 4.0 International License)

approach, their model reached a DSC of 0.910 (Fig. 17.14). Morgan et al. (2022) used a 3D U-Net for maxillary sinus segmentation on CBCT, reporting a DSC of 0.984.

Jung et al. (2021) trained a self-configuring 3D U-Net (nnU-Net; Isensee et al. 2021) to segment the maxillary sinus on CBCT images into 'air' and 'lesion' (Fig. 17.14). They found a DSC of 0.930 for air and 0.760 for lesions. An alternative approach involved CNN-based paranasal sinus segmentation on CT images to determine an opacification score (Humphries et al. 2020); they found a high degree of correlation between this CNN-derived score and the Lund-MacKay visual score, pulmonary function parameters and blood test parameters. Maxillary sinus segmentation has also been explored on panoramic radiographs; the aforementioned panoptic segmentation study by Cha et al. (2021) showed an IoU of 0.898 for the sinus.

As for the upper airways, due to the radiation exposure from CT and CBCT scans, magnetic resonance imaging (MRI) is commonly used; for children in particular, the fact that MRI scanning does not involve ionizing radiation is of particular interest. Accordingly, several studies have explored the use of DL for segmenting the upper airways on MRI. Xie et al. (2022) used two parallel 2D U-Nets to segment the nasal cavity and the remainder of the upper airway on static and dynamic MRI data, with a DSC ranging between 0.84 and 0.89. The same network architecture was used by Bommineni et al. (2023) for segmenting various structures on T1 MRI datasets for the purpose of determining risk factors for OSA. For the retropalatal and retroglossal airway, they found a DSC of 0.63 and 0.73.

Ryu et al. (2021) trained a 3D U-Net for upper airway segmentation on CT data, followed by automated OSA diagnosis using a support vector machine approach applied to several patient features, including flow characteristics. The DSC for segmentation was 0.74 and 0.76 for low- and high-resolution models; the eventual diagnosis was performed with a sensitivity of 0.893, specificity of 0.862, and F1 score of 0.876. Shujaat et al. (2021) also used a 3D U-Net for pharyngeal airway segmentation on a mix of CT and CBCT data, showing an average DSC of 0.97.

Cephalometry

Cephalometric analysis is commonly used to evaluate dental and skeletal relationships, particularly in orthodontics and orthognathic surgery. It relies on detection and various anatomical landmarks, which are used to calculate distances and angles that can be linked to a normal population distribution.

Automatic cephalometric analysis has been a topic of interest for several decades and has recently been revisited owing to developments in the field of deep learning. In this section, a brief overview of DL-based cephalometric landmarking will be given, using a few selected examples of research studies. For a comprehensive overview of the use of deep learning in cephalometry, we refer to the systematic review and meta-analysis by de Queiroz Tavares Borges Mesquita et al. (2023).

Cephalometric Radiographs

Conventional cephalometric analysis is performed on lateral cephalometric radiographs, which are standardized radiographs using a natural head position and a low

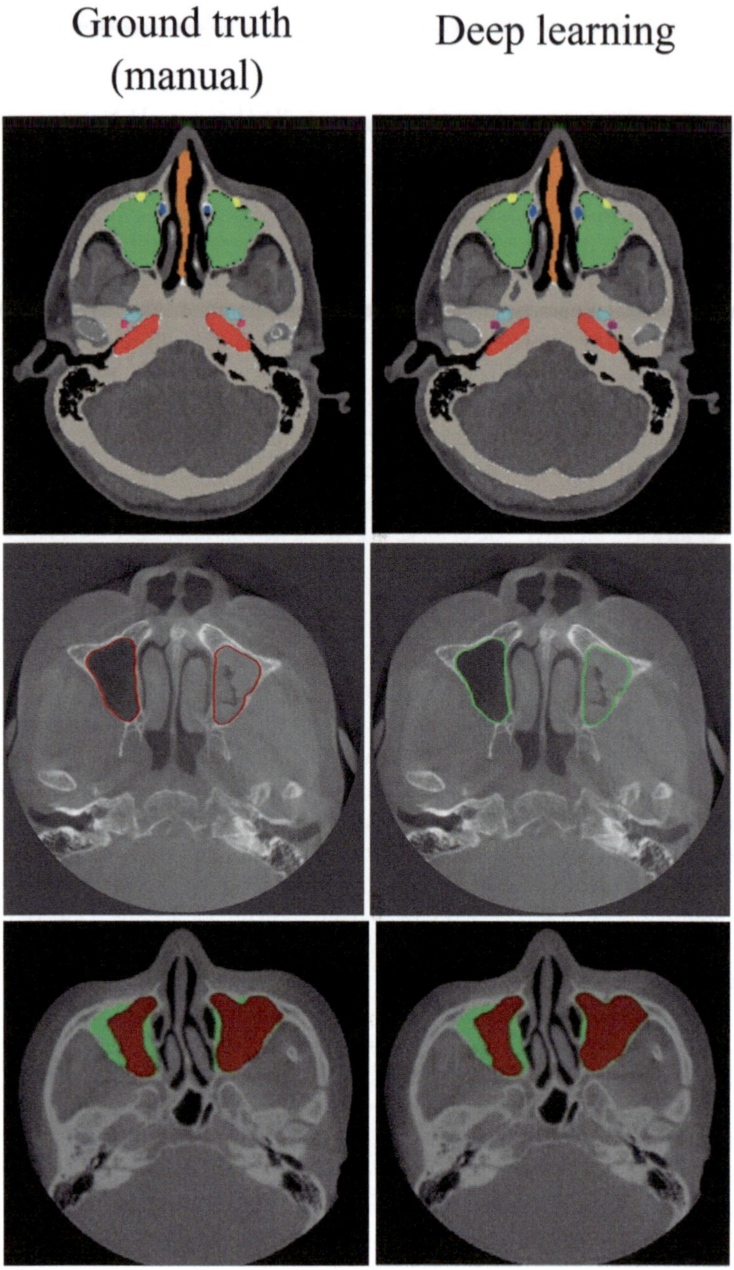

Fig. 17.14 Deep learning-based segmentation of the maxillary sinus. *Top row*: patch-based 3D U-Net, CT data, by Steybe et al. (2022). *Middle row*: slice-based 2D U-Net, CBCT data, by Choi et al. (2022). *Bottom row*: self-configuring 3D U-Net segmenting air space (*red*) and lesions (*green*), CBCT data, by Jung et al. (2021). (Reproduced under a Creative Commons Attribution 4.0 International License; cropped and relabeled versions of original figures)

degree of magnification. Regardless, for structures far removed from the midsagittal plane, magnification plays a role. Furthermore, whereas landmarks on bone-soft tissue or air-soft tissue edges can be ascertained easily, other anatomical landmarks can be difficult to pinpoint due to anatomical overlap.

The commonly used neural network architectures in DL-based 2D cephalometry are variations of ResNet (Chen et al. 2019b; Gilmour and Ray 2020; Muraev et al. 2020; Noothout et al. 2020; Song et al. 2020), U-Net (Zhong et al. 2019; Qian et al. 2020), and YOLO (Park et al. 2019; Hwang et al. 2021). Overall, research studies on AI-based cephalometric landmark detection show an agreement of 79% with the ground truth, considering a 2-mm error threshold (de Queiroz Tavares Borges Mesquita et al. 2023; includes both studies using cephalometric radiographs and CBCT).

(Cone-Beam) Computed Tomography

Although CT and CBCT should not be considered as diagnostic options for routine cephalometry, they are often acquired for particular cases requiring a more comprehensive treatment planning. In the event that these scans are acquired, a 3D cephalometric analysis is possible, which would overcome the distortion and magnification issues posed by 2D radiographs.

As mentioned earlier in this chapter, for deep learning, large-volume 3D data poses a computational challenge, especially for CBCT due to its relatively small voxel size. Therefore, several studies attempted to transform 3D cephalometry to a 2D space. For example, Lee et al. (2019) developed a 3D cephalometry tool for CT, in which the skull is first segmented, after which 2D views are generated using simulated lighting and shadow (Fig. 17.15). Subsequently, a VGG-19 network (i.e., 16 convolutional layers, 3 dense layers) was trained to detect seven landmarks. Their method resulted in an average error of 1.5 mm; for most landmarks located on a bone surface, sub-mm accuracy was reached, but the approach proved to be challenging for determining the center of the foramen magnum (error: 4.6 mm). Yun et al. (2020) used the approach from Lee et al. (2019) as an initial step in their processing pipeline, i.e., to normalize the 3D pose of the skull. Subsequently, they generated a slice in the midsagittal plane with a limited thickness, on which a coarse and patched-based fine detection of 8 landmarks was performed using CNNs. Finally, post-processing involving a variational autoencoder yielded a set of 93 3D landmarks in the original coordinate space (Fig. 17.15). Their approach resulted in an average error of 3.63 mm. In a subsequent study, Yun et al. (2022) modified their pipeline by introducing a 3D patch-based VGGNet-type CNN for mandibular landmark annotation (Fig. 17.15); they found a mean error of 2.88 mm for 90 landmarks using this adapted method.

A more direct combination of DL-based bone segmentation and landmark detection was proposed by Torosdagli et al. (2019), who used a DenseNet for mandible segmentation on CBCT images, followed by a U-Net and long short-term memory recurrent network for landmark identification. Anatomical landmarks were localized with errors generally below 1 mm; for the pogonion, mean errors ranged from 1.36 to 2.4 mm, depending on the choice of pooling function. Zhang et al. (2020)

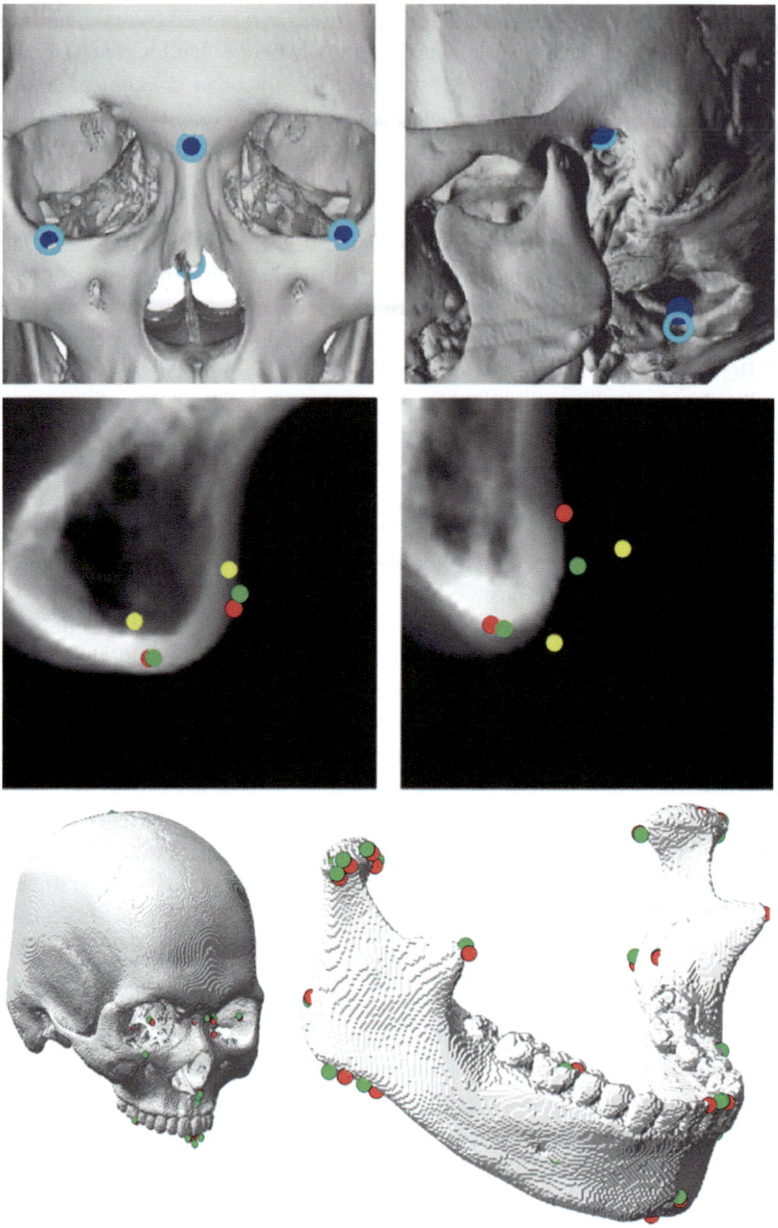

Fig. 17.15 3D cephalometry using deep learning (DL). *Top row*: using 2D views with lighting and shadow (Lee et al. 2019). *Blue dots*: output of DL model. *Cyan dots*: labeled landmark. *Middle row*: using normalized midsagittal slice (Yun et al. 2020). *Yellow dot*: coarse DL landmark detection. *Green dot*: fine DL landmark detection. *Red dot*: ground truth. Note that this step was followed by further processing to yield 3D landmarks. *Bottom row*: using same method as Yun et al. (2020) for cranial landmarks, with the addition of a 3D CNN for mandibular landmarks (Yun et al. 2022). *Green dots*: output of DL model. *Red dots*: ground truth. (Reproduced under a Creative Commons Attribution 3.0/4.0 license; cropped versions of original figures)

also combined CBCT segmentation with landmark identification using context-guided fully convolutional networks with a U-Net-like architecture. Their proposed method outperformed several alternative segmentation/landmarking methods, with a DSC of 0.932 for midface segmentation, a DSC of 0.933 for mandible segmentation, and an average landmark localization error of 1.1 mm.

Recently, a few studies have explored 3D cephalometry that acts directly on the reconstructed CT and CBCT data without generating 2D or pseudo-2D views. Lang et al. (2022) proposed a three-stage coarse-to-fine framework for CBCT images, using a 3D Mask R-CNN approach. Their method resulted in an average error of 1.38 mm. Dot et al. (2022b) used a coarse prediction model on downsampled full-head CT data in order to define five ROIs, followed by five fine prediction models on high-resolution patches for each ROI. All models were based on the same network architecture, combining spatial configuration (i.e., prior knowledge regarding the overall relation between landmarks) with heatmap regression (Payer et al. 2019). This approach resulted in a mean error of 1.0 mm.

Facial Photographs/Scans

Whereas dental treatment mostly involves the hard tissues of the craniomaxillofacial region, soft tissue and facial profile evaluations are often needed during treatment planning and follow-up. In recent years, caliper-based anthropometry has gradually been replaced with digital solutions. In particular, stereophotogrammetry tools as well as facial scanners (e.g., integrated in CBCT units) allow for accurate depiction of the soft tissue surface, as well as a registration of this surface with (CB)CT or MRI data. Several clinical applications of this type of data have been described, including OSA screening (Fernandes Fagundes et al. 2022), soft tissue evaluation of cleft lip and palate patients (Alpagan Ozdemir and Esenlik 2018), symmetry evaluation after reconstructive surgery (Ueda et al. 2021), etc.

While research involving the use of DL on this type of data for dental purposes has been scarce, several models have been established for automated facial landmark analysis on optical data (Böhringer and de Jong 2019). Interestingly, with the increasing availability and quality of smartphone cameras, applications of DL-based facial analysis may go beyond the use of 3D surface scans. For example, the MediaPipe platform by Google (Fig. 17.16) includes a module for real-time face detection on photographs or videos using BlazeFace (Bazarevsky et al. 2019) followed by the detection of 468 pseudo-3D landmarks that can be combined into a mesh representation (Kartynnik et al. 2019), as well as further refinement using an attention-based model (Grishchenko et al. 2020). Although further validation of this approach would be needed regarding applications requiring absolute distance measurements, this approach could serve several clinical roles, particularly as a screening tool or for the planning and follow-up of surgical interventions involving soft tissue displacement.

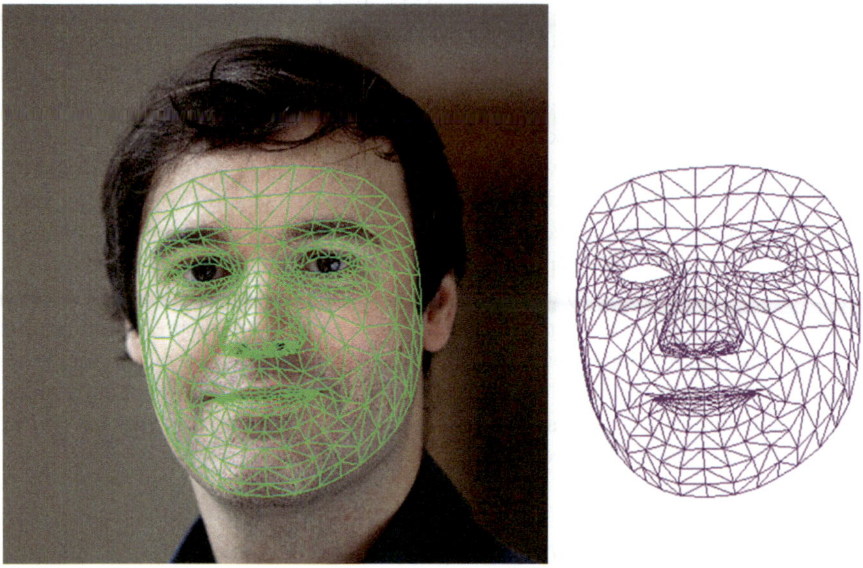

Fig. 17.16 Deep learning for facial mesh estimation using 468 landmarks, applied to the author's headshot. Generated using the MediaPipe Face Mesh tool

Unsupervised Segmentation: Clustering

Clustering is a type of unsupervised learning, in which data is grouped together based on a similarity measure. For segmentation, clustering can be used to group pixels/voxels based on a combination of their intensity and coordinates or by adding additional features such as local gradients. Examples of clustering methods are:

- *K-means clustering*: works by iteratively (1) defining k centroids (i.e., central points of a cluster) in the feature space and (2) reassigning points to the nearest centroids. It is straightforward and relatively fast, but sensitive to the number of clusters and the initial centroid position and tends to perform poorly for irregular distributions (Fig. 17.17).
- *Hierarchical clustering*: as its name implies, this approach progressively combines smaller clusters into larger ones; it starts off by allocating each data point to its own cluster and ultimately results in a single cluster. In each step, the nearest clusters are combined. Several implementations have been described to calculate the distance between clusters, such as single-link (closest points), complete-link (farthest points), average-link (average between all points), and Ward's method (minimizes variance). To obtain a segmentation, a cut-off of the desired number of clusters can be made.

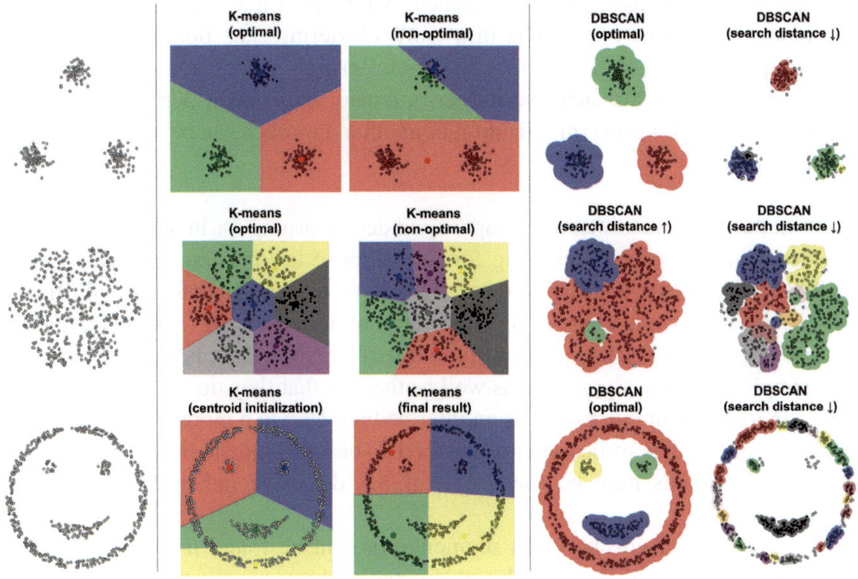

Fig. 17.17 K-means clustering vs. density-based clustering (DBSCAN). *Top row*: densely clustered points, well separated. Although all clustering methods tend to perform well, k-means clustering can fail for certain initial centroid positions, and DBSCAN will require a proper search distance setting. *Middle row*: closely connected circular clusters. K-means clustering can resolve the clusters if initial centroid points are positioned properly, whereas DBSCAN will typically result in over- or under-clustering, depending on the search distance. *Bottom row*: irregular point distribution. K-means clustering will not be able to properly identify the clusters, regardless of initial centroid placement. DBSCAN will perform well if the search distance is selected appropriately. Visualized using Naftali Harris' online tools (www.naftaliharris.com)

- *Density-based clustering:* groups points that are closely located within the feature space. A popular implementation is density-based spatial clustering of applications with noise (DBSCAN). DBSCAN works by iteratively searching an area around each point for nearby points and thereby classifying them as core points, border points, or noise (note: this should not be confused with image noise; it refers to outliers in the distribution of points in the feature space). Although it handles irregular distribution well, it can show limited effectiveness in separating adjacent or overlapping clusters (Fig. 17.17); the fact that the number of desired clusters does not have to be defined acts more as a disadvantage in this case.
- *Gaussian mixture models*: Using this approach, k Gaussian distributions are generated, and the probability for each point is calculated for each Gaussian distribution. Then, the Gaussians' parameters (mean and covariance) as well as the point assignments are iteratively determined using an expectation maximization

algorithm until convergence is reached. Although it is flexible (in terms of the cluster size/shape) and results in a 'soft' clustering (i.e., points can belong to multiple clusters, also known as fuzzy clustering), it does not always reach an optimal solution. To increase its performance, rather than performing manual initialization, k-means initialization or another approach can be used to speed up convergence.

With the increasing interest in supervised deep learning for image segmentation, the use of unsupervised clustering for this purpose has become relatively rare. It should also be noted that, while these algorithms do operate automatically from a certain point, they often require a certain amount of fine-tuning (e.g., proper initialization or parameter selection) for optimal performance. That being said, the relative simplicity of the algorithms as well as the fact that they do not require labeled data can make them interesting as an intermediary step in a more complex pipeline (e.g., as pre- or post-processing tools for DL-based segmentation). Furthermore, clustering methods may be used for pathosis detection rather than anatomical segmentation.

Applications of unsupervised segmentation can be found in fields other than dentistry. For example, Rim et al. (2021) applied k-means clustering as an accessory tool to segment the heart on chest CT images using thresholding. Caballo et al. (2018) also used k-means clustering within an automatic segmentation pipeline; in their case, it was used as a final step after applying region growing and active contour models for breast tissue segmentation on CT images. Chamroukhi et al. (2022) proposed the use of functional mixture models for the segmentation of squamous cell carcinoma on dual-energy CT scans. Their proposed method outperformed conventional Gaussian mixed models, k-means clustering, and selective search algorithms (Fig. 17.18). Zhang et al. (2017) used DBSCAN within a segmentation pipeline for lung nodules on CT, whereas Baumgartner et al. (2005) used both k-means clustering and DBSCAN within a tool to detect acute stroke on CT.

While research on unsupervised segmentation on dental radiographic or tomographic images is scarce, Wongkhuenkaew et al. (2023) used unsupervised fuzzy clustering to identify and classify fluorosis on dental photographs. Their proposed method was able to classify pixels with an accuracy of 79.5% and classify test images correctly in 67.2% of cases (Fig. 17.19).

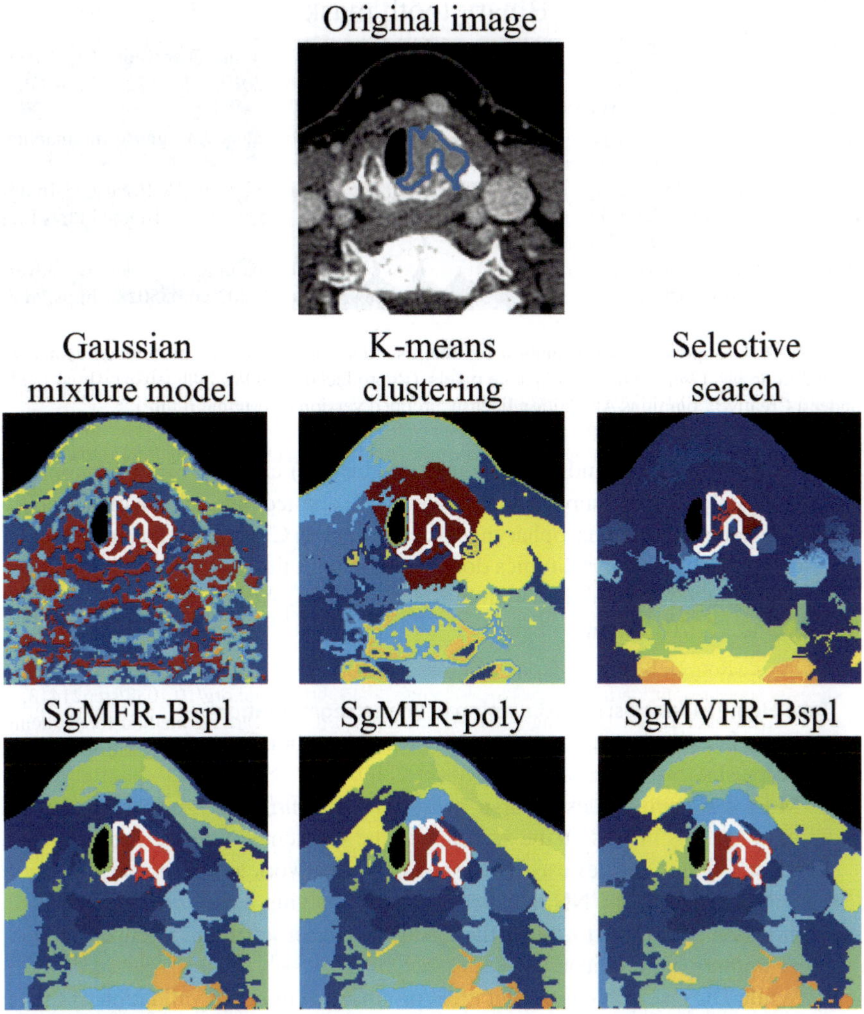

Fig. 17.18 Unsupervised segmentation for squamous cell carcinoma segmentation on dual-energy CT. *Top row & white outline:* ground truth. *Middle row*: conventional methods (for benchmarking). *M(V)FR*: proposed methods, using mixtures of (vectorized) functional regressions. (Reproduced from Chamroukhi et al. 2022 under a Creative Commons Attribution license; cropped and relabeled version of original figure)

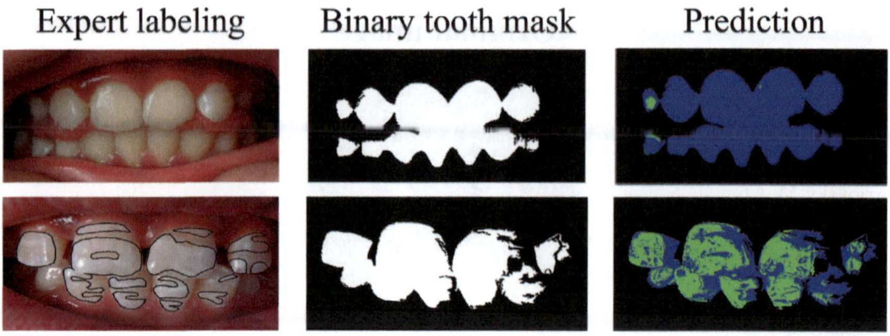

Fig. 17.19 Unsupervised segmentation for fluorosis detection. *Top row*: normal. *Bottom row*: stage 2 fluorosis. *Green:* predicted opaque pixels. (Reproduced from Wongkhuenkaew et al. 2023 under a Creative Commons Attribution license; cropped version of original figure)

Note that clustering (and dimensionality reduction) can also play an important role in radiomics. For example, Liang et al. (2019) applied hierarchical clustering to radiomics parameters for nasopharyngeal carcinoma on CT and MRI data. However, an in-depth discussion of radiomics does not fit in with the topic of this chapter; the interested reader is referred to Lambin et al. (2012), Avanzo et al. (2020), and Rogers et al. (2020), among others.

Take-Home Messages: Deep Learning in Image Segmentation

- Deep learning models can be a *powerful, fast* tool for various segmentation tasks.
- Most research studies involve *supervised learning*; the performance of these models hinges on the accuracy of the segmented training data.
- Most research studies use established neural network architectures such as U-Net or Mask R-CNN. Further research involving *novel, alternative DL methods* is needed to judge their added value in terms of accuracy and computational efficiency.
- While DL research has shown great promise, an in-depth validation of the outcome is often lacking. *Benchmarking* DL models vs. manual experts and/or conventional segmentation methods should be the standard for future research.
- A trained DL model is deterministic and (typically) fully automated. If a segmentation result is suboptimal, extensive *manual correction* may be needed (which would defeat the purpose of using DL). Further work is needed on efficiently implementing an *interactive* aspect to DL-based segmentation.

References

Adnan N, Khalid WB, Umer F. An artificial intelligence model for teeth segmentation and numbering on orthopantomograms. Int J Comput Dent. 2023. https://doi.org/10.3290/j.ijcd.b3840535.

Alpagan Ozdemir S, Esenlik E. Three-dimensional soft-tissue evaluation in patients with cleft lip and palate. Med Sci Monit. 2018;24:8608–20.

Arjovsky M, Chintala S, Bottou L. Wasserstein generative adversarial networks. Int Conf Mach Learn. 2017;70:214–23. https://doi.org/10.48550/arXiv.1701.07875.

Avanzo M, Wei L, Stancanello J, Vallières M, Rao A, Morin O, et al. Machine and deep learning methods for radiomics. Med Phys. 2020;47:e185–202. https://doi.org/10.1002/mp.13678.

Baumgartner C, Gautsch K, Böhm C, Felber S. Functional cluster analysis of CT perfusion maps: a new tool for diagnosis of acute stroke? J Digit Imaging. 2005;18:219–26. https://doi.org/10.1007/s10278-004-1048-9.

Bazarevsky V, Kartynnik Y, Vakunov A, Raveendran K, Grundmann M. BlazeFace: sub-millisecond neural face detection on mobile GPUs. arXiv. 2019:1907.05047. https://doi.org/10.48550/arXiv.1907.05047.

Bilgir E, Bayrakdar İŞ, Çelik Ö, Orhan K, Akkoca F, Sağlam H, et al. An artificial intelligence approach to automatic tooth detection and numbering in panoramic radiographs. BMC Med Imaging. 2021;21:124. https://doi.org/10.1186/s12880-021-00656-7.

Böhringer S, de Jong MA. Quantification of facial traits. Front Genet. 2019;10:397. https://doi.org/10.3389/fgene.2019.00397.

Bommineni VL, Erus G, Doshi J, Singh A, Keenan BT, Schwab RJ, et al. Automatic segmentation and quantification of upper airway anatomic risk factors for obstructive sleep apnea on unprocessed magnetic resonance images. Acad Radiol. 2023;30:421–30. https://doi.org/10.1016/j.acra.2022.04.023.

Bronstein MM, Bruna J, LeCun Y, Szlam A, Vandergheynst P. Geometric deep learning: going beyond Euclidean data. IEEE Signal Process Mag. 2017;34:18–42. https://doi.org/10.1109/MSP.2017.2693418.

Caballo M, Boone JM, Mann R, Sechopoulos I. An unsupervised automatic segmentation algorithm for breast tissue classification of dedicated breast computed tomography images. Med Phys. 2018;45:2542–59. https://doi.org/10.1002/mp.12920.

Cha JY, Yoon HI, Yeo IS, Huh KH, Han JS. Panoptic segmentation on panoramic radiographs: deep learning-based segmentation of various structures including maxillary sinus and mandibular canal. J Clin Med. 2021;10:2577. https://doi.org/10.3390/jcm10122577.

Chamroukhi F, Brivet S, Savadjiev P, Coates M, Forghani R. DECT-CLUST: dual-energy CT image clustering and application to head and neck squamous cell carcinoma segmentation. Diagnostics (Basel). 2022;12:3072. https://doi.org/10.3390/diagnostics12123072.

Chandrashekar G, AlQarni S, Bumann EE, Lee Y. Collaborative deep learning model for tooth segmentation and identification using panoramic radiographs. Comput Biol Med. 2022;148:105829. https://doi.org/10.1016/j.compbiomed.2022.105829.

Chen H, Zhang K, Lyu P, Li H, Zhang L, Wu J, et al. A deep learning approach to automatic teeth detection and numbering based on object detection in dental periapical films. Sci Rep. 2019a;9:3840. https://doi.org/10.1038/s41598-019-40414-y.

Chen R, Ma Y, Chen N, Lee D, Wang W. Cephalometric landmark detection by attentive feature pyramid fusion and regression-voting. arXiv. 2019b:1908.08841. https://doi.org/10.48550/arXiv.1908.08841.

Chen Y, Du H, Yun Z, Yang S, Dai Z, Zhong L, et al. Automatic segmentation of individual tooth in dental CBCT images from tooth surface map by a multi-task FCN. IEEE Access. 2020;8:97296–309. https://doi.org/10.1109/ACCESS.2020.2991799.

Cheng B, Collins MD, Zhu Y, Liu T, Huang TS, Adam H, et al. Panoptic-deeplab: a simple, strong, and fast baseline for bottom-up panoptic segmentation. In: Proc IEEE/CVF Conf Comput Vis Pattern Recognit. 2020. pp. 12475–85. https://doi.org/10.48550/arXiv.1911.10194.

Choi H, Jeon KJ, Kim YH, Ha EG, Lee C, Han SS. Deep learning-based fully automatic segmentation of the maxillary sinus on cone-beam computed tomographic images. Sci Rep. 2022;12:14009. https://doi.org/10.1038/s41598-022-18436-w.

Cordonnier JB, Loukas A, Jaggi M On the relationship between self-attention and convolutional layers. arXiv. 2019:1911.03584. https://doi.org/10.48550/arXiv.1911.03584.

de Queiroz Tavares Borges Mesquita G, Vieira WA, Vidigal MTC, Travençolo BAN, Beaini TL, Spin-Neto R, Paranhos LR, de Brito Júnior RB. Artificial intelligence for detecting cephalometric landmarks: a systematic review and meta-analysis. J Digit Imaging. 2023;36:1158. https://doi.org/10.1007/s10278-022-00766-w.

Dot G, Schouman T, Dubois G, Rouch P, Gajny L. Fully automatic segmentation of craniomaxillofacial CT scans for computer-assisted orthognathic surgery planning using the nnU-Net framework. Eur Radiol. 2022a;32:3639–48. https://doi.org/10.1007/s00330-021-08455-y.

Dot G, Schouman T, Chang S, Rafflenbeul F, Kerbrat A, Rouch P, et al. Automatic 3-dimensional cephalometric landmarking via deep learning. J Dent Res. 2022b;101:1380–7. https://doi.org/10.1177/00220345221112333.

Estai M, Tennant M, Gebauer D, Brostek A, Vignarajan J, Mehdizadeh M, et al. Deep learning for automated detection and numbering of permanent teeth on panoramic images. Dentomaxillofac Radiol. 2022;51:20210296. https://doi.org/10.1259/dmfr.20210296.

Fernandes Fagundes NC, Carlyle T, Dalci O, Darendeliler MA, Kornerup I, Major PW, et al. Use of facial stereophotogrammetry as a screening tool for pediatric obstructive sleep apnea by dental specialists. J Clin Sleep Med. 2022;18:57–66. https://doi.org/10.5664/jcsm.9490.

Gilmour L, Ray N. Locating cephalometric x-ray landmarks with foveated pyramid attention. arXiv. 2020:2008.04428. https://doi.org/10.48550/arXiv.2008.04428.

Girshick R. Fast R-CNN. arXiv. 2015:1504.08083. https://doi.org/10.48550/arXiv.1504.08083.

Girshick R, Donahue J, Darrell T, Malik J. Rich feature hierarchies for accurate object detection and semantic segmentation. arXiv. 2013:1311.2524. https://doi.org/10.48550/arXiv.1311.2524.

Gkioxari G, Malik J, Johnson J. Mesh R-CNN. arXiv. 2019:1906.02739. https://doi.org/10.48550/arXiv.1906.02739.

Görürgöz C, Orhan K, Bayrakdar IS, Çelik Ö, Bilgir E, Odabaş A, et al. Performance of a convolutional neural network algorithm for tooth detection and numbering on periapical radiographs. Dentomaxillofac Radiol. 2022;51:20210246. https://doi.org/10.1259/dmfr.20210246.

Gou M, Rao Y, Zhang M, Sun J, Cheng K. Automatic image annotation and deep learning for tooth CT image segmentation. Lect Notes Comput Sci. 2019;11902:519–28. https://doi.org/10.1007/978-3-030-34110-7_43.

Grishchenko I, Ablavatski A, Kartynnik Y, Raveendran K, Grundmann M. Attention mesh: high-fidelity face mesh prediction in real-time. arXiv. 2020:2006.10962. https://doi.org/10.48550/arXiv.2006.10962.

Hao J, Liao W, Zhang YL, Peng J, Zhao Z, Chen Z, et al. Toward clinically applicable 3-dimensional tooth segmentation via deep learning. J Dent Res. 2022;101:304–11. https://doi.org/10.1177/00220345211040459.

He K, Zhang X, Ren S, Sun J. Deep residual learning for image recognition. In: Proc IEEE Conf Comput Vis Pattern Recognit. 2016:770–778. https://doi.org/10.1109/CVPR.2016.90.

He K, Gkioxari G, Dollar P, Girshick R. Mask R-CNN. IEEE Trans Pattern Anal Mach Intell. 2020;42:386–97. https://doi.org/10.1109/TPAMI.2018.2844175.

Hedegaard L, Bakhtiarnia A, Iosifidis A. Continual transformers: redundancy-free attention for online inference. Int Conf Learn Representations. 2023. https://doi.org/10.48550/arXiv.2201.06268.

Huang G, Liu Z, Van Der Maaten L, Weinberger, KQ. Densely connected convolutional networks. In: Proc IEEE Comput Soc Conf Comput Vis Pattern Recognit. 2017. pp. 2261–2269. https://doi.org/10.1109/CVPR.2017.243.

Humphries SM, Centeno JP, Notary AM, Gerow J, Cicchetti G, Katial RK, et al. Volumetric assessment of paranasal sinus opacification on computed tomography can be automated using a convolutional neural network. Int Forum Allergy Rhinol. 2020;10:1218–25. https://doi.org/10.1002/alr.22588.

Hwang HW, Moon JH, Kim MG, Donatelli RE, Lee SJ. Evaluation of automated cephalometric analysis based on the latest deep learning method. Angle Orthod. 2021;91:329–35. https://doi.org/10.2319/021220-100.1.

Isensee F, Jaeger PF, Kohl SAA, Petersen J, Maier-Hein KH. nnU-Net: a self-configuring method for deep learning-based biomedical image segmentation. Nat Methods. 2021;18:203–11. https://doi.org/10.1038/s41592-020-01008-z.

Isola P, Zhu JY, Zhou T, Efros AA. Image-to-image translation with conditional adversarial networks. arXiv. 2016:1611.07004. https://doi.org/10.48550/arXiv.1611.07004.

Jaskari J, Sahlsten J, Järnstedt J, Mehtonen H, Karhu K, Sundqvist O, et al. Deep learning method for mandibular canal segmentation in dental cone beam computed tomography volumes. Sci Rep. 2020;10:5842. https://doi.org/10.1038/s41598-020-62321-3.

Jung SK, Lim HK, Lee S, Cho Y, Song IS. Deep active learning for automatic segmentation of maxillary sinus lesions using a convolutional neural network. Diagnostics (Basel). 2021;11:688. https://doi.org/10.3390/diagnostics11040688.

Kabir T, Lee CT, Chen L, Jiang X, Shams S. A comprehensive artificial intelligence framework for dental diagnosis and charting. BMC Oral Health. 2022;22:480. https://doi.org/10.1186/s12903-022-02514-6.

Karras T, Aila T, Laine S, Lehtinen J. Progressive growing of GANs for improved quality, stability, and variation. Int Conf Learn Representations. 2018. https://doi.org/10.48550/arXiv.1710.10196.

Kartynnik Y, Ablavatski A, Grishchenko I, Grundmann M. Real-time facial surface geometry from monocular video on mobile GPUs. arXiv. 2019:1907.06724. https://doi.org/10.48550/arXiv.1907.06724.

Kaya E, Gunec HG, Gokyay SS, Kutal S, Gulum S, Ates HF. Proposing a CNN method for primary and permanent tooth detection and enumeration on pediatric dental radiographs. J Clin Pediatr Dent. 2022;46:293–8.

Kılıc MC, Bayrakdar IS, Çelik Ö, Bilgir E, Orhan K, Aydın OB, Kaplan FA, Sağlam H, Odabaş A, Aslan AF, Yılmaz AB. Artificial intelligence system for automatic deciduous tooth detection and numbering in panoramic radiographs. Dentomaxillofac Radiol. 2021;50:20200172. https://doi.org/10.1259/dmfr.20200172.

Kingma DP, Welling M. Auto-encoding variational bayes. arXiv. 2014:1312.6114. https://doi.org/10.48550/arXiv.1312.6114.

Kipf TN, Welling M. Semi-supervised classification with graph convolutional networks. arXiv. 2016:1609.02907. https://doi.org/10.48550/arXiv.1609.02907.

Kirillov A, He K, Girshick R, Rother C, Dollár P. Panoptic segmentation. arXiv. 2018:1801.00868. https://doi.org/10.48550/arXiv.1801.00868.

Kosalagood P, Silkosessak OC, Pittayapat P, Pisarnturakit P, Pauwels R, Jacobs R. Linear measurement accuracy of eight cone beam computed tomography scanners. Clin Implant Dent Relat Res. 2015;17:1217–27. https://doi.org/10.1111/cid.12221.

Kurt Bayrakdar S, Orhan K, Bayrakdar IS, Bilgir E, Ezhov M, Gusarev M, et al. A deep learning approach for dental implant planning in cone-beam computed tomography images. BMC Med Imaging. 2021;21:86. https://doi.org/10.1186/s12880-021-00618-z.

Kwak GH, Kwak EJ, Song JM, Park HR, Jung YH, Cho BH, et al. Automatic mandibular canal detection using a deep convolutional neural network. Sci Rep. 2020;10:5711. https://doi.org/10.1038/s41598-020-62586-8.

Lambin P, Rios-Velazquez E, Leijenaar R, Carvalho S, van Stiphout RG, Granton P, et al. Radiomics: extracting more information from medical images using advanced feature analysis. Eur J Cancer. 2012;48:441–6. https://doi.org/10.1016/j.ejca.2011.11.036.

Lang Y, Lian C, Xiao D, Deng H, Thung KH, Yuan P, et al. Localization of craniomaxillofacial landmarks on CBCT images using 3D mask R-CNN and local dependency learning. IEEE Trans Med Imaging. 2022;41:2856–66. https://doi.org/10.1109/TMI.2022.3174513.

Lee SM, Kim HP, Jeon K, Lee SH, Seo JK. Automatic 3D cephalometric annotation system using shadowed 2D image-based machine learning. Phys Med Biol. 2019;64:055002. https://doi.org/10.1088/1361-6560/ab00c9.

Lee S, Woo S, Yu J, Seo J, Lee J, Lee C. Automated CNN-based tooth segmentation in cone-beam CT for dental implant planning. IEEE Access. 2020;8:50507–18. https://doi.org/10.1109/ACCESS.2020.2975826.

Liang X, Lambrichts I, Sun Y, Denis K, Hassan B, Li L, et al. A comparative evaluation of cone beam computed tomography (CBCT) and multi-slice CT (MSCT). Part II: on 3D model accuracy. Eur J Radiol. 2010;75:270–4. https://doi.org/10.1016/j.ejrad.2009.04.016.

Liang ZG, Tan HQ, Zhang F, Rui Tan LK, Lin L, Lenkowicz J, et al. Comparison of radiomics tools for image analyses and clinical prediction in nasopharyngeal carcinoma. Br J Radiol. 2019;92:20190271. https://doi.org/10.1259/bjr.20190271.

Liu MQ, Xu ZN, Mao WY, Li Y, Zhang XH, Bai HL, et al. Deep learning-based evaluation of the relationship between mandibular third molar and mandibular canal on CBCT. Clin Oral Investig. 2022;26:981–91. https://doi.org/10.1007/s00784-021-04082-5.

Liu Z, He X, Wang H, Xiong H, Zhang Y, Wang G, et al. Hierarchical self-supervised learning for 3D tooth segmentation in intra-oral mesh scans. IEEE Trans Med Imaging. 2023;42:467–80. https://doi.org/10.1109/TMI.2022.3222388.

Luong MT, Pham H, Manning CD. Effective approaches to attention-based neural machine translation. arXiv. 2015:1508.04025. https://doi.org/10.48550/arXiv.1508.04025.

Minnema J, van Eijnatten M, Kouw W, Diblen F, Mendrik A, Wolff J. CT image segmentation of bone for medical additive manufacturing using a convolutional neural network. Comput Biol Med. 2018;103:130–9. https://doi.org/10.1016/j.compbiomed.2018.10.012.

Minnema J, van Eijnatten M, Hendriksen AA, Liberton N, Pelt DM, Batenburg KJ, et al. Segmentation of dental cone-beam CT scans affected by metal artifacts using a mixed-scale dense convolutional neural network. Med Phys. 2019;46:5027–35. https://doi.org/10.1002/mp.13793.

Miyato T, Kataoka T, Koyama M, Yoshida Y. Spectral normalization for generative adversarial networks. Int Conf Learn Representations. 2018. https://doi.org/10.48550/arXiv.1802.05957.

Morgan N, Van Gerven A, Smolders A, de Faria VK, Willems H, Jacobs R. Convolutional neural network for automatic maxillary sinus segmentation on cone-beam computed tomographic images. Sci Rep. 2022;12:7523. https://doi.org/10.1038/s41598-022-11483-3.

Muraev AA, Tsai P, Kibardin I, Oborotistov N, Shirayeva T, Ivanov S, et al. Frontal cephalometric landmarking: humans vs artificial neural networks. Int J Comput Dent. 2020;23:139–48.

Noothout JMH, De Vos BD, Wolterink JM, Postma EM, Smeets PAM, Takx RAP, et al. Deep learning-based regression and classification for automatic landmark localization in medical images. IEEE Trans Med Imaging. 2020;39:4011–22. https://doi.org/10.1109/TMI.2020.3009002.

Orhan K, Bilgir E, Bayrakdar IS, Ezhov M, Gusarev M, Shumilov E. Evaluation of artificial intelligence for detecting impacted third molars on cone-beam computed tomography scans. J Stomatol Oral Maxillofac Surg. 2021;122:333–7. https://doi.org/10.1016/j.jormas.2020.12.006.

Park JH, Hwang HW, Moon JH, Yu Y, Kim H, Her SB, et al. Automated identification of cephalometric landmarks: part 1-comparisons between the latest deep-learning methods YOLOV3 and SSD. Angle Orthod. 2019;89:903–9. https://doi.org/10.2319/022019-127.1.

Park EY, Cho H, Kang S, Jeong S, Kim EK. Caries detection with tooth surface segmentation on intraoral photographic images using deep learning. BMC Oral Health. 2022;22:573. https://doi.org/10.1186/s12903-022-02589-1.

Pauwels R, Beinsberger J, Stamatakis H, Tsiklakis K, Walker A, Bosmans H, et al. Comparison of spatial and contrast resolution for cone-beam computed tomography scanners. Oral Surg Oral Med Oral Pathol Oral Radiol. 2012;114:127–35. https://doi.org/10.1016/j.oooo.2012.01.020.

Pauwels R, Jacobs R, Singer SR, Mupparapu M. CBCT-based bone quality assessment: are Hounsfield units applicable? Dentomaxillofac Radiol. 2015;44:20140238. https://doi.org/10.1259/dmfr.20140238.

Payer C, Štern D, Bischof H, Urschler M. Integrating spatial configuration into heatmap regression based CNNs for landmark localization. Med Image Anal. 2019;54:207–19. https://doi.org/10.1016/j.media.2019.03.007.

Prados-Privado M, García Villalón J, Blázquez Torres A, Martínez-Martínez CH, Ivorra C. A convolutional neural network for automatic tooth numbering in panoramic images. Biomed Res Int. 2021;2021:3625386. https://doi.org/10.1155/2021/3625386.

Preda F, Morgan N, Van Gerven A, Nogueira-Reis F, Smolders A, Wang X, et al. Deep convolutional neural network-based automated segmentation of the maxillofacial complex from cone-beam computed tomography: a validation study. J Dent. 2022;124:104238. https://doi.org/10.1016/j.jdent.2022.104238.

Qian J, Luo W, Cheng M, Tao Y, Lin J, Lin H. CephaNN: a multi-head attention network for cephalometric landmark detection. IEEE Access. 2020;8:112633–41.

Rao Y, Wang Y, Meng F, Pu J, Sun J, Wang Q. A symmetric fully convolutional residual network with DCRF for accurate tooth segmentation. IEEE Access. 2020;8:92028–38. https://doi.org/10.1109/ACCESS.2020.2994592.

Ren S, He K, Girshick R, Sun J. Faster R-CNN: towards real-time object detection with region proposal networks. IEEE Trans Pattern Anal Mach Intell. 2017;39:1137–49. https://doi.org/10.1109/TPAMI.2016.2577031.

Rim B, Lee S, Lee A, Gil HW, Hong M. Semantic cardiac segmentation in chest CT images using K-means clustering and the mathematical morphology method. Sensors (Basel). 2021;21:2675. https://doi.org/10.3390/s21082675.

Rogers W, Thulasi Seetha S, Refaee TAG, Lieverse RIY, Granzier RWY, Ibrahim A, et al. Radiomics: from qualitative to quantitative imaging. Br J Radiol. 2020;93:20190948. https://doi.org/10.1259/bjr.20190948.

Ronneberger O, Fischer P, Brox T. U-Net: convolutional networks for biomedical image segmentation. arXiv. 2015:1505.04597. https://doi.org/10.48550/arXiv.1505.04597.

Ryu S, Kim JH, Yu H, Jung HD, Chang SW, Park JJ, et al. Diagnosis of obstructive sleep apnea with prediction of flow characteristics according to airway morphology automatically extracted from medical images: computational fluid dynamics and artificial intelligence approach. Comput Methods Prog Biomed. 2021;208:106243. https://doi.org/10.1016/j.cmpb.2021.106243.

Shujaat S, Jazil O, Willems H, Van Gerven A, Shaheen E, Politis C, et al. Automatic segmentation of the pharyngeal airway space with convolutional neural network. J Dent. 2021;111:103705. https://doi.org/10.1016/j.jdent.2021.103705.

Song Y, Qiao X, Iwamoto Y, Chen Y. Automatic cephalometric landmark detection on x-ray images using a deep-learning method. Appl Sci. 2020;10:2547. https://doi.org/10.3390/app10072547.

Steybe D, Poxleitner P, Metzger MC, Brandenburg LS, Schmelzeisen R, Bamberg F, et al. Automated segmentation of head CT scans for computer-assisted craniomaxillofacial surgery applying a hierarchical patch-based stack of convolutional neural networks. Int J Comput Assist Radiol Surg. 2022;17:2093–101. https://doi.org/10.1007/s11548-022-02673-5.

Torosdagli N, Liberton DK, Verma P, Sincan M, Lee JS, Bagci U. Deep geodesic learning for segmentation and anatomical landmarking. IEEE Trans Med Imaging. 2019;38:919–31. https://doi.org/10.1109/TMI.2018.2875814.

Tuzoff DV, Tuzova LN, Bornstein MM, Krasnov AS, Kharchenko MA, Nikolenko SI, et al. Tooth detection and numbering in panoramic radiographs using convolutional neural networks. Dentomaxillofac Radiol. 2019;48:20180051. https://doi.org/10.1259/dmfr.20180051.

Ueda N, Imai Y, Yamakawa N, Yagyuu T, Tamaki S, Nakashima C, et al. Assessment of facial symmetry by three-dimensional stereophotogrammetry after mandibular reconstruction: a comparison with subjective assessment. J Stomatol Oral Maxillofac Surg. 2021;122:56–61. https://doi.org/10.1016/j.jormas.2020.04.003.

Uijlings JRR, van de Sande KEA, Gevers T, Smeulders AWM. Selective search for object recognition. Int J Comput Vis. 2013;104:154–71. https://doi.org/10.1007/s11263-013-0620-5.

Veličković P, Cucurull G, Casanova A, Romero A, Liò P, Bengio Y. Graph attention networks. arXiv. 2017:1710.10903. https://doi.org/10.48550/arXiv.1710.10903.

Verhelst PJ, Smolders A, Beznik T, Meewis J, Vandemeulebroucke A, Shaheen E, et al. Layered deep learning for automatic mandibular segmentation in cone-beam computed tomography. J Dent. 2021;114:103786. https://doi.org/10.1016/j.jdent.2021.103786.

Vinayahalingam S, Xi T, Bergé S, Maal T, de Jong G. Automated detection of third molars and mandibular nerve by deep learning. Sci Rep. 2019;9:9007. https://doi.org/10.1038/s41598-019-45487-3.

Vincent P, Larochelle H, Lajoie I, Bengio Y, Manzagol PA. Stacked denoising autoencoders: learning useful representations in a deep network with a local denoising criterion. J Mach Learn Res. 2010;11:3371–408.

Wang Y, Sun Y, Liu Z, Sarma SE, Bronstein MM, Solomon JM. Dynamic graph CNN for learning on point clouds. ACM Trans Graph. 2019a;38:1–12. https://doi.org/10.1145/3326362.

Wang CY, Mark Liao HY, Yeh IH, Wu YH, Chen PY, Hsieh JW. CSPNet: a new backbone that can enhance learning capability of CNN. arXiv. 2019b:1911.11929. https://doi.org/10.48550/arXiv.1911.11929.

Wongkhuenkaew R, Auephanwiriyakul S, Theera-Umpon N, Teeyapan K, Yeesarapat U. Fuzzy K-nearest neighbor based dental fluorosis classification using multi-prototype unsupervised possibilistic fuzzy clustering via cuckoo search algorithm. Int J Environ Res Public Health. 2023;20:3394. https://doi.org/10.3390/ijerph20043394.

Wu TH, Lian C, Lee S, Pastewait M, Piers C, Liu J, et al. Two-stage mesh deep learning for automated tooth segmentation and landmark localization on 3D intraoral scans. IEEE Trans Med Imaging. 2022;41:3158–66. https://doi.org/10.1109/TMI.2022.3180343.

Xie L, Udupa JK, Tong Y, Torigian DA, Huang Z, Kogan RM, et al. Automatic upper airway segmentation in static and dynamic MRI via anatomy-guided convolutional neural networks. Med Phys. 2022;49:324–42. https://doi.org/10.1002/mp.15345.

Xu X, Liu C, Zheng Y. 3D tooth segmentation and labeling using deep convolutional neural networks. IEEE Trans Vis Comput Graph. 2019;25:2336–48. https://doi.org/10.1109/TVCG.2018.2839685.

Yan M, Guo J, Tian W, Yi Z. Symmetric convolutional neural network for mandible segmentation. Knowl Based Syst. 2018;159:63–71. https://doi.org/10.1016/j.knosys.2018.06.003.

Yaren Tekin B, Ozcan C, Pekince A, Yasa Y. An enhanced tooth segmentation and numbering according to FDI notation in bitewing radiographs. Comput Biol Med. 2022;146:105547. https://doi.org/10.1016/j.compbiomed.2022.105547.

Yasa Y, Çelik Ö, Bayrakdar IS, Pekince A, Orhan K, Akarsu S, et al. An artificial intelligence proposal to automatic teeth detection and numbering in dental bite-wing radiographs. Acta Odontol Scand. 2021;79:275–81. https://doi.org/10.1080/00016357.2020.1840624.

Yun HS, Jang TJ, Lee SM, Lee SH, Seo JK. Learning-based local-to-global landmark annotation for automatic 3D cephalometry. Phys Med Biol. 2020;65:085018. https://doi.org/10.1088/1361-6560/ab7a71.

Yun HS, Hyun CM, Baek SH, Lee SH, Seo JK. A semi-supervised learning approach for automated 3D cephalometric landmark identification using computed tomography. PLoS One. 2022;17:e0275114. https://doi.org/10.1371/journal.pone.0275114.

Zhang W, Zhang X, Zhao J, Qiang Y, Tian Q, Tang X. A segmentation method for lung nodule image sequences based on superpixels and density-based spatial clustering of applications with noise. PLoS One. 2017;12:e0184290. https://doi.org/10.1371/journal.pone.0184290.

Zhang J, Liu M, Wang L, Chen S, Yuan P, Li J, et al. Context-guided fully convolutional networks for joint craniomaxillofacial bone segmentation and landmark digitization. Med Image Anal. 2020;60:101621. https://doi.org/10.1016/j.media.2019.101621.

Zhong Z, Li J, Zhang Z, Jiao Z, Gao X. An attention-guided deep regression model for landmark detection in cephalograms. arXiv. 2019:1906.07549. https://doi.org/10.1007/978-3-030-32226-7_60.

Zhu JY, Park T, Isola P, Efros AA. Unpaired image-to-image translation using cycle-consistent adversarial networks. arXiv. 2017:1703.10593. https://doi.org/10.48550/arXiv.1703.10593.

Deep Learning in Image Processing: Part 2—Image Enhancement, Reconstruction and Registration

18

Ruben Pauwels and Alexandros Iosifidis

Introduction

In the previous chapter, *neural networks* (NN) with potential application in image processing were presented, and an overview was given of applications of *deep learning* (DL) as well as unsupervised clustering in image segmentation. The current chapter covers applications of DL for three other types of image processing.

Applications in *image enhancement* and *image reconstruction* attempt to improve one or more of the fundamental image quality properties in medical imaging: sharpness, contrast, noise and artefacts. Such improvements serve several benefits. They can enhance the diagnostic efficacy by improving the visibility of anatomical and (potential) pathological details, thereby affecting the patient's treatment decision (confidence) and/or treatment outcome. Furthermore, for imaging modalities using ionizing radiation, sharpness-preserving noise reduction techniques can allow for acquisition at lower exposure levels. For tomographic imaging modalities, advanced image enhancement or reconstruction can allow for shorter scan times, which can reduce motion artefacts.

Applications in *image registration* can allow for fast and accurate image matching. Seeing as how registration can be a time-consuming component of the clinical workflow, for both manual and (semi-)automatic methods, a quick and fully automated method could be of great benefit. Furthermore, DL could help overcome typical image quality issues that affect the feasibility of conventional registration methods.

R. Pauwels (✉)
Department of Dentistry and Oral Health, Aarhus University, Aarhus, Denmark

Department of Radiology, Faculty of Dentistry, Chulalongkorn University, Bangkok, Thailand
e-mail: ruben.pauwels@dent.au.dk

A. Iosifidis
DIGIT, Department of Electrical and Computer Engineering, Aarhus University, Aarhus, Denmark
e-mail: ai@ece.au.dk

K. Orhan, R. Jagtap (eds.), *Artificial Intelligence in Dentistry*,
https://doi.org/10.1007/978-3-031-43827-1_18

For all of the applications described in this chapter, an exhaustive literature review is beyond the scope of this chapter; in-depth reviews on particular applications will be cited accordingly.

Deep Learning in Image Enhancement

Denoising

Noise is prevalent in any type of medical image. In imaging modalities involving X-rays (incl. tomographic images), several sources of noise can be identified. *Quantum noise* is caused by the stochastic nature of X-ray interactions and is therefore connected to the amount of exposure as well as the pixel or voxel size. *X-ray scattering*, comprising Compton (incoherent) and Rayleigh (coherent) scatter, can be considered as having a pseudo-random behaviour, with the latter having a less homogeneous distribution; thus, they result in both noise and artefacts (Pauwels et al. 2016, 2021). Finally, *electronic noise* is added at the detector side during the digitization of the X-ray signal. In computed tomography (CT) and cone-beam CT (CBCT) reconstructions using backprojection, noise is enhanced (at least for 'bone' kernels) due to the use of 'sharp' *filters* in the frequency domain. *Magnetic resonance imaging* (MRI) has entirely different sources of image noise, both from the patients themselves (who emit small radiofrequency signals from internal thermal motion of charged particles) and from the imaging system (coils, electronics).

Several straightforward techniques can be used to reduce noise. The main challenge is to suppress noise while preserving edges. *Smoothening* operators (e.g. Gaussian filtering) and *downsampling* (incl. increasing the slice thickness in CT/CBCT/MRI) come at the cost of reducing sharpness (Fig. 18.1). While

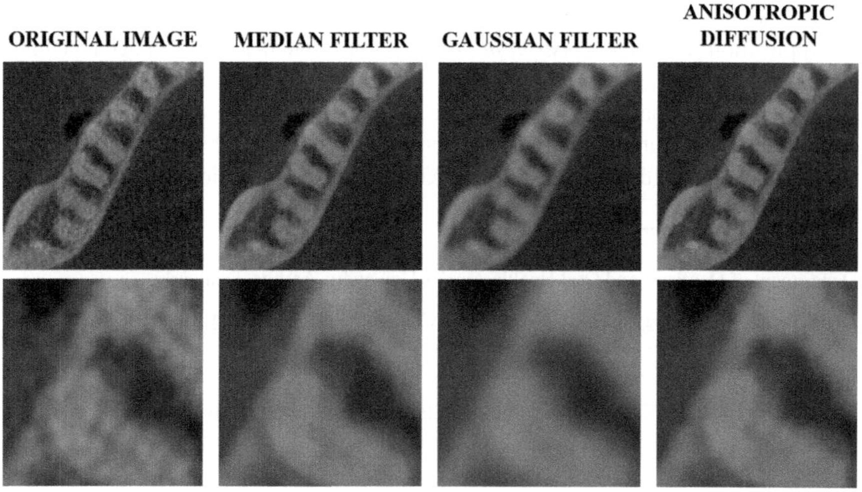

Fig. 18.1 Conventional denoising methods applied to a cone-beam computed tomography image

edge-preserving denoising techniques have been explored through the decades, the use of DL for this purpose has gained increasing attention. Note that the subsequent section "Deep Learning in Image Reconstruction" comprises several noise reduction techniques implemented into a reconstruction pipeline; the current section describes DL-denoising on single images or applied to scans *after* reconstruction. Also note that the following section describes super-resolution techniques that tend to include some form of denoising, albeit from a different perspective (i.e. increasing sharpness while keeping noise low, rather than reducing noise while keeping sharpness high).

The main NN architectures of interest for image denoising are *encoder-decoders, U-Nets* and *generative adversarial networks* (GAN, i.e. conditional GAN for paired data and cycleGAN for unpaired data); see Chap. 17 for a more detailed description of these NN types. Common performance metrics include the peak signal-to-noise ratio (PSNR), structural similarity index (SSIM) and root mean square error (RMSE); ideally, one would also measure some type of sharpness index (e.g. modulation transfer function, edge spread function), although this is often difficult to measure on clinical images. Certain studies have proposed alternative loss functions in low-dose CT denoising to avoid excessive blurring, such as *perceptual feature loss* (Yang et al. 2018), *structure loss* (You et al. 2018) and *sharpness loss* (Yi and Babyn 2018).

Training data can be obtained in several ways. Often, one would start from a high-quality image set and add *artificial* (e.g. Poisson) *noise*. However, this does not represent the actual noise distribution on clinical images. Fu et al. (2022) addressed this issue by training a GAN to learn realistic noise distributions on CT images of single teeth and transferring this noise distribution to other types of CT images to generate training data for a denoising CNN including an attention module. Other studies that focused on simulating realistic noise for other types of images include Guo et al. (2019), Zhuo et al. (2019) and Yue et al. (2019).

An alternative approach would be to acquire actual sets of *high- and low-dose images*, which would ensure realistic noise depiction. However, this approach is usually not feasible for clinical data, as it would require unjustified repeated exposures to patients. Furthermore, the image sets would have to be registered with pixel- or perfect-voxel accuracy in order for the denoising model to be effective (unless an unpaired NN approach is used).

Denoising is also of relevance for mesh-type data; however, the abovementioned CNN architectures cannot be readily used on data that does not adhere to a Euclidean grid structure (see Chap. 17). Armando et al. 2022 proposed a multi-resolution graph convolutional network, which outperformed state-of-the-art methods at a reasonable computational time (24–160 s, for models ranging between 20 000 and 171 000 faces).

Medical Image Denoising

Apart from studies mentioned earlier, this section will highlight selected research studies on medical image denoising. The overwhelming majority of studies involve tomographic imaging (e.g. CT and MRI); although research involving radiography is scarce, CNN-based denoising can be found on commercial radiographic systems (Toepfer et al. 2020). Hariharan et al. (2022) applied a U-Net-type denoising model on *radiographs* that were normalized using a generalized Anscombe transform; this approach accounted for the fact that noise patterns in X-ray imaging consist of a mixture of different sources of noise. Wu et al. (2022) included known, trainable filters within a deep learning pipeline that also included a deep image prior generator; their method (Masked Joint Bilateral Filtering; MJBF) outperformed other denoising models/algorithms on different types of radiographs. Jiang et al. (2021) used an attention-based multi-resolution residual CNN for denoising chest radiographs for the purpose of optimizing COVID-19 detection.

CT denoising has been a pertinent research topic for several decades due to the continuous challenge to lower patient doses as much as possible. DL models that operate on reconstructed CT images are not necessarily different from those that denoise other types of images, especially when the model only considers one slice at a time. Whereas a DL model that considers the local 3D region may be more effective in retaining structural information, this comes with computational challenges. This section will highlight a few recent studies on CT denoising using DL; see the review by Li et al. (2022) for a more exhaustive overview of the developments in this field. Wong et al. (2021) compared different approaches for denoising non-contrast head CT images: (1) BM3D, a commonly used denoising method using block-matching, 3D transforms and principal component analysis (Dabov et al. 2009); (2) RED-CNN, a residual convolutional neural network (Chen et al. 2017); (3) SRED-GCNN, their proposed model, which is an adapted version of the latter using skip connections and group convolutions (Cohen and Welling 2016). While RED-CNN showed the highest degree of noise reduction among the three methods, this came at the cost of a visibly reduced sharpness; their proposed method (SRED-GCNN) was able to retain sharpness while reducing noise at a significantly higher degree than BM3D. Azour et al. (2023) used a U-Net variant to denoise low-dose chest CT scans, showing good quantitative and quality image quality for mA reductions up to 80%. Lee and Jeong (2021) proposed a method called Interdependent Self-Cooperative Learning, based on cycleGAN and self-supervised residual learning. They tested their approach on various types of unpaired biomedical images; for low-dose CT data, the method outperformed other unpaired methods in terms of PSNR. Finally, Wang et al. (2023) tested a convolution-free approach using a vision transformer on the AAPM Low-Dose CT Grand Challenge dataset; their proposed model outperformed alternative DL approaches at a similar image throughput (Fig. 18.2). They also showed how transformer models are more efficient at feature extraction, as CNN models can be prone to having 'inactive' features that do not actually contribute to its output (Fig. 18.3).

Various studies focused on *MRI denoising*; see, e.g., the review on brain MRI by Mishro et al. (2022). Aetesam and Maji (2023) trained a Wasserstein GAN (WGAN) with perceptual loss, batch normalization and a global feature attention module on simulated MRI datasets with varying noise levels; their model was able to improve the PSNR by 22–87%. Kojima et al. (2022) applied the Noise2Void method (Krull et al. 2018), which does not require low-noise/noiseless training data, to low-field

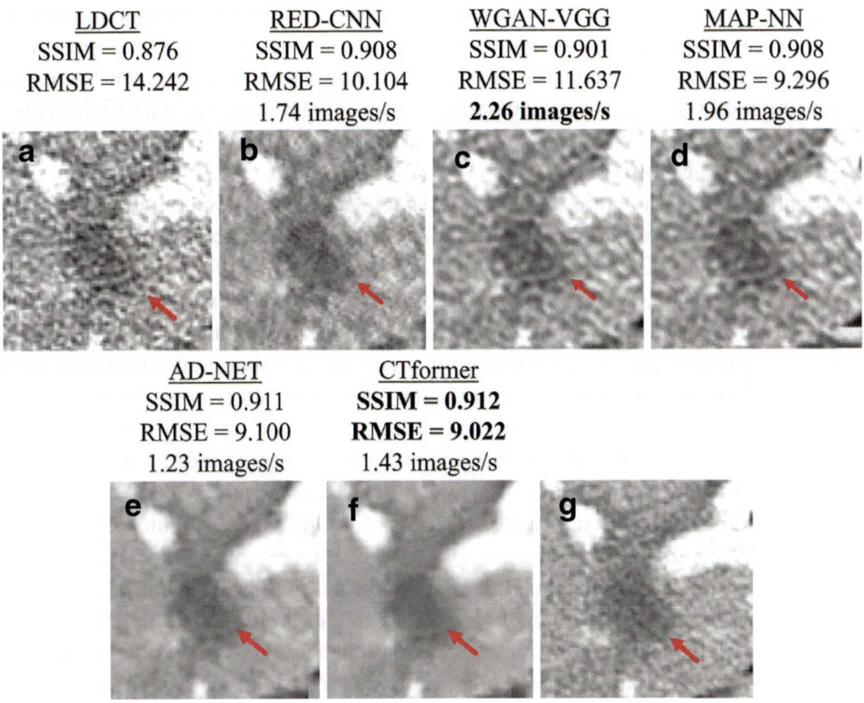

Fig. 18.2 Low-dose CT denoising using deep learning. Small region of interest of an abdominal CT scan. (**a**) Original low-dose CT, (**b**) RED-CNN (Chen et al. 2017), (**c**) WGAN-VGG (Yang et al. 2018), (**d**) MAP-NN (Shan et al. 2019), (**e**) AD-NET (Tian et al. 2020), (**f**) CTformer (Wang et al. 2023), (**g**) Normal-dose CT. *Red arrow* shows a liver metastasis. *SSIM,* structural similarity index measure. *RMSE,* root mean squared error. *Images/s,* data throughput. For each metric, the best-performing denoising method is highlighted in bold. (Reproduced from Wang et al. 2023 under a Creative Commons Attribution 4.0 license; relabeled version of original figure)

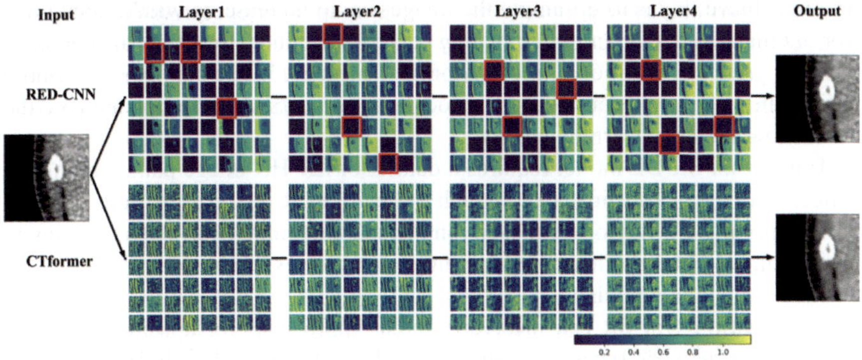

Fig. 18.3 Feature maps of a convolutional neural network (RED-CNN) vs. a transformer model (CTformer) trained for denoising low-dose CT images. *Red outlines* denote 'inactive' features within the CNN model; note that several other features within RED-CNN show a lower activation level than those for the transformer model. (Reproduced from Wang et al. 2023 under a Creative Commons Attribution 4.0 license)

MRI scans at 0.35 T. They showed a considerable SNR improvement while retaining contrast and sharpness. With the advent of dental-dedicated MRI scanners with relatively low magnetic field strengths (Fischel and Eriksen 2022), it is possible that denoising methods will have to be optimized for images acquired with such fields.

Dental Image Denoising

Denoising studies on dental images are scarce at the time of writing, although one can expect that several of the published models are generic enough to be applied on dental radiographs, CT or MRI data.

Hegazy et al. (2020) used a WGAN for noise reduction of low-dose dental CBCT scans after reconstruction, using skulls phantoms scanned at high and low (−60%) doses. A 'conventional' WGAN was compared with one that used a U-Net as generator (U-WGAN) and an end-to-end U-Net. While the latter showed good performance according to metrics like PSNR and SSIM, it appeared to result in oversmoothing. WGAN and U-WGAN showed comparable performance, with the latter having a much faster execution speed (9 ms/slice for U-WGAN vs 106 ms/slice for WGAN). This is particularly relevant for CBCT scans, which can consist of >500 slices.

For denoising and Hounsfield Unit (HU) calibration of CBCT scans in particular, CT scans can be used as training data/labels. Kang et al. (2023) trained a GAN on CBCT and CT data acquired from the same patient sample, using a combination of loss functions aimed at sharpness preservation. PSNR increased by 20.6%, while HU error reduced by almost 60%. See section "CT/CBCT Reconstruction" for more examples of inter-modality conversion using DL.

Super-Resolution

In general, super-resolution (SR) refers to a method for producing a high-resolution (HR) image from a low-resolution (LR) one (Bashir et al. 2021). The most basic way to achieve this is to upsample the image, i.e. to increase its width, height and (for 3D images) depth, and interpolating each pixel value. However, this approach does not yield any additional information in the image. While several more elaborate SR methods have been proposed throughout the years, the attention has recently shifted towards deep learning methods.

Training an SR DL model requires a dataset of LR-HR image pairs. Often, one collects an HR dataset first, from which the paired LR data can be derived using downsampling, blurring operators, etc. In medical imaging, it can be challenging to obtain clinical HR data; therefore, training often involves *ex vivo* (e.g. micro-CT) or *in silico* (i.e. simulated) data.

Deep learning for SR can involve different approaches for upsampling, along with various network types, algorithms, etc. Furthermore, SR can be applied on single images such as radiographs or reconstructed CT data, or implemented within a reconstruction technique such as in CT or MRI. Within this section, single-image

SR approaches are summarized; the use of DL in reconstruction is discussed in the section "CT/CBCT Reconstruction".

One approach for upsampling using DL involves a *subpixel layer*, which generates additional channels and reorganizes these channels to increase the image dimensions by a certain scaling factor in an end-to-end manner (Shi et al. 2016). An alternative approach is through the use of a *deconvolution layer* (Hugelier et al. 2016), which is equivalent to expanding the input image by multiplying each pixel with learned filters of suitable size over the channels dimension. Recently, a method using arbitrary scaling factors called *Meta-Upscale Module* was proposed, which has shown great performance up to a given magnification level (Hu et al. 2019). Even more recently, a *Local Texture Estimator* (LTE) model was proposed by Lee and Jin (2021), which operates on the amplitude, frequency and phase spaces of an encoded LR image and can be coupled to a decoder to yield an HR image at an arbitrary resolution.

As for the network architectures used in SR, methods based on recursive learning, residual learning, dense learning, multi-path learning, other convolution-based learning (e.g. group convolution, dilated convolution) and attention-based learning have been proposed, as well as several others. Furthermore, a variety of loss functions have been used for this purpose. Another way to distinguish SR method is based on the chronology of image processing, i.e. whether the upsampling precedes or succeeds the convolutions or whether some iterative or progressive process is used.

A recent review compared several state-of-the-art supervised SR methods on benchmark datasets in terms of signal-to-noise ratio and computational cost. Note that the test images are not medical images in this case, but photographs and drawings of various objects such as buildings, faces and animals. Some of the 'older' (2014–2017) models included, ordered from higher to lower signal-to-noise ratio:

- LapSRN, a cascaded CNN (Lai et al. 2017)
- FSRCNN, a lightweight approach towards SR (Dong et al. 2016)
- SRCNN, the first SR model using deep learning (Dong et al. 2014)
- SRResNet, a subpixel approach using a GAN and a perceptual loss function (Ledig et al. 2017)
- ESPCN, another subpixel approach (Shi et al. 2016)

The best-performing models were, from higher to lower signal-to-noise ratio:

- WRAN, a wavelet-based residual attention network (Xue et al. 2020)
- RCAN, a residual channel attention network (Zhang et al. 2018)
- SAN, a second-order attention network (Dai et al. 2019)
- Meta-RDN, a residual dense network with arbitrary magnification as described above (Hu et al. 2019)
- EDSR, an enhanced deep residual network (Lim et al. 2017)

In addition to supervised SR methods, several unsupervised or weakly supervised (using unpaired LR and HR data) methods have been proposed, including the use of cycleGANs (Yuan et al. 2018), 'zero-shot' or 'blind' SR (Shocher et al. 2018; Michaeli and Irani 2013) and the use of randomly initialized CNNs as an image prior (Ulyanov et al. 2020).

Many examples can be found of SR methods applied to various medical imaging modalities, including but not limited to CT (Umehara et al. 2018), MRI (Chaudhari et al. 2018), mammograms (Umehara et al. 2017), angiograms (Siow et al. 2023), ultrasound scans (Chen et al. 2021) and positron emission tomography (Pain et al. 2022). However, research regarding its use in dental imaging is still scarce. Moran et al. (2021) used a GAN-based SR model on periapical radiographs, showing improved objective and subjective image quality over the use of interpolation. Mohammad-Rahimi et al. (2023) compared various SR models on panoramic radiographs; the abovementioned LTE model performed best in terms of signal-to-noise ratio and subjective image quality assessment (Fig. 18.4).

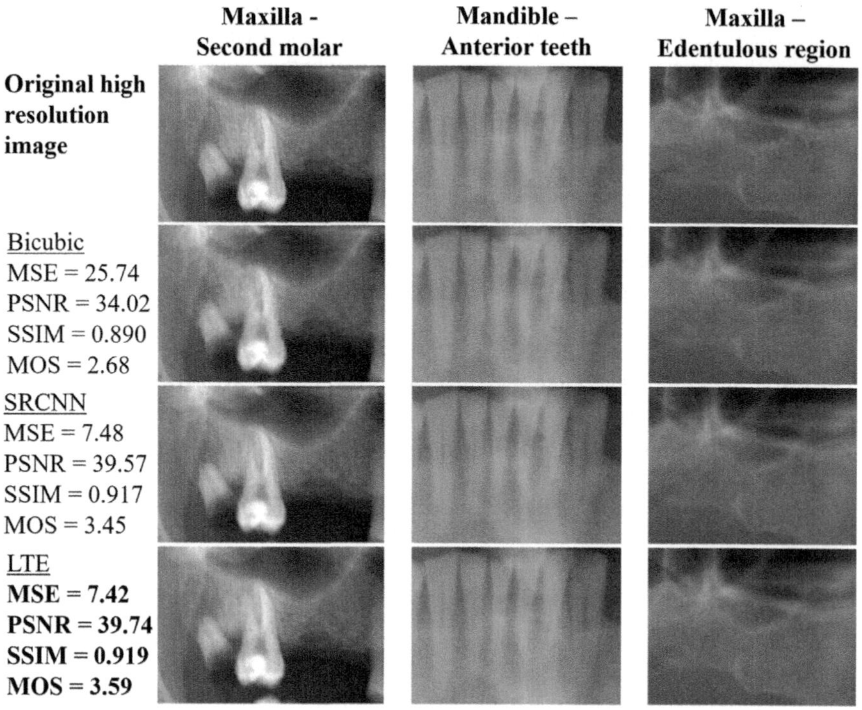

Fig. 18.4 Application of deep learning-based super-resolution models to dental radiographs. The two best-performing models (LTE and SRCNN) are shown, along with bicubic interpolation. *MSE* mean squared error, *PSNR* peak signal-to-noise ratio, *SSIM* structural similarity index measure, *MOS* mean opinion score (i.e. subjective evaluation). For each metric, the best performance among denoising methods is highlighted in bold. (Reproduced from Mohammad-Rahimi et al. 2023 under a Creative Commons Attribution license; cropped and relabeled version of original figure)

Image Correction

The use of deep learning for image correction is mainly of interest in photography; several models have been proposed for applications such as image colorization, restoration and inpainting.

In medical imaging, there is considerable potential for the use of deep learning in artefact correction of any type of reconstructed image (e.g. CT, CBCT, MRI); this will be covered in section "Deep Learning in Image Reconstruction". For the correction of radiographic or photographic images, applications with clinical relevance are relatively scarce. For example, while deep learning models could be trained to clean up artefacts from intra-oral radiographs, this is unlikely to yield a diagnostic benefit. Another example would be the removal of text overlays (Ulyanov et al. 2020); while one could see an application for radiographs with hardcoded text overlays in clinical regions of interest, it cannot be expected that the inpainted data is of diagnostic value.

One particular use of DL-based image correction is in the removal of compression artefacts. JPEG lossy image compression is commonly used to reduce image file sizes with little perceptual change, but it can impair the visualization of small details in some cases. While radiographic images are often stored as JPEGs, CT and CBCT data are sometimes exported in a compressed DICOM format, which may or may not be lossy. The clinical potential of generic compression artefact removal methods using DL, such as those by Svoboda et al. (2016) and Cavigelli et al. (2017), or dedicated models for specific medical imaging modalities, could be explored further.

Take-Home Messages: Deep Learning in Image Enhancement

- DL-based denoising and super-resolution methods both address the inherent balance between image sharpness and noise, but from a different perspective: the former attempts to suppress noise while retaining sharpness, and the latter attempts to boost sharpness without increasing noise.
- Many DL models were trained on diverse set of (mostly) non-medical images; retraining the models on specific medical image datasets may result in better performance than using pretrained models directly.
- One should be aware that image quality degradation caused by physical limitations of the imaging system may be difficult to overcome, even with a highly elaborate DL approach. Any newly gained information should be carefully assessed, as it may not reflect reality. This is especially the case for image restoration methods, where the restored portion should be considered as a 'best guess'.

Deep Learning in Image Reconstruction

Within this section, several applications of deep learning related to medical image reconstruction will be described. Due to the distinct way in which image formation and reconstruction happens in CT and CBCT vs. MRI, the manner(s) in which DL models are incorporated vary between these modalities; thus, they will be discussed separately. Regardless, the ultimate goal is the same: ensuring that the image quality is sufficient for a given diagnostic task. This can be boiled down to the optimization of four image quality metrics: sharpness, contrast, noise and artefacts. Whereas previous sections have focused on DL models aimed at increasing resolution, reducing noise or correcting artefacts on single images, the implementation of such models within a reconstruction pipeline could allow for a more robust and image quality enhancement that is truer to reality and may therefore augment the diagnostic performance.

CT/CBCT Reconstruction

Although CT and CBCT have some distinct differences in terms of exposure geometry and imaging hardware, the principles of reconstruction are largely the same. In both cases, reconstruction is an inverse problem, in which a voxelized representation of the scanned object is estimated based on a series of *projections* that are acquired over a certain angular range.

Several challenges can be found in tomographic reconstruction. First, there is the finite data sampling. A limited set of projections is available for the reconstruction of a given slice or volume; for the purpose of radiation protection, the number of projections is minimized according to the diagnostic task. Second, the discrepancy between the physics of the image acquisition process and the assumptions made during reconstruction:

- The *focal spot* has a finite size as well as a non-zero depth; thus, X-rays do not all originate from the same exact point.
- X-rays do not all have the same energy; the *X-ray spectrum* is defined by the tube voltage (kV), filtration and anode angle.
- Incoherent/coherent *scattering* as well as *beam hardening* occurs when X-rays traverse matter. The former contributes to a corrupted fraction of the detector signal, whereas the latter results in non-linear attenuation behaviour of an X-ray beam.
- X-ray interactions have a *stochastic* nature; at low exposure levels, this results in *quantum noise*.
- The source-object-detector system is *not perfectly stationary*; there is patient motion ranging from imperceptible micro-movements (e.g. breathing, muscle tremor or blood flow) to severe movements, as well as mechanical jittering of the source-detector assembly during its rotation.

Finally, the detector has a finite pixel size, limited efficiency and adds a degree of electronic noise to the signal. All of these factors cause different types and degrees of degradation of the image quality after reconstruction.

For several decades, the standard reconstruction algorithm used in CT was based on *filtered backprojection* (FBP). To this day, a modified version of FBP (Feldkamp et al. 1984) is by far the most used reconstruction technique in dental CBCT (Pauwels et al. 2015). Based on a mathematical description provided by Johann Radon in 2017, FBP is considered a computationally fast method that yields an adequate image quality in most situations. Furthermore, it is somewhat flexible in the sense that the choice of filter can be adapted towards higher sharpness or smoothness, depending on the diagnostic task. However, FBP has several flaws, many of which are the same for CT and CBCT; some issues are particular to the adaptation of FBP to a cone-beam geometry (Schulze et al. 2011). As a result, CT and CBCT scans are subject to different types of artefacts.

In CT, although FBP remains available on current-generation scanners, the use of *iterative reconstruction* (IR) has become more common. IR can be considered as an umbrella term, which covers a multitude of methods. IR algorithms incorporated in CT scanners are typically referred to as either statistical or model-based IR techniques (Stiller 2018; Pelc and Wang 2020). IR algorithms have shown impressive performance, e.g. for low-dose scans with high degrees of noise, allowing for noise suppression while retaining sharpness and contrast (Widmann et al. 2016, 2017, 2023). However, a complete and accurate modelling of the physics behind the imaging process, including all effects described above, remains a computational challenge. This is where the potential benefit of DL comes into play.

The use of DL in CT/CBCT reconstruction can be categorized in different ways. Although one can look at the neural network architecture (e.g. GAN, U-Net), a more intuitive way to distinguish the applications would be based on in which phase of image reconstruction they take place: preprocessing, reconstruction or postprocessing (Fig. 18.5).

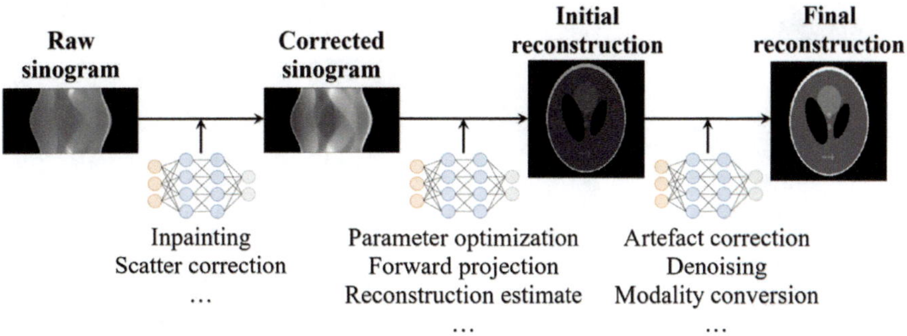

Fig. 18.5 Deep learning can be implemented into the reconstruction process by (1) preprocessing projection data, (2) integration into the reconstruction algorithm, (3) post-processing of reconstructed data. The example shows a CT/CBCT-type reconstruction process, but the distinction applies to MRI reconstruction as well

Preprocessing of Projection Data

Projections themselves are corrupted in several ways. DL models can be trained to *correct projections* for several causes of image quality degradation (e.g. denoising, scatter correction, motion correction), after which conventional reconstruction algorithms can be used. Also, missing projections (or parts of projections) can be estimated for *sparse-view* (i.e. low-dose) or *limited-angle* (e.g. tomosynthesis or discarded projections due to metal/motion/…) situations.

Maier et al. (2019) developed a U-Net-type DL model for scatter correction on CBCT projection data and applied it to simulated and experimental scans. They found that DL could estimate the scatter distribution within 2% for head scans, whereas alternative scatter correction methods (kernel-based and hybrid) showed errors of 14.5% and 6.2%, respectively, on the same data. This improvement in scatter estimation by the DL model results in more accurate reconstructed grey values as well, with deviations of 6 HU for the DL-corrected data vs. 278 HU for uncorrected data, 123 HU for kernel-based correction and 65 HU for hybrid correction. The same U-Net architecture was adapted by Pauwels et al. (2019) for the correction of scatter, beam hardening and truncation (i.e. exomass) on simulated CBCT data. Preliminary results showed that these effects are difficult to address in combination using a single DL model, due to stark differences in spatial frequency between them (Fig. 18.6). Furthermore, for beam hardening and truncation in particular, a naïve correction based on individual projections may not be the most ideal

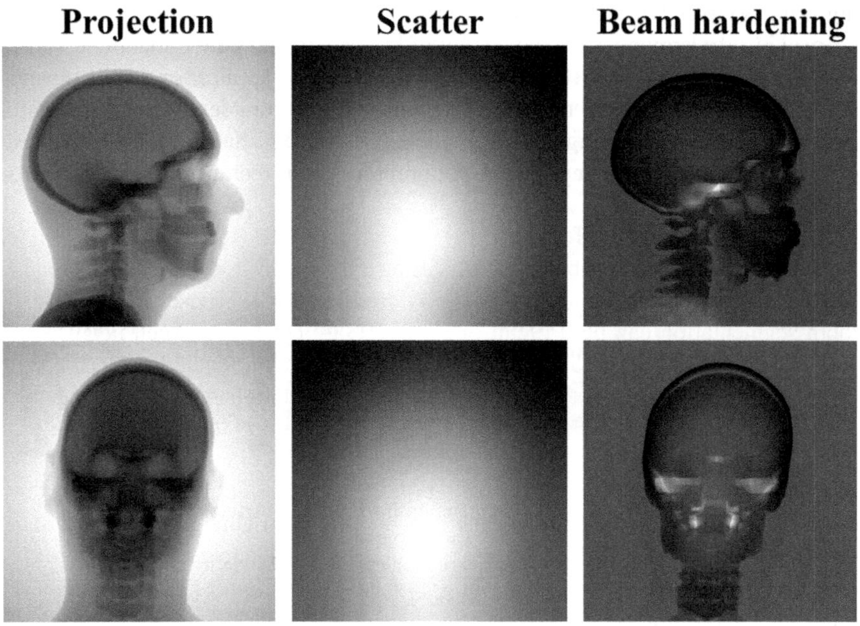

Fig. 18.6 Simulation of CBCT projections using simplified ICRP AM mesh-type phantom. Note the different appearance between scatter and beam hardening effects, which can complicate simultaneous correction

approach compared with a model that exploits the complementary information from multiple projection angles or a model that is incorporated in an iterative reconstruction process.

Several studies have explored the use of DL in situations with sparse and/or limited-view projections. For a more exhaustive literature review, the reader is referred to Minnema et al. (2022). Dong et al. (2019) trained a U-Net that acts on a forward-projected sinogram obtained from an initial FBP reconstruction; the model completes the sinogram, after which FBP can be used to yield the final result. Their approach can be applied in situations with either sparse (down to 60 projections) or limited-angle (down to 90°) situations. For head CT data, their approach improved the PSNR considerably compared with an uncorrected FBP reconstruction (Fig. 18.7), with an inference time of 1 s. GAN-based sinogram inpainting has also shown promising results, e.g. for limited-angle situations using a U-Net as generator and a discriminator to judge whether the inpainted data is real or fake (Li et al. 2019a; Fig. 18.8).

DL has also been explored to address metal artefact reduction (MAR) at the level of the projection data. The challenge is similar to the sparse- and limited-view situations, in the sense that gaps in the sinogram need to be filled; in this case, the gap only corresponds to the section of the projection corresponding to the metal object. While interpolation has been commonly used for the inpainting of projections affecting by metals, the use of DL for inpainting has been shown to lead to an improved image quality (Liang et al. 2019). Another study on MAR in dental CT used two CNNs, one of which applied an initial correction in the projection domain,

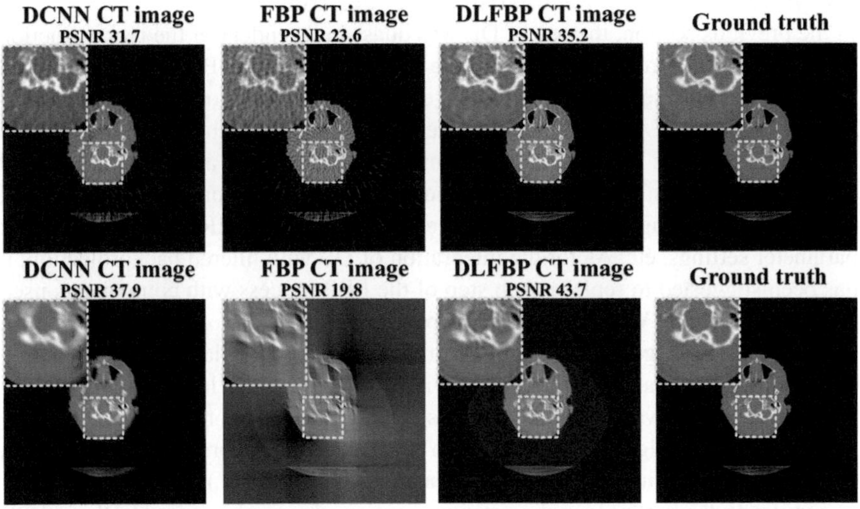

Fig. 18.7 Deep learning-based sinogram completion for sparse (*top*) and limited-angle (*bottom*) CT scans. *DCNN* deep convolutional neural network (Jin et al. 2017), *FBP* filtered backprojection, *DLFBP* deep learning filtered backprojection (Dong et al. 2019), *PSNR* peak signal-to-noise ratio. (Reproduced from Dong et al. 2019 under a Creative Commons Attribution License)

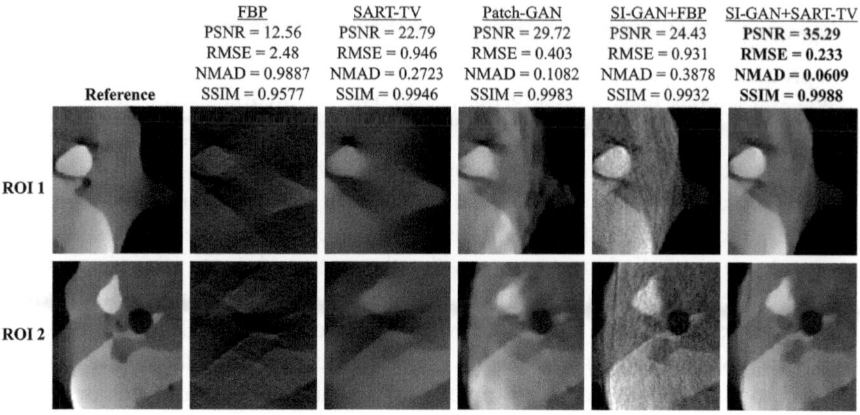

Fig. 18.8 Region of interest (*ROI*) within a limited-angle (80°) head CT scan, reconstructed with different methods. *FBP* filtered backprojection, *SART-TV* simultaneous algebraic reconstruction technique with total variation (Yu and Wang 2009). *patch-GAN* (Li et al. 2019b) and *SI-GAN* (Li et al. 2019a): generative adversarial network-based sinogram inpainting. Reference images were reconstructed with a full sinogram using SART-TV. *PSNR* peak signal-to-noise ratio, *RMSE* root mean squared error ($\times 10^{-3}$), *NMAD* normalized mean absolute distance, *SSIM* structural similarity index measure. For each metric, the best-performing method is highlighted in bold. (Reproduced from Li et al. 2019a under a Creative Commons Attribution License)

followed by an FBP reconstruction and a second correction in the image domain (Lee et al. 2020).

Integrated Within the Reconstruction Algorithm

In the previous section, the use of DL was quasi-independent of the reconstruction technique; after correcting or inpainting a sinogram, either FBP or IR could be used in principle. This section mostly involves the combination of DL with IR techniques, in which DL is integrated into the reconstruction pipeline. The overall goal of these methods is to overcome the limitations of IR, such as the computational demands of using an elaborate physics model during forward projection, the overall difficulty in reaching convergence, the sensitivity of certain IR techniques to their parameter settings, etc. As for the integration of DL with filtered backprojection, it has been suggested to replace each step of the FBP process with components used in neural networks (Würfl et al. 2016). Specifically, pixel or voxel weights used for fan- or cone-beam geometries could be replaced with a 1:1 layer, filtering with a convolutional layer and backprojection with a fully connected layer. Finally, a rectified linear unit activation can be used as a non-negativity constraint. It would be interesting to investigate whether such an approach could improve image quality in CBCT, particularly in regions closer to the field of view (FOV) periphery.

Similar to the methods in the previous section, the combination of DL with IR tends to focus on specific situations that cause image degradation, i.e. sparse-view and limited-view scans, metal artefacts, scatter, beam hardening, etc. An example is the use of a CNN to mimic an iteration in compressed sensing, which overcomes the issue of adaptive parameter selection (Chen et al. 2018). CNNs have also been used to replace the penalty function in proximal gradient descent for CT (Wu et al. 2019). Chen et al. (2020) developed a DL model (AirNet) aimed primarily at sparse-view situations in which total variation reconstruction methods are challenging. Their approach combines analytical and iterative reconstruction, using a residual learning-based NN for regularization; they also explored the use of dense connectivity between iterations, optimizing the number of prior iterations to be used at $n = 20$. The optimized version of AirNet outperformed other methods for sparse (down to 30 projections) and limited-angle (90°) conditions on prostate CT scans. Cheng et al. (2017) explored a different approach towards combining iterative reconstruction and DL, which they referred to as 'leapfrogging'. The similarity with the previous study is that information from a certain number of prior iterations is combined; in this case, the aim is to predict an image that corresponds to a future iteration. This approach could save computational time by ensuring a faster convergence of the iterative algorithm. While the authors evaluated this concept on positron emission tomography (PET) using an image-to-image CNN without pooling layers, they emphasized its potential for other imaging modalities, including model-based iterative reconstruction (MBIR) for CT.

Recently, a Grand Challenge from the American Association of Physicists in Medicine boosted research efforts on sparse-view CT reconstruction using DL (Sidky and Pan 2022). A summary of the best-performing submissions indicated a very high overall reconstruction accuracy, with improvements of up to two orders of magnitude compared with a benchmark CNN-based method (Sidky et al. 2021), as well as a high degree of robustness as indicated by worst-case test data results. The methods used varied considerably, although out of the top-five methods, most approaches involved deriving the forward model from the sinogram. The winning method involved an iterative network (ItNet) containing a pretrained U-Net and a data consistency layer that ensures agreement between the predicted and true sinograms (Genzel et al. 2022). The computational efficiency of their approach allows them to use the average of an ensemble of ten networks for increased consistency.

An example of a method that combines DL with IR for the purpose of metal artefact reduction is the approach proposed by Park et al. (2022). They used an encoder-decoder network, similar to a U-Net but using wavelets for down- and upsampling, which was integrated into an iterative MAR algorithm for dental CBCT. This approach lowered the quantitative effect of metal artefacts, expressed by the standard deviation of voxel values, compared with conventional MAR techniques.

Post-processing of Reconstructed Data

Certain studies attempt to train DL models to correct CT/CBCT scans that were reconstructed using a conventional algorithm. While the efficacy of such an approach may be somewhat more limited, the models are relatively easy to develop (as one can use reconstruction algorithms available on the scanners themselves), and training data is more readily available (as one does not require access to projection data and calibration info).

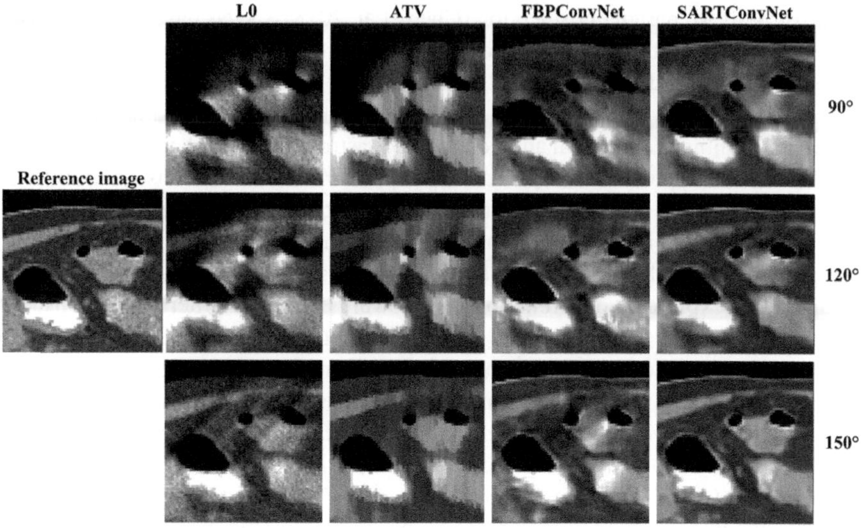

Fig. 18.9 Deep learning-based post-processing of computed tomography (CT) images. Zoomed-in regions of interest of an abdominal limited-angle CT scan. *Reference image*: full-angle reconstruction. *L0* Regularized gradient prior reconstruction (Yu et al. 2017), *ATV* Anisotropic total variation (Jin et al. 2010), *FBPConvNet* & *SARTConvNet* Convolutional neural network applied after filtered backprojection and simultaneous algebraic reconstruction technique, respectively (Wang et al. 2020). (Reproduced from Wang et al. 2020 under a Creative Commons Attribution License; relabeled version of original figure)

Previous sections have covered super-resolution and denoising methods, which largely use the same approach for radiographs, reconstructed scans or other images. For CT, reconstruction techniques such as SART and ART can be used instead of post-processing techniques for denoising, but these algorithms do not perform well in situations with incomplete data. To address this issue, Wang et al. (2020) used a U-Net for artefact correction of SART-reconstructed limited-angle CT scans. This approach improved image quality compared with alternative methods, including one where a CNN is combined with FBP rather than SART (Fig. 18.9).

Other applications of DL that operate after reconstruction include the correction of *metal artefacts.* A DL reconstruction technique was recently developed by one of the major CT manufacturers, which aims to reach high-dose model-based image reconstruction quality using a linear ten-layer CNN that incorporates advanced physics models (Tatsugami et al. 2019). Sakai et al. (2021) evaluated this reconstruction mode on a mandibular phantom with metal components, showing improvements in terms of both subjective image quality and technical image quality metrics compared with a hybrid iterative reconstruction technique. Huang et al. (2018) used deep residual learning using a modified VGG architecture, which provided an artefact map that can be subtracted from reconstructed CT data in a patch-based slice-by-slice manner (Fig. 18.10). Zhang and Yu (2018) proposed an approach in which an original FBP reconstruction is combined with two rudimentary MAR-corrected

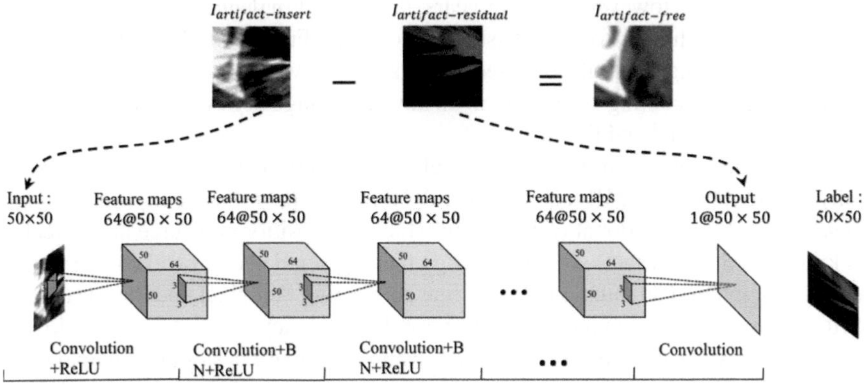

Fig. 18.10 Deep residual learning for estimating artefacts on reconstructed CT images (Huang et al. 2018). Two-dimensional patches of 50 × 50 pixels are used as input for a convolutional neural network. Image resolution is retained throughout the network (i.e. no down- or upsampling is performed, unlike a U-Net). The resulting output estimates the artefact intensity for each pixel, which can be combined with the input to yield an artefact-free image. (Reproduced from Huang et al. 2018 under a Creative Commons Attribution 4.0 International License)

reconstructions (i.e. beam hardening correction and linear interpolation) as a three-channel image, which is used as input for a five-layer CNN. The number of channels could be further expanded by incorporating additional MAR techniques. Their approach showed improved artefact suppression and anatomical visibility compared with conventional MAR methods, including for CT scans of the dental region. The aforementioned study by Lee et al. (2020) uses two CNNs, one of which operates in the projection domain to perform a preliminary MAR, followed by FBP and a second CNN that performs a final MAR in the image domain.

An interesting approach for MAR in dental CBCT, in which an intra-oral scan is used as additional input data, was suggested by Hyun et al. (2022). Specifically, the fact that intra-oral scans provide accurate boundaries of the crowns was exploited to suppress artefacts from fillings and other metal objects in that region.

Note that the expected image quality improvement for any image processing method applied to a reconstructed CT/CBCT scan is limited, especially in the presence of severe streaking with saturation of grey values. While the missing values are filled in in a somewhat 'smarter' way than what is used in interpolation-based projection completion methods, i.e. using expected structural information rather than nearby pixels/voxels, they should still be considered as a 'best guess'. It remains to be seen if diagnostic information can be restored through post-processing.

MRI Reconstruction

MRI has been traditionally used as an advanced imaging modality in dentistry, used in cases where conventional radiography does not suffice and when the main focus is on soft tissues. However, in recent years, the interest in dental MRI has increased considerably, including for hard-tissue applications (Fuglsig et al. 2021, 2023). At the time of writing, 'dental-dedicated' MRI scanners with a smaller physical footprint and built-in cooling system are in an advanced stage of development and (clinical) testing (Fischel and Eriksen 2022).

The image acquisition principle, as well as its underlying physics, is fundamentally different between MRI and CT (or CBCT). CT acquisition occurs within *image space,* as it is a projectional technique in which the position of source and detector is known throughout the scan. Thus, a signal at a given detector pixel can be attributed to the integral attenuation along a line connecting that pixel and the focal spot. MRI, however, uses a magnetic field and radiofrequency (RF) pulses that do not inherently have spatial attributes. Instead, using different types of *encoding,* data is acquired in a *k-space*. Reconstruction can be seen as a decoding of the k-space into image space (Hansen and Kellman 2015). The main similarity with CT reconstruction is that both are *inverse* problems; in MRI, prior knowledge regarding the forward model (i.e. the manner in which the k-space is filled) is used to yield an image. Reconstruction can be either direct (e.g. Fast Fourier Transform) or iterative (e.g. compressed sensing).

As with every medical imaging modality, image quality of MRI can be expressed using four fundamental parameters: sharpness, contrast, noise and artefacts. However, because MRI scans involve magnetic fields and non-ionizing radiation as opposed to X-rays, sources and effects of image degradation vary considerably between CT and MRI. Sources of noise in MRI include thermal effects within the patient, the bandwidth and 'detector' noise from the RF coil elements and analogue-digital converter. Several sources of artefacts can be noted, including but not limited to aliasing (for small FOVs) and imperfections in the magnetic field or gradients that lead to mismatches between encoding and decoding. Dental MRI is particularly susceptible to metal artefacts due to the frequent presence of objects with ferromagnetic properties, such as orthodontic appliances and prostheses (Johannsen et al. 2023). Furthermore, the image acquisition time is relatively long in MRI, resulting in an increased susceptibility for motion artefacts; whereas high-bandwidth protocols can lead to shorter acquisitions, this comes at the cost of increased noise.

An overview of the use of *DL in MRI reconstruction* can be found in the reviews by Lin et al. (2021), Pal and Rathi (2022), and Chandra et al. (2021). Similar to the use of DL in different phases of CT reconstruction, for MRI, a distinction can be made between DL methods that operate within the k-space only, that are involved in the mapping between the k-space and reconstructed image, and post-processing methods. Furthermore, distinctions can be made based on the neural network architecture, e.g. encoder-decoder networks and GANs. Some of the situations for which DL models are training include sparse sampling, motion correction, eddy current correction, metal/susceptibility artefacts as well as generic denoising and super-resolution. Figure 18.11 shows a comparison between several conventional and DL-based methods for accelerated MRI acquisitions.

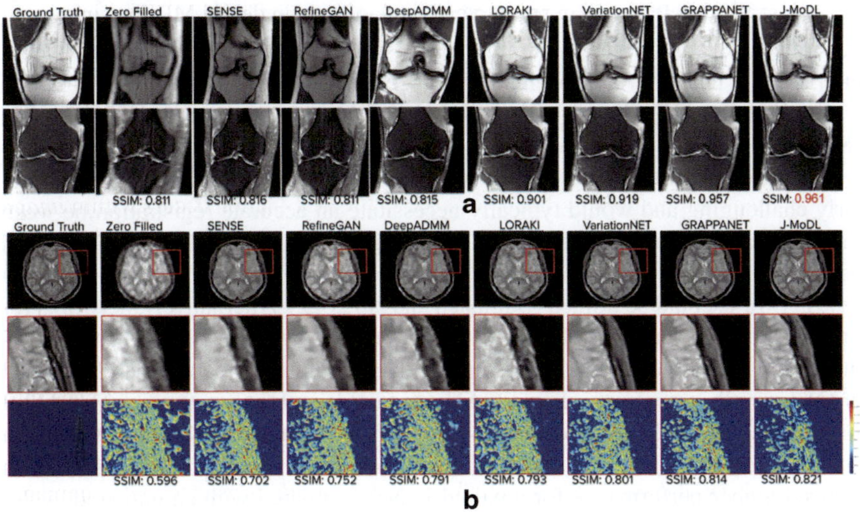

Fig. 18.11 Comparison between conventional and deep learning-based reconstruction for an 8× acceleration protocol for (**a**) knee and (**b**) brain fast MRI datasets. Apart from a basic '*zero filled*' approach, the following methods were evaluated: *SENSE* (Pruessmann et al. 1999), *DeepADMM* (Yang et al. 2016), *LORAKI* (Kim et al. 2019), *RefineGAN* (Quan et al. 2018), *VariationNET* (Sriram et al. 2020a), *GrappaNet* (Sriram et al. 2020b), *J-MoDL* (Aggarwal and Jacob 2020). Apart from a qualitative comparison, corresponding structural similarity index measure (SSIM) scores are shown as well. (Reproduced from Pal and Rathi 2022 under a CC-BY 4.0 license)

Inter-modality Conversion

Finally, DL can be trained to perform inter-modality conversion, e.g. MRI-to-CT (for radiotherapy planning or bone segmentation) or CBCT-to-CT (for Hounsfield unit calibration and contrast-to-noise ratio improvement). As mentioned in section "Deep Learning in Image Registration", inter-modality conversion can also facilitate multi-modal registration.

Similar to other applications covered in this and the previous chapter, the training of DL methods that operate on 3D images can be challenging due to memory limitations. On the other hand, a slice-by-slice 2D DL model could lead to discrepancies between adjacent slices. A common solution is the use of a patch-based 3D CNN: for example, a 3D U-Net using patches of 48 × 48 × 48 voxels has been used for MRI-CT conversion to allow for dose calculations in head and neck radiotherapy (Dinkla et al. 2019). Another study used 32 × 32 × 32 voxel MRI patches as input for a GAN, which yielded 16 × 16 × 16 voxel pseudo-CT patches as output (Nie et al. 2017). A comparison between 2D and 3D U-Nets for pseudo-CT generation from T1 MRI scans, also for the purpose of dose calculation in radiotherapy, showed a slightly better performance using a 2D approach; note that the 3D U-Net was in fact a 3D-to-2D architecture, in which a single slice was generated as output based on an input consisting of 32 consecutive slices (Neppl et al. 2019). The latter approach has also been explored for cycleGANs, in which 3 consecutive MRI slices were used as a '2.5D' input for pseudo-CT synthesis (Sun et al. 2023).

For inter-modality conversion, obtaining adequately paired data can be particularly challenging and would typically necessitate an accurate registration between input and labels. For example, a study involving head and neck MRI-CT conversion used an affine registration to pair the data, after which different encoder-decoder-type networks could be trained (Bambach and Ho 2022). Alternatively, networks for unpaired images can be used. For the conversion of low-dose CBCT to pseudo-CT in order to perform dose calculation in adaptive radiotherapy, between a conditional GAN (paired), a cycle-consistent GAN (unpaired) and an attention-guided GAN (unpaired), the latter showed the best outcome (Gao et al. 2021). Conversely, a study on MRI-CT conversion for the purpose of enhanced bone visualization showed higher performance for a paired U-Net compared with an unpaired cycle-GAN (Song et al. 2021). Indeed, unpaired approaches for inter-modality conversion could lead to inconsistencies at edges, especially due to the varying contrast in MRI vs. CT. To improve the performance of MRI-to-CT cycleGANs in boundary regions, the use of gradient consistency loss has been proposed (Hiasa et al. 2018). Note that, due to the differences in image appearance between MRI protocols (e.g. T1 vs. T2, post-contrast, fluid-attenuated inversion recovery), it can be difficult to train generalizable DL models for pseudo-CT synthesis, and retraining may be necessary (Li et al. 2021). To facilitate MRI-CT conversion, intensity normalization can be performed first (Hou et al. 2021).

When considering conversion from CBCT to pseudo-CT, one has to be mindful of the difference in sharpness between the two modalities and ensure that the method is geared towards achieving the contrast, noise and HU accuracy of CT while retaining the sharpness of CBCT.

Take-Home Messages: Deep Learning in Image Reconstruction

- DL-based reconstruction is an umbrella term, covering a wide variety of methods that operate on raw data, facilitate the reconstruction process itself or perform post-processing.
- Most research studies evaluate the performance of DL reconstruction methods at Level 1 of the Fryback and Thornbury (1991) diagnostic efficacy scale (e.g. noise, sharpness); further evidence is needed regarding higher-level efficacy of these methods (e.g. diagnostic accuracy, effect on treatment planning/outcome).

Deep Learning in Image Registration

Introduction

Registration refers to the spatial alignment of two or more images. In a medical context, many applications of registration can be found. As the definition is rather broad, there are several ways to categorize medical image registration (Fu et al. 2020):

- *Unimodal* vs. *multimodal*. In general, unimodal registration is more straightforward, as the source and target images would have highly similar properties. Multimodal registration can be 2D-to-2D, 3D-to-3D, 2D-to-3D, etc.
- *Inter-patient* vs. *intra-patient*. The former would typically be unimodal; for the latter, same-day multimodal acquisitions or different-day unimodal acquisitions can be distinguished.
- *Rigid* vs. *similarity* vs. *affine* vs. *deformable* (Fig. 18.12). A rigid registration involves translation and rotation of the image; for 3D images, this corresponds to six degrees of freedom. A similarity transform also includes an isotropic scaling factor; this can be of use if one of the images is not geometrically calibrated. Affine registration adds non-isotropic scaling and skewing (shearing), thereby doubling the degrees of freedom compared with rigid registration. Deformable (non-rigid) registration, as its name implies, involves curved transformation matrices (e.g. B-splines), allowing for images that represent objects of different shape to be aligned (e.g. inter-patient, intra-patient in the presence of tissue deformation due to surgery, weight loss or motion).
- *Voxel-based* vs. *surface-based* vs. *landmark-based*. Voxel-based registration (or pixel-based for 2D images) attempts to find pairwise correspondence between original intensities of each image element. Surface-based registration is used for matching mesh-type data (e.g. a segmented CT/CBCT scan with an intra-oral or face scan). Landmark-based registration minimizes the distance between a set of, often manually placed, landmarks at distinct anatomical locations.

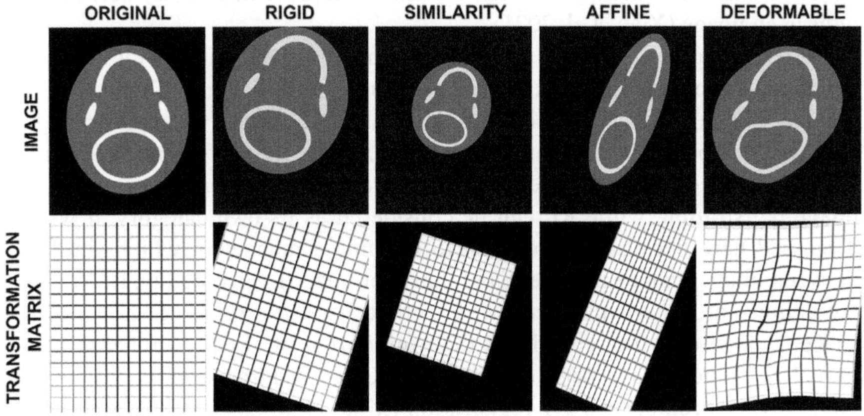

Fig. 18.12 Types of transformations used in image registration

Throughout the years, several algorithms have been proposed for generic or modality/application-specific image registration (Fu et al. 2020). A general challenge is to assure high accuracy and robustness at a reasonable computational time, especially for 3D registration of high-resolution images. Therefore, recent research has explored the use of deep learning as an optimization tool for image registration. This section will describe the applications of DL in image registration; for an exhaustive literature review, the reader is referred to the work of Fu et al. (2020), Xiao et al. (2021) and, for deformable registration in particular, Zou et al. (2022).

Types of DL Registration Methods

The use of DL in image registration can be categorized in different ways. Fu et al. (2020) suggested six general (non-exclusive) categories of methods, in which some type of (convolutional) neural network is almost always used, plus 'other' methods using different machine learning algorithms (e.g. random forest, support vector machine). Xiao et al. (2021) proposed three main categories: (1) deep iterative registration (incl. deep similarity and reinforcement learning), (2) supervised registration and (3) unsupervised registration (incl. GAN-based registration). A modified version of these two categorizations will be presented in this section.

Deep Similarity (incl. Reinforcement Learning)

Image registration outcome is highly dependent on the metric that is used to express *similarity* between two or more images. Depending on the type of metric, an algorithm attempts to minimize or maximize its value in order to reach an optimal alignment. Deep similarity methods attempt to go beyond conventional metrics for image similarity based on intensity, such as mean square error and mutual information. While these conventional metrics have shown good performance, especially for unimodal registration, there are a few common limitations, such as sensitivity to noise and artefacts, and the fact that they are calculated at the level of individual pixels or voxels, and do not naturally take into account the relative importance between features in an image (Xiao et al. 2021).

Different studies proposed the use of trainable deep similarity classifiers, in which the alignment can be expressed as a binary outcome, i.e. 'aligned' or 'not aligned' (Cheng et al. 2018; Simonovsky et al. 2016). Using an appropriate loss function, this outcome can then be optimized. While the aforementioned studies used supervised learning, others have explored *reinforcement learning* (RL) in image registration; while RL can be considered as its own category, it will be discussed here because it also aims to redefine a manner in which similarity between images can be assessed (and thus, optimized). Specifically, RL requires the definition of a *reward function*, a method for *exploration* of the parameter space to maximize the reward and the *exploitation* of already-gained information. RL methods have been described for CBCT-CT registration (Liao et al. 2016), 2D-3D radiograph-CT registration (Miao et al. 2017) MRI-CT registration (Sun et al. 2019; Fig. 18.13), etc. For optimal performance and high

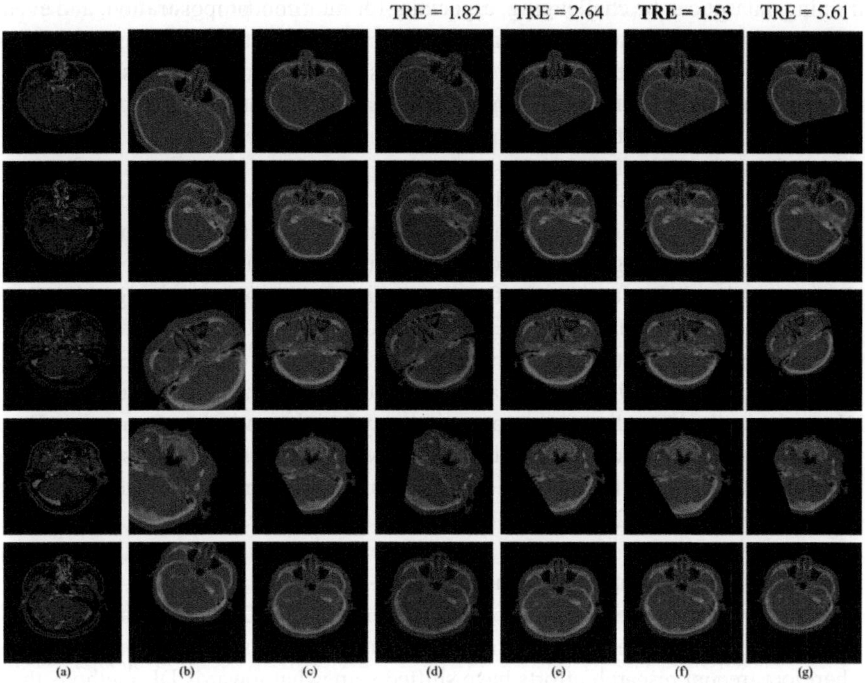

Fig. 18.13 Comparison of MRI-CT registration results for different methods. (**a**) Fixed image, (**b**) initial moving image, (**c**) ground truth registration for moving image, (**d**) conventional registration algorithm (elastix; advanced Mattes mutual information), (**e**) supervised learning using transformation matrix, (**f**) deep recurrent reinforcement learning with landmark error, (**g**) same network as 'f' with supervised learning (mean square error). The mean target registration error (TRE) for two test cases is shown above each method; the best-performing method is highlighted in bold. (Reproduced from Sun et al. 2019 with permission by Springer Nature)

computational efficiency, RL methods need to be tailored to a given task, and random/brute-force searching should be avoided. It has been noted that training time to reach convergence for RL methods can be an issue (Xiao et al. 2021). This implies that RL is mainly of interest for rigid registration problems due to the limited degrees of freedom that are involved (i.e. translation and rotation), although methods for deformable registration have also been proposed, in which the reward function is trained in a supervised manner (Krebs et al. 2017). Alternatively, RL methods with DL components have been developed for 3D landmark detection (Ghesu et al. 2016), which could then be used for landmark-based registration.

An entirely different approach involves the use of machine learning to combine different metrics for an increased robustness; Ferrante et al. (2019) trained a support vector machine that considers various similarity features, which outperformed methods based on individual metrics.

A challenge for deep similarity methods with some form of supervised or reinforcement learning is the need for accurately aligned image pairs. Obtaining such a training dataset can be challenging, especially for multimodal registration, and even more so if the goal is to outperform conventional registration methods. Although other DL methods have addressed this issue, several deep similarity studies have tried to overcome this challenge, e.g. using particular data augmentation techniques (Sedghi et al. 2018) or using autoencoders that learn low-level features in an unsupervised manner (Wu et al. 2016).

While deep similarity methods have shown good performance in several situations, often outperforming traditional metrics, they do not overcome the computational challenge in image registration as they still require an iterative process. The metrics are also difficult to interpret, and assessing or improving training/validation performance can be challenging. Furthermore, optimization algorithms based on deep similarity require these metrics to have a smooth first derivative. Even if deep similarity methods can lead to increased registration outcome or faster convergence, DL methods that use a direct transformation may be inherently more attractive. Due to the ever-improving accuracy of the latter type of methods, it can be seen that the interest in deep similarity and (especially) RL methods waned in the late 2010s (Fu et al. 2020; Xiao et al. 2021).

One-Shot Transformation (Supervised)

As mentioned in the previous section, despite the fact that DL can enhance the performance of iterative registration methods, computational speed remains an issue. Therefore, recent research efforts have shifted somewhat towards DL methods that provide a one-shot prediction of the optimal transformation. While this approach is interesting from the point of view of clinical implementation, potentially speeding up a laborious process, it is considered more challenging as well.

For supervised one-shot transformation, as with all other methods that require ground truth data, training performance hinges on image pairs with known transformations. Such image pairs are often generated during the training process itself, e.g. using randomly imposed transformations, traditional registration methods or model-based transformations (Fu et al. 2020).

The supervision approach can vary as well. Traditional supervised learning considers the final output of a model during training and minimizes the loss with the expected output. Certain registration methods are considered *weakly supervised*, as they do not look at similarities between the entire, original images, but at specific representations such as anatomical masks or landmarks. Others are *deeply supervised*, as they consider the output for individual layers rather than a singular final output. *Dual supervised* approaches, using both supervised and unsupervised loss, have also been explored.

Performance of one-shot transformation methods has been somewhat limited due to the exploratory nature of most studies; in many cases, they have not (yet) outperformed traditional registration methods (Fu et al. 2020). Issues that were noted include overfitting, image downsampling or patching needed due to GPU memory limits and pre-registration being needed (Sun and Zhang 2018; Sokooti et al. 2019; Eppenhof and Pluim 2019). While some of the limitations of this approach are addressed through unsupervised learning (see next section), interest in further development of supervised methods is expected to remain high.

One-Shot Transformation (Unsupervised)

Whereas unsupervised transformations do not rely on training datasets, their performance relies on a suitable network design and loss function. A specific method that has shown potential in this context is the spatial transformer network (Jaderberg et al. 2015), which can be used as a module within CNN architectures such as autoencoders (Yoo et al. 2017) and U-Net variants (Balakrishnan et al. 2018, 2019), from which a similarity loss value can be derived.

Interestingly, several studies combined segmentation and registration (Balakrishnan et al. 2019; Qin et al. 2018; Mahapatra et al. 2018). Indeed, it makes sense that these are two complementary (and mutually reinforcing) functions, which rely on similar features.

Unsupervised transformation approaches have been arguably more popular than supervised ones, mainly due to a lack of suitable training data for the latter. While results have shown promising performance, most studies involve unimodal registration; its application for the registration of images from different modalities is likely to be more challenging. Research interest in unsupervised one-shot registration is expected to remain high (Fu et al. 2020).

Generative Adversarial Networks in Registration

GANs have been described in previous sections as polyvalent tools for various types of image processing, such as denoising, super-resolution, projection completion and artefact correction. Within the context of image registration, they can be used as an accessory method for:

- *Regularizing the transformation:* there are different manners in which to use a GAN-discriminator and adversarial loss to verify the registration outcome. Whereas the most obvious application is to verify whether or not images are aligned (Fan et al. 2019), it can also be used to ensure that the transformation still results in a realistic image (Lei et al. 2020), which is relevant for deformable registration in particular. This application of GANs can be considered as a particular case of the deep similarity approach described above.
- *Generating pseudo-unimodal images*: for multimodal registration tasks, DL registration can be particularly challenging. Therefore, GANs can be useful as a preprocessing step to map images from one modality to the other (see section "Inter-modality Conversion"), essentially turning the registration into a unimodal one.

Registration Validation

Fu et al. (2020) distinguished a group of methods used in *registration validation*, which are not necessarily used in the registration process itself (unlike conventional or deep similarity metrics) but provide a more interpretable and relevant performance evaluation compared with such metrics.

Dental Applications of DL Registration

As DL registration is a relatively new field, arguably even more so than other DL applications in medical imaging, research involving dental applications has been somewhat scarce. Of course, several of the previously described approaches are expected to be applicable to dental images, either directly (unsupervised) or after a certain degree of adaptation/retraining on dental data (supervised/reinforcement).

A potential application is in the registration of CBCT (or CT) data with intra-oral scans (Fig. 18.14). A recent study compared a DL registration tool with two

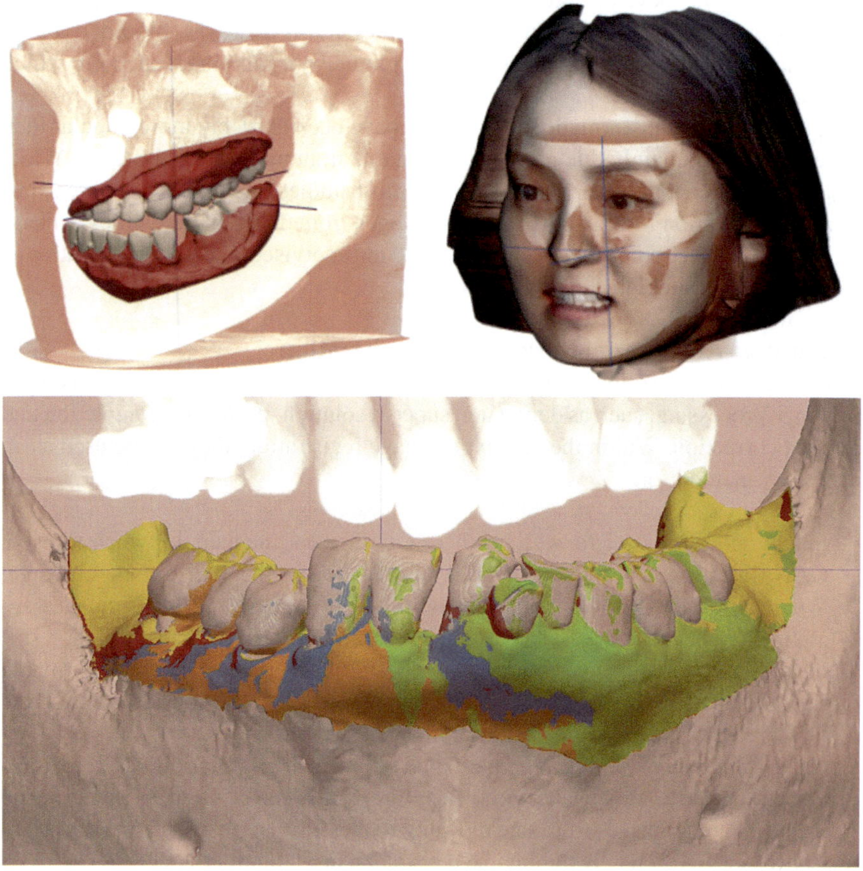

Fig. 18.14 *Top:* automatic registration of intra-oral (*left*) and facial scan (*right*) with cone-beam computed tomography scans using deep learning. *Bottom:* Comparison between different registration methods. *Red*: deep learning registration. *Orange*: manual registration. *Yellow*: surface-based registration. *Green* and *blue*: landmark-based registration. In accordance with the high degree of visual overlap shown in this figure, the mean error between the methods was not significantly different. (*Top:* Reproduced with permission by Dentbird, Seoul, Republic of Korea (http://dentbird.com). *Bottom:* Reproduced from Piao et al. 2022 with permission by Springer Nature; cropped version of original figure)

landmark-based, one surface-based, and one manual method found in various software packages (Piao et al. 2022). Although details regarding the DL tool in question were proprietary, results showed that it performed similarly to the other methods in terms of registration accuracy, with a mean error of ca. 0.3 mm for each method. However, the time needed for registration was greatly reduced using DL, with a mean time of 12 s (note: the DL tool is cloud-based) vs. 416 s for manual registration, 230 s for surface-based registration and 93–125 s for landmark-based registration. DL registration proved to be sensitive to the amount of dental restorations, which was also the case for the other non-manual registration methods. A different approach, which attempts to overcome the issue with artefacts from dental restorations, was proposed by Kim et al. (2023). They used a 2D CNN to determine a plane that separates upper and lower teeth on lateral maximum intensity projections from CT scans, after which the tooth surfaces are determined by determining the nearest 'hard-tissue' voxels along vertical lines through each point of the separation plane. For registration, they proposed a method called curvature variance of neighbourhood, which is linked to strong local variations in surface smoothness that correspond either to artefacts or to naturally changing surfaces such as incisal edges. Although their method outperformed alternative approaches, it was shown to be sensitive to the choice of an HU threshold value; thus, it remains to be seen if this approach can be readily applied to CBCT data as well. Another method for registering CT to optical scans, which does not rely on prior segmentation of the CT image, was proposed by Chung et al. (2020). Similar to the research by Kim et al. (2023), they reduced the 3D voxel-based data of CT to a lateral maximum intensity projection; subsequently, two VGG-16 CNNs operated in parallel to determine a corresponding point and line on both datasets, which are then used for initial alignment. The registration was then refined by matching similarities using clustering.

Another potential application is in the registration of unimodal CT or CBCT scans acquired throughout a treatment process in order to evaluate hard- and soft-tissue changes. Note that cephalometric landmark identification, which is an application of DL described in the previous chapter, can be used as an initial step in automated landmark-based registration of large-volume CBCT or CT scans. However, clinical applications in which this could be of use would likely involve a growing patient and/or surgical intervention which alters certain aspects of the patient's morphology, which would limit the relevance of landmark-based image superposition. Likely, a regional rigid registration (voxel-based or surface-based) using anatomical features with a fixed morphology would be of more use for those cases (Cevidanes et al. 2009); further research is needed to evaluate the use of DL for this purpose.

As for other dental applications, it will be interesting to see whether DL will open the door towards novel clinical uses of registration, including 2D-to-3D registration.

Take-Home Messages: Deep Learning in Image Registration

- Registration using DL covers a wide variety of methods: some are generic, and others are highly tailored to specific registration tasks.
- Unlike other applications of DL in image processing, in which DL often outperforms alternative methods, DL registration involving a 'one-shot' transformation was not found to consistently outperform conventional registration techniques (yet).
- Research interest in this field is expected to remain high, with the main focus likely being on supervised/unsupervised methods that do not need an iterative process and pipelines in which segmentation and registration are combined.

References

Aetesam H, Maji SK. Perceptually motivated generative model for magnetic resonance image denoising. J Digit Imaging. 2023;36:725–38. https://doi.org/10.1007/s10278-022-00744-2.

Aggarwal HK, Jacob M. J-MoDL: joint model-based deep learning for optimized sampling and reconstruction. IEEE J Sel Top Signal Process. 2020;14:1151–62. https://doi.org/10.1109/jstsp.2020.3004094.

Armando M, Franco JS, Boyer E. Mesh denoising with facet graph convolutions. IEEE Trans Vis Comput Graph. 2022;28:2999–3012. https://doi.org/10.1109/TVCG.2020.3045490.

Azour L, Hu Y, Ko JP, Chen B, Knoll F, Alpert JB, et al. Deep learning denoising of low-dose computed tomography chest images: a quantitative and qualitative image analysis. J Comput Assist Tomogr. 2023;47:212–9. https://doi.org/10.1097/RCT.0000000000001405.

Balakrishnan G, Zhao A, Sabuncu MR, Guttag J, Dalca AV. An unsupervised learning model for deformable medical image registration. In: Proc IEEE/CVF Conf Comput Vis Pattern Recognit. 2018. pp. 9252–9260. https://doi.org/10.1109/CVPR.2018.00964.

Balakrishnan G, Zhao A, Sabuncu MR, Guttag J, Dalca AV. VoxelMorph: a learning framework for deformable medical image registration. IEEE Trans Med Imaging. 2019;38:1788–800. https://doi.org/10.1109/TMI.2019.2897538.

Bambach S, Ho ML. Deep learning for synthetic CT from bone MRI in the head and neck. AJNR Am J Neuroradiol. 2022;43:1172–9. https://doi.org/10.3174/ajnr.A7588.

Bashir SMA, Wang Y, Khan M, Niu Y. A comprehensive review of deep learning-based single image super-resolution. PeerJ Comput Sci. 2021;7:e621. https://doi.org/10.7717/peerj-cs.621.

Cavigelli L, Hager P, Benini L. CAS-CNN: a deep convolutional neural network for image compression artifact suppression. Int Jt Conf Neural Netw. 2017;752–759. https://doi.org/10.1109/IJCNN.2017.7965927.

Cevidanes LH, Heymann G, Cornelis MA, DeClerck HJ, Tulloch JF. Superimposition of 3-dimensional cone-beam computed tomography models of growing patients. Am J Orthod Dentofac Orthop. 2009;136:94–9. https://doi.org/10.1016/j.ajodo.2009.01.018.

Chandra SS, Bran Lorenzana M, Liu X, Liu S, Bollmann S, Crozier S. Deep learning in magnetic resonance image reconstruction. J Med Imaging Radiat Oncol. 2021;65:564–77. https://doi.org/10.1111/1754-9485.13276.

Chaudhari AS, Fang Z, Kogan F, Wood J, Stevens KJ, Gibbons EK, et al. Super-resolution musculoskeletal MRI using deep learning. Magn Reson Med. 2018;80:2139–54. https://doi.org/10.1002/mrm.27178.

Chen H, Zhang Y, Kalra MK, Lin F, Chen Y, Liao P, et al. Low-dose CT with a residual encoder-decoder convolutional neural network. IEEE Trans Med Imaging. 2017;36:2524–35. https://doi.org/10.1109/TMI.2017.2715284.

Chen H, Zhang Y, Chen Y, Zhang J, Zhang W, Sun H, et al. LEARN: learned experts' assessment-based reconstruction network for sparse-data CT. IEEE Trans Med Imaging. 2018;37:1333–47. https://doi.org/10.1109/TMI.2018.2805692.

Chen G, Hong X, Ding Q, Zhang Y, Chen H, Fu S, et al. AirNet: fused analytical and iterative reconstruction with deep neural network regularization for sparse-data CT. Med Phys. 2020;47:2916–30. https://doi.org/10.1002/mp.14170.

Chen Q, Song H, Yu J, Kim K. Current development and applications of super-resolution ultrasound imaging. Sensors (Basel). 2021;21:2417. https://doi.org/10.3390/s21072417.

Cheng L, Ahn S, Ross SG, Qian H, De Man B. Accelerated iterative image reconstruction using a deep learning based leapfrogging strategy. In: Proc Int Conf Fully Three-Dimensional Image Reconstr Radiol Nucl Med. 2017. https://doi.org/10.13140/RG.2.2.32134.88647.

Cheng X, Zhang L, Zheng Y. Deep similarity learning for multimodal medical images. Comput Methods Biomech Biomed Engin. 2018;6:248–52. https://doi.org/10.1080/21681163.2015.1135299.

Chung M, Lee J, Song W, Song Y, Yang IH, Lee J, Shin YG. Automatic registration between dental cone-beam CT and scanned surface via deep pose regression neural networks and clustered similarities. IEEE Trans Med Imaging. 2020;39:3900–9. https://doi.org/10.1109/TMI.2020.3007520.

Cohen T, Welling M. Group equivariant convolutional networks. In: Proc Int Conf Mach Learn. 2016;48:2990–9. https://doi.org/10.48550/arXiv.1602.07576.

Dabov K, Foi A, Katkovnik V, Egiazarian K. BM3D image denoising with shape-adaptive principal component analysis. 2009.

Dai T, Cai J, Zhang Y, Xia ST, Zhang L. Second-order attention network for single image superresolution. In: Proc IEEE Comput Soc Conf Comput Vis Pattern Recognit. 2019. pp. 11065–11074. https://doi.org/10.1109/CVPR.2019.01132.

Dinkla AM, Florkow MC, Maspero M, Savenije MHF, Zijlstra F, Doornaert PAH, et al. Dosimetric evaluation of synthetic CT for head and neck radiotherapy generated by a patch-based three-dimensional convolutional neural network. Med Phys. 2019;46:4095–104. https://doi.org/10.1002/mp.13663.

Dong C, Loy CC, He K, Tang X. Learning a deep convolutional network for image super-resolution. Lect Notes Comput Sci. 2014;8692:184–99. https://doi.org/10.1007/978-3-319-10593-2_13.

Dong C, Loy CC, Tang X. Accelerating the super-resolution convolutional neural network. Lect Notes Comput Sci. 2016;9906:391–407. https://doi.org/10.1007/978-3-319-46475-6_25.

Dong J, Fu J, He Z. A deep learning reconstruction framework for X-ray computed tomography with incomplete data. PLoS One. 2019;14:e0224426. https://doi.org/10.1371/journal.pone.0224426.

Eppenhof KAJ, Pluim JPW. Pulmonary CT registration through supervised learning with convolutional neural networks. IEEE Trans Med Imaging. 2019;38:1097–105. https://doi.org/10.1109/TMI.2018.2878316.

Fan J, Cao X, Wang Q, Yap PT, Shen D. Adversarial learning for mono- or multi-modal registration. Med Image Anal. 2019;58:101545. https://doi.org/10.1016/j.media.2019.101545.

Feldkamp LA, Davis LC, J. W. Kress JW. Practical cone-beam algorithm. J Opt Soc Am A 1984;1:612–9. https://doi.org/10.1364/JOSAA.1.000612.

Ferrante E, Dokania PK, Silva RM, Paragios N. Weakly supervised learning of metric aggregations for deformable image registration. IEEE J Biomed Health Inform. 2019;23:1374–84. https://doi.org/10.1109/JBHI.2018.2869700.

Fischel S, Eriksen LW. I was so excited that I was hardly able to sleep last night. 2022. https://dent.au.dk/en/display/artikel/jeg-er-saa-spaendt-at-jeg-naesten-ikke-har-sovet-i-nat. Accessed 23 Apr 2023.

Fryback DG, Thornbury JR. The efficacy of diagnostic imaging. Med Decis Mak. 1991;11:88–94. https://doi.org/10.1177/0272989X9101100203.

Fu Y, Lei Y, Wang T, Curran WJ, Liu T, Yang X. Deep learning in medical image registration: a review. Phys Med Biol. 2020;65:20TR01. https://doi.org/10.1088/1361-6560/ab843e.

Fu B, Zhang X, Wang L, Ren Y, Thanh DNH. A blind medical image denoising method with noise generation network. J Xray Sci Technol. 2022;30:531–47. https://doi.org/10.3233/XST-211098.

Fuglsig JMCES, Wenzel A, Hansen B, Lund TE, Spin-Neto R. Magnetic resonance imaging for the planning, execution, and follow-up of implant-based oral rehabilitation: systematic review. Int J Oral Maxillofac Implants. 2021;36:432–41. https://doi.org/10.11607/jomi.8536.

Fuglsig JMCES, Hansen B, Schropp L, Nixdorf DR, Wenzel A, Spin-Neto R. Alveolar bone measurements in magnetic resonance imaging compared with cone beam computed tomography: a pilot, ex-vivo study. Acta Odontol Scand. 2023;81:241–8. https://doi.org/10.1080/00016357.2022.2121321.

Gao L, Xie K, Wu X, Lu Z, Li C, Sun J, et al. Generating synthetic CT from low-dose cone-beam CT by using generative adversarial networks for adaptive radiotherapy. Radiat Oncol. 2021;16:202. https://doi.org/10.1186/s13014-021-01928-w.

Genzel M, Gühring I, Macdonald J, März M. Near-exact recovery for tomographic inverse problems via deep learning. arXiv. 2022:2206.07050. https://doi.org/10.48550/arXiv.2206.07050.

Ghesu FC, Georgescu B, Mansi T, Neumann D, Hornegger J, Comaniciu D. An artificial agent for anatomical landmark detection in medical images. Lect Notes Comput Sci. 2016;9902:229–37. https://doi.org/10.1007/978-3-319-46726-9_27.

Guo S, Yan Z, Zhang K, Zuo W, Zhang L. Toward convolutional blind denoising of real photographs. Proc IEEE Conf Comput Vis Pattern Recognit. 2019:1712–1722. https://doi.org/10.1109/CVPR.2019.00181.

Hansen MS, Kellman P. Image reconstruction: an overview for clinicians. J Magn Reson Imaging. 2015;41:573–85. https://doi.org/10.1002/jmri.24687.

Hariharan SG, Kaethner C, Strobel N, Kowarschik M, Fahrig R, Navab N. Robust learning-based x-ray image denoising-potential pitfalls, their analysis and solutions. Biomed Phys Eng Express. 2022;8. https://doi.org/10.1088/2057-1976/ac3489.

Hegazy MAA, Cho MH, Lee SY. Image denoising by transfer learning of generative adversarial network for dental CT. Biomed Phys Eng Express. 2020;6:055024. https://doi.org/10.1088/2057-1976/abb068.

Hiasa Y, Otake Y, Takao M, Matsuoka T, Takashima K, Carass A, et al. Cross-modality image synthesis from unpaired data using CycleGAN. Lect Notes Comput Sci. 2018;11037:31–41. https://doi.org/10.1007/978-3-030-00536-8_4.

Hou KY, Lu HY, Yang CC. Applying MRI intensity normalization on non-bone tissues to facilitate pseudo-CT synthesis from MRI. Diagnostics (Basel). 2021;11:816. https://doi.org/10.3390/diagnostics11050816.

Hu X, Mu H, Zhang X, Wang Z, Tan T, Sun J. Meta-SR: a magnification-arbitrary network for super-resolution. Proc IEEE Comput Soc Conf Comput Vis Pattern Recognit. 2019:1575–1584. https://doi.org/10.1109/CVPR.2019.00167.

Huang X, Wang J, Tang F, Zhong T, Zhang Y. Metal artifact reduction on cervical CT images by deep residual learning. Biomed Eng Online. 2018;17:175. https://doi.org/10.1186/s12938-018-0609-y.

Hugelier S, de Rooi JJ, Bernex R, Duwé S, Devos O, Sliwa M, et al. Sparse deconvolution of high-density super-resolution images. Sci Rep. 2016;6:21413. https://doi.org/10.1038/srep21413.

Hyun CM, Bayaraa T, Yun HS, Jang TJ, Park HS, Seo JK. Deep learning method for reducing metal artifacts in dental cone-beam CT using supplementary information from intra-oral scan. Phys Med Biol. 2022;67. https://doi.org/10.1088/1361-6560/ac8852.

Jaderberg M, Simonyan K, Zisserman A, Kavukcuoglu K. Spatial transformer networks. arXiv. 2015:1506.02025. https://doi.org/10.48550/arXiv.1506.02025.

Jiang X, Zhu Y, Zheng B, Yang D. Images denoising for COVID-19 chest X-ray based on multi-resolution parallel residual CNN. Mach Vis Appl. 2021;32:100. https://doi.org/10.1007/s00138-021-01224-3.

Jin X, Li L, Chen Z, Zhang L, Xing Y. Anisotropic total variation for limited-angle CT reconstruction. IEEE Nucl Sci Symp Med Imaging Conf. 2010:2232–38. https://doi.org/10.1109/NSSMIC.2010.5874180.

Jin KH, McCann MT, Froustey E, Unser M. Deep convolutional neural network for inverse problems in imaging. IEEE Trans Image Process. 2017;26:4509–22. https://doi.org/10.1109/TIP.2017.2713099.

Johannsen KM, de Carvalho E, Silva Fuglsig JM, Hansen B, Wenzel A, Spin-Neto R. Magnetic resonance imaging artefacts caused by orthodontic appliances and/or implant-supported prosthesis: a systematic review. Oral Radiol. 2023;39:394–407. https://doi.org/10.1007/s11282-022-00652-9.

Kang SR, Shin W, Yang S, Kim JE, Huh KH, Lee SS, et al. Structure-preserving quality improvement of cone beam CT images using contrastive learning. Comput Biol Med. 2023;158:106803. https://doi.org/10.1016/j.compbiomed.2023.106803.

Kim TH, Garg P, Haldar JP. LORAKI: Autocalibrated recurrent neural networks for autoregressive MRI reconstruction in k-space. arXiv. 2019:1904.09390. https://doi.org/10.48550/arXiv.1904.09390.

Kim M, Chung M, Shin YG, Kim B. Automatic registration of dental CT and 3D scanned model using deep split jaw and surface curvature. Comput Methods Prog Biomed. 2023;233:107467. https://doi.org/10.1016/j.cmpb.2023.107467.

Kojima S, Ito T, Hayashi T. Denoising using Noise2Void for low-field magnetic resonance imaging: a phantom study. J Med Phys. 2022;47:387–93. https://doi.org/10.4103/jmp.jmp_71_22.

Krebs J, Mansi T, Delingette H, Zhang L, Ghesu FC, Miao S, et al. Robust non-rigid registration through agent-based action learning. Lect Notes Comput Sci. 2017;10433:344–52. https://doi.org/10.1007/978-3-319-66182-7_40.

Krull A, Buchholz TO, Jug F. Noise2Void - Learning Denoising from Single Noisy Images. arXiv 2018:1811.10980. https://doi.org/10.48550/arXiv.1811.10980.

Lai WS, Bin Huang J, Ahuja N, Yang MH. Deep Laplacian pyramid networks for fast and accurate super-resolution. Proc IEEE Conf Comput Vis Pattern Recognit. 2017:624–632. https://doi.org/10.1109/CVPR.2017.618.

Ledig C, Theis L, Huszár F, Caballero J, Cunningham A, Acosta A, et al. Photo-realistic single image super-resolution using a generative adversarial network. Proc IEEE Conf Comput Vis Pattern Recognit. 2017:4681–4690. https://doi.org/10.1109/CVPR.2017.19.

Lee K, Jeong WK. ISCL: interdependent self-cooperative learning for unpaired image denoising. IEEE Trans Med Imaging. 2021;40:3238–48. https://doi.org/10.1109/TMI.2021.3096142.

Lee J, Jin KH. Local texture estimator for implicit representation function. arXiv. 2021:2111.08918. https://doi.org/10.48550/arXiv.2111.08918.

Lee D, Park C, Lim Y, Cho H. A metal artifact reduction method using a fully convolutional network in the Sinogram and image domains for dental computed tomography. J Digit Imaging. 2020;33:538–46. https://doi.org/10.1007/s10278-019-00297-x.

Lei Y, Fu Y, Wang T, Liu Y, Patel P, Curran WJ, Liu T, Yang X. 4D-CT deformable image registration using multiscale unsupervised deep learning. Phys Med Biol. 2020;65:085003. https://doi.org/10.1088/1361-6560/ab79c4.

Li Z, Cai A, Wang L, Zhang W, Tang C, Li L, et al. Promising generative adversarial network based Sinogram inpainting method for ultra-limited-angle computed tomography imaging. Sensors (Basel). 2019a;19:3941. https://doi.org/10.3390/s19183941.

Li Z, Zhang W. Wang L, Cai A, Li L. A Sinogram inpainting method based on generative adversarial network for limited-angle computed tomography. Proc Int Meeting Fully Three-Dimensional Image Reconstr Radiol Nucl Med. 2019b. https://doi.org/10.1117/12.2533757.

Li W, Kazemifar S, Bai T, Nguyen D, Weng Y, Li Y, et al. Synthesizing CT images from MR images with deep learning: model generalization for different datasets through transfer learning. Biomed Phys Eng Express. 2021;7. https://doi.org/10.1088/2057-1976/abe3a7.

Li D, Ma L, Li J, Qi S, Yao Y, Teng Y. A comprehensive survey on deep learning techniques in CT image quality improvement. Med Biol Eng Comput. 2022;60:2757–70. https://doi.org/10.1007/s11517-022-02631-y.

Liang K, Zhang L, Yang H, Yang Y, Chen Z, Xing Y. Metal artifact reduction for practical dental computed tomography by improving interpolation-based reconstruction with deep learning. Med Phys. 2019;46:e823–34. https://doi.org/10.1002/mp.13644.

Liao R, Miao S, Tournemire P, Grbic S, Kamen A, Mansi T et al. An artificial agent for robust image registration. arXiv. 2016:1611.10336. https://doi.org/10.48550/arXiv.1611.10336.

Lim B, Son S, Kim H, Nah S, Lee KM. Enhanced deep residual networks for single image SuperResolution. IEEE Comput Soc Conf Comput Vis Pattern Recognit Work. 2017:136–144. https://doi.org/10.1109/CVPRW.2017.151.

Lin DJ, Johnson PM, Knoll F, Lui YW. Artificial intelligence for MR image reconstruction: an overview for clinicians. J Magn Reson Imaging. 2021;53:1015–28. https://doi.org/10.1002/jmri.27078.

Mahapatra D, Ge ZY, Sedai S, Chakravorty R. Joint registration and segmentation of x-ray images using generative adversarial networks. Lect Notes Comput Sci. 2018;11046:73–80. https://doi.org/10.1007/978-3-030-00919-9_9.

Maier J, Eulig E, Vöth T, Knaup M, Kuntz J, Sawall S, et al. Real-time scatter estimation for medical CT using the deep scatter estimation: method and robustness analysis with respect to different anatomies, dose levels, tube voltages, and data truncation. Med Phys. 2019;46:238–49. https://doi.org/10.1002/mp.13274.

Miao S, Piat S, Fischer PW, Tuysuzoglu A, Mewes PW, Mansi T et al. Dilated FCN for multi-agent 2D/3D medical image registration. arXiv. 2017:1712.01651. https://doi.org/10.48550/arXiv.1712.01651.

Michaeli T, Irani M. Nonparametric blind super-resolution. Proc IEEE Int Conf Comput Vis. 2013:945–952. https://doi.org/10.1109/ICCV.2013.121.

Minnema J, Ernst A, van Eijnatten M, Pauwels R, Forouzanfar T, Batenburg KJ, et al. A review on the application of deep learning for CT reconstruction, bone segmentation and surgical planning in oral and maxillofacial surgery. Dentomaxillofac Radiol. 2022;51:20210437. https://doi.org/10.1259/dmfr.20210437.

Mishro PK, Agrawal S, Panda R, Abraham A. A survey on state-of-the-art denoising techniques for brain magnetic resonance images. IEEE Rev Biomed Eng. 2022;15:184–99. https://doi.org/10.1109/RBME.2021.3055556.

Mohammad-Rahimi H, Vinayahalingam S, Mahmoudinia E, Soltani P, Bergé SJ, Krois J, et al. Super-resolution of dental panoramic radiographs using deep learning: a pilot study. Diagnostics (Basel). 2023;13:996. https://doi.org/10.3390/diagnostics13050996.

Moran MBH, Faria MDB, Giraldi GA, Bastos LF, Conci A. Using super-resolution generative adversarial network models and transfer learning to obtain high resolution digital periapical radiographs. Comput Biol Med. 2021;129:104139. https://doi.org/10.1016/j.compbiomed.2020.104139.

Neppl S, Landry G, Kurz C, Hansen DC, Hoyle B, Stöcklein S, et al. Evaluation of proton and photon dose distributions recalculated on 2D and 3D Unet-generated pseudoCTs from T1-weighted MR head scans. Acta Oncol. 2019;58:1429–34. https://doi.org/10.1080/0284186X.2019.1630754.

Nie D, Trullo R, Lian J, Petitjean C, Ruan S, Wang Q, et al. Medical image synthesis with context-aware generative adversarial networks. Med Image Comput Comput Assist Interv. 2017;10435:417–25. https://doi.org/10.1007/978-3-319-66179-7_48.

Pain CD, Egan GF, Chen Z. Deep learning-based image reconstruction and post-processing methods in positron emission tomography for low-dose imaging and resolution enhancement. Eur J Nucl Med Mol Imaging. 2022;49:3098–118. https://doi.org/10.1007/s00259-022-05746-4.

Pal A, Rathi Y. A review and experimental evaluation of deep learning methods for MRI reconstruction. J Mach Learn Biomed Imaging. 2022. https://doi.org/10.48550/arXiv.2109.08618.

Park HS, Seo JK, Hyun CM, Lee SM, Jeon K. A fidelity-embedded learning for metal artifact reduction in dental CBCT. Med Phys. 2022;49:5195–205. https://doi.org/10.1002/mp.15720.

Pauwels R, Araki K, Siewerdsen JH, Thongvigitmanee SS. Technical aspects of dental CBCT: state of the art. Dentomaxillofac Radiol. 2015;44:20140224. https://doi.org/10.1259/dmfr.20140224.

Pauwels R, Jacobs R, Bogaerts R, Bosmans H, Panmekiate S. Reduction of scatter-induced image noise in cone beam computed tomography: effect of field of view size and position. Oral Surg Oral Med Oral Pathol Oral Radiol. 2016;121:188–95. https://doi.org/10.1016/j.oooo.2015.10.017.

Pauwels R, Oliveira-Santos C, Oliveira ML, Watanabe PCA, Faria VA, Jacobs R, Bosmans H, et al. Artefact reduction in cone-beam CT through deep learning: a pilot study using neural networks in the projection domain. Proc Int Congr Dentomaxillofac Radiol. 2019.

Pauwels R, Pittayapat P, Sinpitaksakul P, Panmekiate S. Scatter-to-primary ratio in dentomaxillofacial cone-beam CT: effect of field of view and beam energy. Dentomaxillofac Radiol. 2021;50:20200597. https://doi.org/10.1259/dmfr.20200597.

Pelc NJ, Wang A. CT statistical and iterative reconstructions and post processing. In: Samei E, Pelc N, editors. Computed tomography. Cham: Springer; 2020. p. 45–59. https://doi.org/10.1007/978-3-030-26957-9_4.

Piao XY, Park JM, Kim H, Kim Y, Shim JS. Evaluation of different registration methods and dental restorations on the registration duration and accuracy of cone beam computed tomography data and intraoral scans: a retrospective clinical study. Clin Oral Investig. 2022;26:5763–71. https://doi.org/10.1007/s00784-022-04533-7.

Pruessmann KP, Weiger M, Scheidegger MB, Boesiger P. SENSE: sensitivity encoding for fast MRI. Magn Reson Med. 1999;42:952–62.

Qin C, Bai W, Schlemper J, Petersen SE, Piechnik SK, Neubauer S, et al. Joint learning of motion estimation and segmentation for cardiac MR image sequences. arXiv. 2018:1806.04066. https://doi.org/10.1007/978-3-030-00934-2_53.

Quan TM, Nguyen-Duc T, Jeong WK. Compressed sensing MRI reconstruction using a generative adversarial network with a cyclic loss. IEEE Trans Med Imaging. 2018;37:1488–97. https://doi.org/10.1109/TMI.2018.2820120.

Sakai Y, Kitamoto E, Okamura K, Tatsumi M, Shirasaka T, Mikayama R, et al. Metal artefact reduction in the oral cavity using deep learning reconstruction algorithm in ultra-high-resolution computed tomography: a phantom study. Dentomaxillofac Radiol. 2021;50:20200553. https://doi.org/10.1259/dmfr.20200553.

Schulze R, Heil U, Gross D, Bruellmann DD, Dranischnikow E, Schwanecke U, et al. Artefacts in CBCT: a review. Dentomaxillofac Radiol. 2011;40:265–73. https://doi.org/10.1259/dmfr/30642039.

Sedghi A, Luo J, Mehrtash A, Pieper SD, Tempany CM, Kapur T, et al. Semi-supervised deep metrics for image registration. arXiv. 2018:1804.01565. https://doi.org/10.48550/arXiv.1804.01565.

Shan H, Padole A, Homayounieh F, Kruger U, Khera RD, Nitiwarangkul C, et al. Competitive performance of a modularized deep neural network compared to commercial algorithms for low-dose CT image reconstruction. Nat Mach Intell. 2019;1:269–76. https://doi.org/10.1038/s42256-019-0057-9.

Shi W, Caballero J, Huszar F, Totz J, Aitken AP, Bishop R, et al. Real-time single image and video super-resolution using an efficient sub-pixel convolutional neural network. Proc IEEE Comput Soc Conf Comput Vis Pattern Recognit. 2016:1874–1883. https://doi.org/10.1109/CVPR.2016.207.

Shocher A, Cohen N, Irani M. Zero-shot super-resolution using deep internal learning. Proc IEEE Comput Soc Conf Comput Vis Pattern Recognit. 2018:3118–3126. https://doi.org/10.1109/CVPR.2018.00329.

Sidky EY, Pan X. Report on the AAPM deep-learning sparse-view CT grand challenge. Med Phys. 2022;49:4935–43. https://doi.org/10.1002/mp.15489.

Sidky EY, Lorente I, Brankov JG, Pan X. Do CNNs solve the CT inverse problem? IEEE Trans Biomed Eng. 2021;68:1799–810. https://doi.org/10.1109/TBME.2020.3020741.

Simonovsky M, Gutiérrez-Becker B, Mateus D, Navab N, Komodakis N. A deep metric for multimodal registration. Lect Notes Comput Sci. 2016;9902:10–8. https://doi.org/10.1007/978-3-319-46726-9_2.

Siow TY, Ma CY, Toh CH. Angular super-resolution in X-ray projection radiography using deep neural network: implementation on rotational angiography. Biomed J. 2023;46(1):154–62. S2319-4170(22)00001-4. https://doi.org/10.1016/j.bj.2022.01.001.

Sokooti H, de Vos B, Berendsen F, Ghafoorian M, Yousefi S, Lelieveldt BPF, et al. 3D convolutional neural networks image registration based on efficient supervised learning from artificial deformations. arXiv. 2019:1908.10235. https://doi.org/10.48550/arXiv.1908.10235.

Song L, Li Y, Dong G, Lambo R, Qin W, Wang Y, et al. Artificial intelligence-based bone-enhanced magnetic resonance image-a computed tomography/magnetic resonance image composite image modality in nasopharyngeal carcinoma radiotherapy. Quant Imaging Med Surg. 2021;11:4709–20. https://doi.org/10.21037/qims-20-1239.

Sriram A, Zbontar J, Murrell T, Defazio A, Zitnick CL, Yakubova N, et al. End-to-end variational networks for accelerated MRI reconstruction. Lect Notes Comput Sci. 2020a;12262:64–73. https://doi.org/10.1007/978-3-030-59713-9_7.

Sriram A, Zbontar J, Murrell T, Zitnick CL, Defazio A, Sodickson DK. GrappaNet: combining parallel imaging with deep learning for multi-coil MRI reconstruction. Proc IEEE/CVF Conf Comput Vis Pattern Recognit. 2020b:14315–14322. https://doi.org/10.1109/CVPR42600.2020.01432.

Stiller W. Basics of iterative reconstruction methods in computed tomography: a vendor-independent overview. Eur J Radiol. 2018;109:147–54. https://doi.org/10.1016/j.ejrad.2018.10.025.

Sun L, Zhang S. Deformable MRI-ultrasound registration using 3D convolutional neural network. Lect Notes Comput Sci. 2018;11042:152–8. https://doi.org/10.1007/978-3-030-01045-4_18.

Sun S, Hu J, Yao M, Hu J, Yang X, Song Q, et al. Robust multimodal image registration using deep recurrent reinforcement learning. Lect Notes Comput Sci. 2019;11362:511–26. https://doi.org/10.1007/978-3-030-20890-5_33.

Sun B, Jia S, Jiang X, Jia F. Double U-Net CycleGAN for 3D MR to CT image synthesis. Int J Comput Assist Radiol Surg. 2023;18:149–56. https://doi.org/10.1007/s11548-022-02732-x.

Svoboda P, Hradis M, Barina D, Zemcik P. Compression artifacts removal using convolutional neural networks. J WSCG. 2016;24:63–72. https://doi.org/10.48550/arXiv.1605.00366.

Tatsugami F, Higaki T, Nakamura Y, Yu Z, Zhou J, Lu Y, et al. Deep learning-based image restoration algorithm for coronary CT angiography. Eur Radiol. 2019;29:5322–9. https://doi.org/10.1007/s00330-019-06183-y.

Tian C, Xu Y, Li Z, Zuo W, Fei L, Liu H. Attention-guided CNN for image denoising. Neural Netw. 2020;124:117–29. https://doi.org/10.1016/j.neunet.2019.12.024.

Toepfer K, Barski L, Vogelsang L, Sehnert W. Denoising in digital radiographic images using a deep convolutional neural network. Carestream Health. 2020. https://www.carestream.com/en/us/medical/software/~/media//publicSite/Resources/Smart%20Noise%20Cancellation%20%20Technical%20Paper%20%20Dec%202020.pdf. Accessed 14 Apr 2023.

Ulyanov D, Vedaldi A, Lempitsky V. Deep image prior. Int J Comput Vis. 2020;128:1867–88. https://doi.org/10.1007/s11263-020-01303-4.

Umehara K, Ota J, Ishida T. Super-resolution imaging of mammograms based on the super-resolution convolutional neural network. Open J Med Imaging. 2017;7:180–95. https://doi.org/10.4236/ojmi.2017.74018.

Umehara K, Ota J, Ishida T. Application of super-resolution convolutional neural network for enhancing image resolution in chest CT. J Digit Imaging. 2018;31:441–50. https://doi.org/10.1007/s10278-017-0033-z.

Wang J, Liang J, Cheng J, Guo Y, Zeng L. Deep learning based image reconstruction algorithm for limited-angle translational computed tomography. PLoS One. 2020;15:e0226963. https://doi.org/10.1371/journal.pone.0226963.

Wang D, Fan F, Wu Z, Liu R, Wang F, Yu H. CTformer: convolution-free Token2Token dilated vision transformer for low-dose CT denoising. Phys Med Biol. 2023;68:065012. https://doi.org/10.1088/1361-6560/acc000.

Widmann G, Bischel A, Stratis A, Kakar A, Bosmans H, Jacobs R, et al. Ultralow dose dentomaxillofacial CT imaging and iterative reconstruction techniques: variability of Hounsfield units and contrast-to-noise ratio. Br J Radiol. 2016;89:20151055. https://doi.org/10.1259/bjr.20151055.

Widmann G, Bischel A, Stratis A, Bosmans H, Jacobs R, Gassner EM, et al. Spatial and contrast resolution of ultralow dose dentomaxillofacial CT imaging using iterative reconstruction technology. Dentomaxillofac Radiol. 2017;46:20160452. https://doi.org/10.1259/dmfr.20160452.

Widmann G, Schönthaler H, Tartarotti A, Degenhart G, Hörmann R, Feuchtner G, et al. As low as diagnostically acceptable dose imaging in maxillofacial trauma: a reference quality approach. Dentomaxillofac Radiol. 2023;52:20220387. https://doi.org/10.1259/dmfr.20220387.

Wong KK, Cummock JS, He Y, Ghosh R, Volpi JJ, Wong STC. Retrospective study of deep learning to reduce noise in non-contrast head CT images. Comput Med Imaging Graph. 2021;94:101996. https://doi.org/10.1016/j.compmedimag.2021.101996.

Wu G, Kim M, Wang Q, Munsell BC, Shen D. Scalable high-performance image registration framework by unsupervised deep feature representations learning. IEEE Trans Biomed Eng. 2016;63:1505–16. https://doi.org/10.1109/TBME.2015.2496253.

Wu D, Kim K, Li Q. Computationally efficient deep neural network for computed tomography image reconstruction. Med Phys. 2019;46:4763–76. https://doi.org/10.1002/mp.13627.

Wu Q, Tang H, Liu H, Chen YC. Masked joint bilateral filtering via deep image prior for digital X-ray image denoising. IEEE J Biomed Health Inform. 2022;26:4008–19. https://doi.org/10.1109/JBHI.2022.3179652.

Würfl T, Ghesu FC, Christlein V, Maier A. Deep learning computed tomography. Lect Notes Comput Sci. 2016;9902:432–40. https://doi.org/10.1007/978-3-319-46726-9_50.

Xiao H, Teng X, Liu C, Li T, Ren G, Yang R, Shen D, Cai J. A review of deep learning-based three-dimensional medical image registration methods. Quant Imaging Med Surg. 2021;11:4895–916. https://doi.org/10.21037/qims-21-175.

Xue S, Qiu W, Liu F, Jin X. Wavelet-based residual attention network for image super-resolution. Neurocomputing. 2020;382:116–26. https://doi.org/10.1016/j.neucom.2019.11.044.

Yang Y, Sun J, Li H, Xu Z. Deep ADMM-net for compressive sensing MRI. Proc Int Conf Neural Inf Processing Syst. 2016;10–18. https://doi.org/10.48550/arXiv.1705.06869.

Yang Q, Yan P, Zhang Y, Yu H, Shi Y, Mou X, et al. Low-dose CT image denoising using a generative adversarial network with Wasserstein distance and perceptual loss. IEEE Trans Med Imaging. 2018;37:1348–57. https://doi.org/10.1109/TMI.2018.2827462.

Yi X, Babyn P. Sharpness-aware low-dose CT denoising using conditional generative adversarial network. J Digit Imaging. 2018;31:655–69. https://doi.org/10.1007/s10278-018-0056-0.

Yoo I, Hildebrand DGC, Tobin WF, Lee WCA, Jeong WK. ssEMnet: serial-section electron microscopy image registration using a spatial transformer network with learned features. Lect Notes Comput Sci. 2017;10553:249–57. https://doi.org/10.1007/978-3-319-67558-9_29.

You C, Yang Q, Shan H, Gjesteby L, Li G, Ju S, et al. Structurally-sensitive multi-scale deep neural network for low-dose CT denoising. IEEE Access. 2018;6:41839–55. https://doi.org/10.1109/ACCESS.2018.2858196.

Yu H, Wang G. Compressed sensing based interior tomography. Phys Med Biol. 2009;54:2791–805. https://doi.org/10.1088/0031-9155/54/9/014.

Yu W, Wang C, Huang M. Edge-preserving reconstruction from sparse projections of limited-angle computed tomography using ℓ0-regularized gradient prior. Rev Sci Instrum. 2017;88:043703. https://doi.org/10.1063/1.4981132.

Yuan Y, Liu S, Zhang J, Zhang Y, Dong C, Lin L. Unsupervised image super-resolution using cycle-in-cycle generative adversarial networks. IEEE Comput Soc Conf Comput Vis Pattern Recognit Work. 2018:701–710. https://doi.org/10.1109/CVPRW.2018.00113.

Yue Z, Yong H, Zhao Q, Zhang L, Meng D. Variational denoising network: toward blind noise modeling and removal. Proc Conf Neural Inf Processing Syst. 2019:1690–701. https://doi.org/10.48550/arXiv.1908.11314.

Zhang Y, Yu H. Convolutional neural network based metal artifact reduction in X-ray computed tomography. IEEE Trans Med Imaging. 2018;37:1370–81. https://doi.org/10.1109/TMI.2018.2823083.

Zhang Y, Li K, Li K, Wang L, Zhong B, Fu Y. Image super-resolution using very deep residual channel attention networks. Lect Notes Comput Sci. 2018;11211:294–310. https://doi.org/10.1007/978-3-030-01234-2_18.

Zhuo S, Jin Z, Zou W, Li X. RIDNet: recursive information distillation network for color image denoising. Proc IEEE/CVF Int Conf Comput Vision Workshop. 2019:3896–3903. https://doi.org/10.1109/ICCVW.2019.00483.

Zou J, Gao B, Song Y, Qin J. A review of deep learning-based deformable medical image registration. Front Oncol. 2022;12:1047215. https://doi.org/10.3389/fonc.2022.1047215.

Future Perspectives of Artificial Intelligence in Dentistry

19

Gürkan Ünsal and Kaan Orhan

Introduction

In terms of adopting new technologies to enhance patient care and outcomes, dentistry has always been at the forefront. Dental professionals have been creating and using new instruments and methods to enhance the diagnosis and care of dental issues since the early days of dentistry. The use of artificial intelligence (AI) and machine learning (ML) technologies is currently one of the most exciting and quickly developing areas of dentistry.

AI is transforming dentistry in a number of ways, from enhancing diagnosis speed and accuracy to treatment precision and efficacy. Dental professionals can provide better patient care for their patients by using AI algorithms to analyze massive amounts of data, such as patient records, diagnostic images, and treatment outcomes.

The field of diagnostics is among the critical areas in dentistry where AI is having a significant impact. X-rays, CT scans, and other diagnostic images can be analyzed by AI algorithms to find anomalies and potential problems that might not be visible to the naked eye. These algorithms can improve their analysis over time by utilizing machine learning, producing diagnoses that are more precise and trustworthy. The creation of novel treatment modalities and technologies is another area in which AI is transforming dentistry. Dentists can develop individualized treatment plans that are tailored to each patient using AI-powered tools. AI is enabling dentists to deliver more precise and effective treatments that produce better results for patients in a variety of dental specialties, from orthodontics to restorative dentistry.

G. Ünsal
Faculty of Dentistry, Department of Dentomaxillofacial Radiology, Near East University, Nicosia, Cyprus

K. Orhan (✉)
Faculty of Dentistry, Department of Dentomaxillofacial Radiology, Ankara University, Ankara, Turkey

K. Orhan, R. Jagtap (eds.), *Artificial Intelligence in Dentistry*,
https://doi.org/10.1007/978-3-031-43827-1_19

Please refer to "Chap. 4: Application of AI in Dentistry" for additional applications of AI currently being used in dentistry.

Future applications of AI in dentistry have almost limitless potential. As AI technologies develop and become more sophisticated, dentists will be able to use them to provide even more individualized and effective care for their patients. AI has the potential to completely transform dentistry, from predicting and preventing dental issues before they occur to developing brand-new methods of providing dental care.

We'll examine the prospects for AI in dentistry in this chapter as well as the difficulties and possibilities that lie ahead. We will also discuss ways that dentists can get around these challenges and provide the best care for their patients. Finally, we'll discuss the exciting potential applications of AI in dentistry and explore their broader implications for the field.

Opportunities of AI in the Future

Accurate Diagnosis

Accurate diagnosis is crucial in dentistry as it forms the basis for effective treatment planning and disease management. The ability of AI to make accurate diagnoses in the field of dentistry is one of its most intriguing applications. AI systems can identify patterns and make accurate diagnoses by analyzing and learning from large amounts of data. Dental imaging, including X-rays, CT scans, and intraoral images, can be analyzed using artificial intelligence to detect dental conditions such as caries, periodontal disease, and oral cancers. AI can also examine patient information, such as medical history, family history, and lifestyle factors, to pinpoint dental disease risk factors.

One of AI's key advantages in dental diagnosis is its ability to detect minute changes in dental images that a human eye might miss. AI systems can quickly and accurately analyze large amounts of data, which can speed up diagnosis and save time and money. However, there are some challenges that need to be resolved to ensure the accuracy of AI in dental diagnosis. One of the main challenges is the quality of the data used to train the AI system. Incomplete or biased data may prevent the system from accurately diagnosing a patient. Because dental data is not standardized, it may be difficult for AI systems to learn and create accurate predictions.

To overcome these obstacles, it is critical to ensure that high-quality data is used to train AI systems and that dental data is standardized. Another challenge is the need for human supervision of AI systems. Although AI is capable of making precise diagnoses, a dentist or other dental specialist should review the findings and provide a final diagnosis and treatment plan to prevent overtreatment and patient anxiety. AI systems could be unreliable or give false positive results.

Personalized Treatment Planning

A vital component of dental practice is treatment planning, which entails creating a personalized treatment plan for every patient. Treatment planning's objective is to determine the most effective and efficient course of action for the patient's particular dental condition while taking into account their special traits, preferences, and objectives. By analyzing patient data and offering insights into the most effective and efficient treatment options, artificial intelligence (AI) has the potential to enhance treatment planning in dentistry. In order to identify risk factors, forecast disease progression, and create individualized treatment plans, AI can analyze vast amounts of patient data, including dental imaging, medical history, and lifestyle factors.

AI has the capability to analyze dental imaging, enabling the identification of optimal orthodontic care for each patient. Additionally, it can assess periodontal data to recommend personalized treatment plans based on individual risk factors and the severity of the disease. The significant advantage of AI in treatment planning lies in its ability to deliver tailored care that aligns with each patient's unique needs. By considering specific traits, preferences, and treatment goals, AI can formulate treatment plans that are highly likely to achieve the desired results.

To guarantee the precision of AI in treatment planning, a number of issues must be resolved. The quality of the data used to train the AI system is one of the major obstacles. The system might not be able to offer accurate treatment recommendations if the data is biased or insufficient. The patient's unique preferences and treatment objectives must also be taken into account by the AI system because they can significantly affect the course of treatment. The requirement for human oversight of AI systems presents another difficulty. A dentist or other dental professional should review the treatment plan and make any final recommendations, even though AI can offer useful insights into treatment planning. This is due to the possibility that AI systems may err or produce false positives, which may result in unnecessary treatment and patient anxiety.

Predictive Analysis

In predictive analytics, a large amount of data is analyzed in order to find patterns and trends that can be used to forecast future events. Predictive analytics can be used in dentistry to identify patients who are more likely to develop specific diseases or conditions of the mouth. Machine learning algorithms can be trained to recognize patterns and associations that are predictive of particular conditions by examining patient factors like age, gender, lifestyle, and medical history.

For instance, based on a patient's age, smoking history, and previous dental history, an AI system may be trained to predict their risk of developing periodontitis. The system can determine factors that are linked to an increased risk of periodontitis and use this information to predict the likelihood of the patient developing the condition in the future by analyzing large amounts of data from patients with similar characteristics. Clinicians can use this predictive model to help them plan treatments and provide preventive care in a more informed way. Additionally, oral cancer, dental caries, and other oral health conditions can be predicted in patients using predictive analytics. Clinicians can focus on preventive measures like fluoride treatments or oral cancer screenings by identifying patients who are at a higher risk, potentially lowering the incidence and severity of these conditions.

Overall, the application of predictive analytics in dentistry has the potential to enhance patient outcomes by allowing clinicians to spot patients who are at an increased risk of developing oral health issues and take early preventive action. Dental practices can offer care that is more individualized and efficient by utilizing the power of AI algorithms, improving the outcomes for their patients' oral health.

Patient Engagement

Patient engagement, which involves involving patients in their own care and encouraging them to take an active role in their treatment process, is a crucial component of dental practice. By giving patients individualized education and feedback and by improving communication between patients and dental professionals, the use of AI has the potential to increase patient engagement within dentistry. In order to identify risk factors and offer individualized instruction and feedback, AI can be used to analyze patient data, including dental imaging, medical history, and lifestyle factors. AI, for example, can examine dental imaging to spot problem areas and give patients advice on how to improve their oral hygiene routines.

In order to make personalized recommendations for treatment and follow-up care, AI can also analyze patient data. The ability of AI to provide personalized instruction and feedback that is suited to each patient's particular needs and preferences is one of its key advantages in patient engagement. In order to create educational materials and feedback that are most likely to connect with patients and encourage their active participation in their own care, AI can take into account the patient's particular traits, preferences, and treatment goals. To guarantee the success of AI in patient engagement, however, a number of issues must be resolved.

The requirement for patient trust and acceptance of AI technology is one of the major challenges. Patients might be wary of entrusting AI systems with their private medical data or uncertain of the advantages AI technology can offer. Dental professionals must inform patients about the advantages of AI technology and how it can enhance their treatment. Effective communication between patients and dental professionals is a further challenge. Although AI can offer insightful feedback, it is crucial for dental professionals to explain these findings to patients in a straightforward manner. Additionally, dental professionals must be accessible to patients so they can ask questions and get the help they need.

Integrative Data Analysis

The collection and interpretation of patient data, including dental imaging, medical history, and lifestyle factors, is a crucial component of dentistry. Artificial intelligence (AI) has the potential to enhance data analysis in dentistry by analyzing vast amounts of patient data and offering insightful information on patient care and outcomes. In order to identify risk factors, forecast disease progression, and create individualized treatment plans, AI can analyze patient data. AI, for instance, can analyze dental imaging to spot problem areas and create treatment strategies that are customized to each patient's requirements. AI can also examine patient data to find patterns and trends in the development of diseases, which can assist dental professionals in creating more efficient treatment plans.

The ability of AI to accurately and quickly analyze vast amounts of patient data is one of the major benefits of AI in data analysis. By using AI to analyze patient data, dental professionals can identify patterns and trends in patient outcomes and care that may not be readily apparent with conventional methods of analysis. Dental professionals can improve patient outcomes and satisfaction by identifying areas for improvement in patient care with the aid of AI. To ensure the precision and efficacy of AI in data analysis, however, a number of issues must be resolved. The quality of the data used to train the AI system is one of the major obstacles. The system might not be able to provide accurate insights into patient care and outcomes if the data is incomplete or biased. It is crucial to ensure that the AI system can account for the patient's unique traits and preferences, as these can significantly affect the success of a treatment. The requirement for human oversight of AI systems presents another difficulty. A dental professional should review the findings and make any final recommendations, even though AI can offer useful insights into patient care and outcomes. This is so that unnecessary treatment and patient anxiety are avoided. AI systems have the potential to be inaccurate or to produce false positives.

Federated Learning

Due to the sensitivity of health data, it is frequently dispersed across numerous institutions. For effective model training, more varied data are preferred. Even with sluggish and unreliable network connections, federated learning can help solve this problem by training a centralized model using distributed training data from multiple clients. This is especially important for patient-generated data that patients might be hesitant to share on a public cloud, like data from wearables or mobile phones. Users can download the most recent model version with federated learning, update it with their own local data locally, and then send a targeted update back to the cloud using encrypted communication. The model is then improved by averaging these updates, ensuring that all data stays secure on local devices and that individual updates are not kept in the cloud. The quality of patient similarity measures can be maintained by using privacy-preserving techniques like homomorphic encryption, which are crucial but difficult to develop for federated health AI technologies.

Model Transparency

The debate over the interpretability of AI models revolves around the idea that older rule-based systems are more transparent than more recent deep learning models. Interpretability, according to some, is not crucial because users' trust in transparent models and black-box models does not differ noticeably, and increased transparency may even make it harder for users to spot errors. Others defend black-box models by drawing parallels between them and human decision-making. Interpretability is essential in the healthcare industry, where human clinicians frequently make the final decisions and AI algorithms only support them. To make clinicians feel more at ease, AI algorithms should provide specific justifications for their claims. They should also be incorporated into routine clinical workflows to maximize their usefulness.

Black-box models can be interpreted using post-hoc explanation techniques like knowledge distillation. However, there is a propensity for opaque, exclusive algorithms, which raises worries about possible harm in clinical practice. In the same way that clinical therapeutics and prognostic biomarkers must meet recognized standards of clinical use, regulatory and professional bodies should make sure that innovative algorithms do as well. Even though black-box models might perform better, healthcare requires interpretability to ensure safe and effective use.

Robotic Dentistry

Multiple aspects, including technical, psychological, and physical ones, can affect how well a surgery goes. However, there are some benefits to using traditional surgical robots, such as tremor and fatigue resistance. These robots may be able to produce better results, minimize procedural errors, and provide more access to body parts that are difficult to reach when used in conjunction with AI control algorithms. Additionally, autonomous surgical robots have the potential to democratize surgical care and standardize surgical outcomes, making them accessible in settings with limited access to healthcare, such as war zones or missions to Mars. Control algorithms, robotics, computer vision, and smart sensor technology must all be developed and integrated in order to produce an autonomous surgical device that is both versatile and clinically viable. The robot will successfully complete its surgical mission thanks to its capacity to map sensory inputs and gauge environmental conditions. Robots can predict outcomes and carry out tasks in real time by using machine learning algorithms to help them learn from previous experiences. Autonomous surgical robots can be particularly helpful in the field of dentistry. In order to place a titanium post and attach a crown to a dental implant, for instance, a robot would need to drill a hole in the jawbone. An autonomous surgical robot could increase the likelihood of success in a procedure like this, which would require extreme precision and accuracy. The infected pulp would need to be removed, and the space would need to be filled with a biocompatible material, in a similar way that a robot could be used to perform a root canal procedure. An autonomous surgical robot could carry out these tasks more accurately and effectively than a human dentist, and by the end of the twenty-first century, clinically viable dentist robots could be available.

Possible Challenges of AI in the Future

Data Quality

When creating AI systems for dentistry, data quality is essential because it affects the precision and dependability of the systems' outputs. AI systems in dentistry can be trained on a variety of data, such as patient records, medical images, and data from clinical research. For instance, large datasets of dental image data can be used to train AI systems to better recognize and identify dental diseases like periodontitis and cavities. The AI system's ability to provide accurate diagnoses or treatment recommendations, however, may be hampered if the data used to train it contains biases or lacks diversity. An AI system may not be able to generalize to other populations, for instance, if it is trained on a dataset that primarily consists of patients from a particular demographic or geographic area. This could result in predictions that are inaccurate or biased leading to inaccurate diagnoses or inadequate treatment recommendations. Researchers and developers must ensure that the training data for AI systems is representative and diverse, gathered from a variety of sources and populations. To maintain the accuracy and currency of the training data, it is crucial for researchers and developers to regularly review and update it.

Data Privacy and Security

Dental information demands stringent protection due to its sensitive nature. For the assurance of private and secure patient data, AI systems must strictly adhere to privacy and security regulations. It is imperative to remain vigilant about potential security risks as AI models become more prevalent in healthcare. Adversarial attacks, wherein data is manipulated to deceive the model and generate inaccurate outcomes, pose a significant concern. For example, subtle alterations in lab results could impact mortality predictions, while external factors like pollution on traffic signs might confuse autonomous driving systems. To uphold the confidentiality of patient data and ensure precise decision-making, healthcare professionals, AI researchers, and policymakers must remain cognizant of these risks and take necessary measures. For a deeper exploration of ethical concerns, refer to "Chap. 16: Medico-Legal Issues in AI." .

Lack of Standardization

To enable AI systems to effectively learn from diverse data and deliver precise diagnoses, standardization of dental data is imperative. This involves not only establishing guidelines for data collection, management, and sharing but also creating universal terminologies and vocabularies for dental conditions and treatments. Notably, the International Organization for Standardization (ISO) has developed standards for dental imaging, ensuring uniform and comparable images across various imaging technologies. Standardizing dental data not only enhances the quality and diversity of training data for AI systems but also facilitates easier sharing among researchers and dental practices. This concerted effort could lead to the development of more precise and efficient AI systems for dental diagnosis and care.

Cost

Cost considerations are pivotal in determining the feasibility of integrating AI systems into dentistry. The development of algorithms, procurement of hardware and software, and the hiring of staff for system management constitute substantial upfront expenses. Additionally, ongoing costs for maintenance, upgrades, and data management can impose further financial burdens.

Smaller dental practices or those with limited financial resources may encounter challenges in adopting AI due to these high implementation costs. However, a comprehensive cost-benefit analysis is essential, weighing the potential advantages that AI can bring to dentistry. AI systems hold the promise of enhancing the precision and efficacy of dental diagnoses and treatments, potentially leading to improved patient outcomes and reduced long-term healthcare costs.

Exploring cost-effective approaches, some AI systems can integrate seamlessly with existing tools and technology, mitigating the need for significant investments in hardware and software. Cloud-based AI systems offer smaller practices more flexible and affordable options.

AI systems tailored for the dental industry have already been developed, performing tasks like dental image analysis, patient risk assessment, and treatment planning. These systems carry the potential to elevate patient satisfaction, decrease reliance on manual labor, and elevate the overall standard of dental care. Despite these benefits, the financial burden may pose a barrier for some dental practices in implementing such advanced systems.

Future Directions of AI

Changes in Machine Learning

Machine learning is rapidly evolving in the healthcare industry, and the future will look vastly different from the present. Currently, the sample size for data is usually less than 2000 instances/images and is mainly derived from information on individual hospitals or insurance claims. However, in the future, the data sources will change to federated learning, where data will be gathered from several institutions, resulting in millions of multi-level linked instances. This change will provide a more comprehensive understanding of healthcare, improving diagnostics and treatment choices.

Additionally, there will be a significant shift in how machine learning is used in healthcare. The main emphasis right now is on association modeling and detecting structures in imagery. Future research will focus on detecting multiple types of pathology, predictive modeling, and decision support. With this shift in focus, machine learning algorithms will be able to make more informed decisions about patient care, resulting in better outcomes and a higher standard of care.

The training mode is another significant distinction between machine learning in healthcare today and in the future. Currently, supervised learning is the predominant training mode, where a machine learning algorithm learns from a labeled dataset. However, in the future, the ability for machine learning algorithms to learn from unlabeled data will come from the use of unsupervised or semi-supervised learning techniques. With this change, machine learning algorithms will be able to identify new patterns and trends that may not have been apparent in the past.

In addition, the testing method for machine learning in healthcare will soon change. Currently, cross-validation is used to evaluate the precision of machine learning algorithms. In the future, algorithms will be evaluated on their performance using independent datasets and hold-out test sets. With this modification, it will be easier to gauge how well the machine learning algorithm works in practical situations.

For machine learning algorithms to be effective, their accuracy must be measured. Currently, accuracy is primarily assessed using metrics like accuracy, area-under-the-curve, F1-score, segment overlap, and others. In the future, the primary focus will shift to measuring value and include elements like impact on treatment decisions, clinical and patient-reported outcomes, and cost-effectiveness. Furthermore, credibility will be a crucial metric, with explainable AI playing a significant role in determining the algorithm's accuracy.

The types of studies used to assess machine learning algorithms will also change. Currently, the most common study type used to assess the efficacy of a machine learning algorithm is diagnostic accuracy studies on retrospectively collected data. In the future, the main study design used to assess machine learning algorithms will be randomized controlled trials or sizable cohort studies collecting data prospectively. This modification will make it possible for researchers to evaluate the algorithm's performance in practical situations, improving patient outcomes.

Artificial General Intelligence and Artificial Super Intelligence

Three main categories of AI that are commonly discussed in relation to the future of AI are Artificial Narrow Intelligence (ANI), Artificial General Intelligence (AGI), and Artificial Super Intelligence (ASI). A sort of AI system called ANI, commonly referred to as weak-AI, is created with a specific job in mind. Playing games like chess or go are examples of these activities, as well as tasks like facial recognition and speech recognition. In order to increase the precision and effectiveness of some jobs, ANI, the most common type of AI currently in use, is already being employed in the dental industry to increase the precision and effectiveness of certain tasks, such as designing and making dental restorations. Computer-aided design and manufacturing (CAD/CAM) systems, which are employed in dentistry, use artificial intelligence (ANI). These methods have a great degree of efficiency and accuracy when designing and making dental restorations, such as crowns or bridges (see Chap. 4: Application of AI in Dentistry).

The use of CAD/CAM technologies to design and create dental restorations like crowns and bridges is one example of ANI being utilized in dentistry. These devices analyze digital photos of a patient's teeth using AI algorithms to produce a 3D model of the restoration that has to be made. The AI system can then employ this model to control a milling machine precisely and effectively while it fabricates the restoration.

Contrarily, AGI is a type of AI system that is capable of carrying out any intellectual work that a person can. AGI is mostly still a theoretical idea that has not yet been completely realized. Artificial General Intelligence (AGI) is the term used to describe an AI system that, without being specifically trained for each task, is capable of carrying out a wide range of intellectual tasks that a human can. Researchers and developers in the field of AI are working to construct AGI systems that can learn and reason in a way that is comparable to human cognition, although the development of such systems is still in its early phases. AGI has a wide range of possible uses in the realm of dentistry. AGI may be particularly helpful in the diagnosis of problems affecting oral health. In order to effectively detect and identify patients' oral health issues, an AGI system might be trained on a sizable dataset of dental photos and medical records. Similar to this, a patient's treatment plan might be created by an AGI system based on their unique dental requirements and medical background. Additionally, difficult dental procedures like root canal therapy and tooth extraction could be carried out using AGI equipment. AGI systems might be designed to carry out these treatments with a high level of precision and accuracy, potentially lowering the risk of errors and complications, thanks to their capacity to reason and learn like a person.

There are two new advances in AI technology on the horizon. The first is the integration of many information types, including textual and visual data, to enhance reasoning skills. Visual question-and-answer systems, for instance, can respond to inquiries concerning images using free text. Some AI models can even pass tests for medical licenses, proving they have good reasoning skills. The second advancement is embodied AI, which entails systems having the capacity to not only sense and reason but also plan interactions with their surroundings. Instead of focusing on narrow problems like today's limited AI systems, embodied AI seeks to solve complex problems like humans do. While there has been advancement in some areas necessary for creating embodied AI, such as multi-task learning and continuous learning, a complete general AI system is still not yet a reality. The ASI, commonly referred to as the "singularity," is an AI system that is capable of outperforming human intelligence and creativity and performing activities that are currently beyond the capabilities of humans. ASI is still mostly a theoretical idea that is not yet technologically feasible. According to some analysts, the development of ASI may occur within the next several decades. Dentistry is one of the many industries that ASI has the potential to change. Creating predictive models that can recognize patients who are at a high risk of contracting specific dental disorders or diseases is one example of how ASI could be utilized in dentistry. Dental professionals would be able to give preventive treatment and therapies that were catered to the individual needs of each patient thanks to these models, which would take a variety of characteristics like genetics, lifestyle, and medical history into account. The creation of ASI also prompts questions about the moral ramifications of such a potent technology and the requirement for controls to ensure its responsible and safe use.

Bibliography

Alam MK, Abutayyem H, Kanwal B, Shayeb MAL. Future of orthodontics—A systematic review and meta-analysis on the emerging trends in this field. J Clin Med. 2023;12(2):532. https://doi.org/10.3390/jcm12020532.

Alawi F. Artificial intelligence: the future might already be here. Oral Surg Oral Med Oral Pathol Oral Radiol. 2023;135(3):313–5. https://doi.org/10.1016/j.oooo.2023.01.002.

Aminoshariae A, Kulild J, Nagendrababu V. Artificial intelligence in endodontics: current applications and future directions. J Endod. 2021;47(9):1352–7. https://doi.org/10.1016/j.joen.2021.06.003.

Carrillo-Perez F, Pecho OE, Morales JC, Paravina RD, Della Bona A, Ghinea R, Pulgar R, Perez MDM, Herrera LJ. Applications of artificial intelligence in dentistry: a comprehensive review. J Esthet Restor Dent. 2022;34(1):259–80. https://doi.org/10.1111/jerd.12844.

Chen YW, Stanley K, Att W. Artificial intelligence in dentistry: current applications and future perspectives. Quintessence Int. 2020;51(3):248–57. https://doi.org/10.3290/j.qi.a43952.

Denecke K, Gabarron E. How artificial intelligence for healthcare look like in the future? Stud Health Technol Inform. 2021;281:860–4. https://doi.org/10.3233/SHTI210301.

Howard J. Algorithms and the future of work. Am J Ind Med. 2022;65(12):943–52. https://doi.org/10.1002/ajim.23429.

Hung KF, Yeung AWK, Bornstein MM, Schwendicke F. Personalized dental medicine, artificial intelligence, and their relevance for dentomaxillofacial imaging. Dentomaxillofac Radiol. 2023;52(1):20220335. https://doi.org/10.1259/dmfr.20220335.

Joshi S, Vibhute G, Ayachit A, Ayachit G. Big data and artificial intelligence—tools to be future ready? Indian J Ophthalmol. 2021;69(7):1652–3. https://doi.org/10.4103/ijo.IJO_514_21.

Karger E, Kureljusic M. Artificial intelligence for cancer detection—a bibliometric analysis and avenues for future research. Curr Oncol. 2023;30(2):1626–47. https://doi.org/10.3390/curroncol30020125.

Kolluri S, Lin J, Liu R, Zhang Y, Zhang W. Machine learning and artificial intelligence in pharmaceutical research and development: a review. AAPS J. 2022;24(1):19. https://doi.org/10.1208/s12248-021-00644-3.

Kulkarni S, Seneviratne N, Baig MS, Khan AHA. Artificial intelligence in medicine: where are we now? Acad Radiol. 2020;27(1):62–70. https://doi.org/10.1016/j.acra.2019.10.001.

Laur O, Wang B. Musculoskeletal trauma and artificial intelligence: current trends and projections. Skeletal Radiol. 2022;51(2):257–69. https://doi.org/10.1007/s00256-021-03824-6.

Lopez-Jimenez F, Attia Z, Arruda-Olson AM, Carter R, Chareonthaitawee P, Jouni H, Kapa S, Lerman A, Luong C, Medina-Inojosa JR, Noseworthy PA, Pellikka PA, Redfield MM, Roger

VL, Sandhu GS, Senecal C, Friedman PA. Artificial intelligence in cardiology: present and future. Mayo Clin Proc. 2020;95(5):1015–39. https://doi.org/10.1016/j.mayocp.2020.01.038.

Malamateniou C, Knapp KM, Pergola M, Woznitza N, Hardy M. Artificial intelligence in radiography: where are we now and what does the future hold? Radiography (Lond). 2021;27(Suppl 1):S58–62. https://doi.org/10.1016/j.radi.2021.07.015.

Morch CM, Atsu S, Cai W, Li X, Madathil SA, Liu X, Mai V, Tamimi F, Dilhac MA, Ducret M. Artificial intelligence and ethics in dentistry: a scoping review. J Dent Res. 2021;100(13):1452–60. https://doi.org/10.1177/00220345211013808.

Muresanu S, Almasan O, Hedesiu M, Diosan L, Dinu C, Jacobs R. Artificial intelligence models for clinical usage in dentistry with a focus on dentomaxillofacial CBCT: a systematic review. Oral Radiol. 2023;39(1):18–40. https://doi.org/10.1007/s11282-022-00660-9.

Niu PH, Zhao LL, Wu HL, Zhao DB, Chen YT. Artificial intelligence in gastric cancer: application and future perspectives. World J Gastroenterol. 2020;26(36):5408–19. https://doi.org/10.3748/wjg.v26.i36.5408.

Noorbakhsh-Sabet N, Zand R, Zhang Y, Abedi V. Artificial intelligence transforms the future of health care. Am J Med. 2019;132(7):795–801. https://doi.org/10.1016/j.amjmed.2019.01.017.

Orhan K, Yazici G, Kolsuz ME, Kafa N, Bayrakdar IS, Çelik Ö. An artificial intelligence hypothetical approach for masseter muscle segmentation on ultrasonography in patients with bruxism. J Adv Oral Res. 2021;12(2):206–13. https://doi.org/10.1177/23202068211005611.

Ossowska A, Kusiak A, Swietlik D. Artificial intelligence in dentistry—narrative review. Int J Environ Res Public Health. 2022;19(6) https://doi.org/10.3390/ijerph19063449.

Panesar S, Cagle Y, Chander D, Morey J, Fernandez-Miranda J, Kliot M. Artificial intelligence and the future of surgical robotics. Ann Surg. 2019;270(2):223–6. https://doi.org/10.1097/SLA.0000000000003262.

Rekawek P, Rajapakse CS, Panchal N. Artificial intelligence: the future of maxillofacial prognosis and diagnosis? J Oral Maxillofac Surg. 2021;79(7):1396–7. https://doi.org/10.1016/j.joms.2021.02.031.

Rowe SP, Soyer P, Fishman EK. The future of radiology: what if artificial intelligence is really as good as predicted? Diagn Interv Imaging. 2022;103(9):385–6. https://doi.org/10.1016/j.diii.2022.04.006.

Savadjiev P, Chong J, Dohan A, Vakalopoulou M, Reinhold C, Paragios N, Gallix B. Demystification of AI-driven medical image interpretation: past, present and future. Eur Radiol. 2019;29(3):1616–24. https://doi.org/10.1007/s00330-018-5674-x.

Schwendicke F, Samek W, Krois J. Artificial intelligence in dentistry: chances and challenges. J Dent Res. 2020;99(7):769–74. https://doi.org/10.1177/0022034520915714.

Shu LQ, Sun YK, Tan LH, Shu Q, Chang AC. Application of artificial intelligence in pediatrics: past, present and future. World J Pediatr. 2019;15(2):105–8. https://doi.org/10.1007/s12519-019-00255-1.

Sunarti S, Fadzlul Rahman F, Naufal M, Risky M, Febriyanto K, Masnina R. Artificial intelligence in healthcare: opportunities and risk for future. Gac Sanit. 2021;35(Suppl 1):S67–70. https://doi.org/10.1016/j.gaceta.2020.12.019.

Tandon D, Rajawat J. Present and future of artificial intelligence in dentistry. J Oral Biol Craniofac Res. 2020;10(4):391–6. https://doi.org/10.1016/j.jobcr.2020.07.015.

Tekkesin AI. Artificial intelligence in healthcare: past, present and future. Anatol J Cardiol. 2019;22(Suppl 2):8–9. https://doi.org/10.14744/AnatolJCardiol.2019.28661.

Wang F, Preininger A. AI in health: state of the art, challenges, and future directions. Yearb Med Inform. 2019;28(1):16–26. https://doi.org/10.1055/s-0039-1677908.

GPSR Compliance

The European Union's (EU) General Product Safety Regulation (GPSR) is a set of rules that requires consumer products to be safe and our obligations to ensure this.

If you have any concerns about our products, you can contact us on ProductSafety@springernature.com

In case Publisher is established outside the EU, the EU authorized representative is:

Springer Nature Customer Service Center GmbH
Europaplatz 3
69115 Heidelberg, Germany

Batch number: 10726058

Printed by Printforce, the Netherlands